COGNITIVE HYPNOTHERAPY

COGNITIVE HYPNOTHERAPY

An Integrated Approach to the Treatment of
Emotional Disorders

Assen Alladin

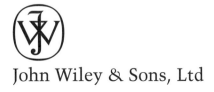

John Wiley & Sons, Ltd

Other Wiley Editorial Offices

John Wiley & Sons Inc., 111 River Street, Hoboken, NJ 07030, USA

Jossey-Bass, 989 Market Street, San Francisco, CA 94103-1741, USA

Wiley-VCH Verlag GmbH, Boschstr. 12, D-69469 Weinheim, Germany

John Wiley & Sons Australia Ltd, 42 McDougall Street, Milton, Queensland 4064, Australia

John Wiley & Sons (Asia) Pte Ltd, 2 Clementi Loop #02-01, Jin Xing Distripark, Singapore 129809

John Wiley & Sons Canada Ltd, 6045 Freemont Blvd, Mississauga, ONT, L5R 4J3, Canada

Wiley also publishes its books in a variety of electronic formats. Some content that appears in print
may not be available in electronic books.

Library of Congress Cataloging in Publication Data

Alladin, Assen.
  Cognitive hypnotherapy : an integrated approach to the treatment of emotional
  disorders / Assen Alladin.
    p. ; cm.
  Includes bibliographical references and index.
  ISBN 978-0-470-03251-0 (cloth : alk. paper) — ISBN 978-0-470-03247-3 (pbk. : alk. paper)
  1. Hypnotism—Therapeutic use. 2. Cognitive therapy. 3. Affective disorders—Treatment.
  I. Title. [DNLM: 1. Cognitive Therapy—methods. 2. Hypnosis. WM 415 A416c 2008]
  RC497.A45 2008
  615.8′512—dc22

                                                                          2008002739

British Library Cataloguing in Publication Data

A catalogue record for this book is available from the British Library

ISBN 978-0-470-03251-0 (hbk)
ISBN 978-0-470-03247-3 (pbk)

Typeset in 10/12pt Palatino by Integra Software Services Pvt. Ltd, Pondicherry, India
Printed and bound in Great Britain by T. J. International, Padstow, Cornwall.

CONTENTS

ABOUT THE AUTHOR

Dr Assen Alladin is a Clinical Psychologist and Adjunct Assistant Professor at Foothills Medical Centre and Department of Psychiatry and Psychology at the University of Calgary Medical School. He has been practicing and teaching hypnosis and clinical psychology for over 25 years. He served as Secretary of the British Society of Experimental and Clinical Hypnosis for many years and currently he is the President of the Canadian Federation of Clinical Hypnosis-Alberta Society. He was Fellow of the Royal Society of Medicine and Associate Fellow of the British Psychological Society.

Dr Alladin has published many chapters and papers on clinical hypnosis and is the author of *Handbook of Cognitive-Hypnotherapy for Depression: An Evidence-Based Approach* (Lippincott, Williams & Wilkins, 2007) and *Hypnotherapy Explained* (Radcliffe Publishing, 2008). He served as Guest Editor for Special Issues in Hypnotherapy for the *Journal of Preventive Neurology and Psychiatry* (1992), the *Journal of Cognitive Psychotherapy: An International Quarterly* (1994), and the *International Journal of Clinical and Experimental Hypnosis* (April 2007 & July 2007).

He is interested in the empirical validation of clinical hypnosis and the integration of hypnosis with other forms of psychotherapy. He is the 2005 recipient of the Best Research Paper from Division 30 of the American Psychological Association

Dr Alladin comes from the island of Mauritius and he completed all his studies in England. He was initially trained as a Registered Nurse and a Social Worker before taking Psychology and Clinical Psychology. Dr. Alladin has two adult children and lives in Calgary, Alberta, Canada. He loves teaching, and traveling with his wife of 27 years. He has presented addresses and workshops on clinical hypnosis at national and international conferences.

FOREWORD

Many years ago, I had occasion to observe Dr. Aaron T. Beck, widely considered the father of modern cognitive therapy, conduct a most interesting therapy session with a young man who was anxious and depressed. Dr. Beck encouraged the man to first recognize errors in his thinking and then deliberately and consciously refute the flood of negative automatic thoughts that, by non-critically believing them, obviously contributed to his difficulties. The man responded quite favorably to Dr. Beck's instructions; he seemed to grasp both the ideas and methods he was being taught for regulating his thoughts and feelings. Then, Dr. Beck did something particularly interesting: He instructed the man to close his eyes and engage in an exercise in imagination. The man was told to visualize himself in a variety of situations that had previously been stressful. Dr. Beck suggested that he see himself in these familiar situations thinking and doing things differently, focusing on how his newly corrected thoughts and revised self-talk would lead him to handle the previously troublesome situations skillfully and successfully. The young man absorbed Dr. Beck's suggestions to associate new thoughts and feelings to those situations, and reported feeling that he could now handle those situations in much improved ways. His broad smile and apparent comfort suggested he was sincere in saying this.

Following this session, I asked Dr. Beck about the last step of his intervention. I asked him what he called this visualization procedure. He replied, 'A success imagery.' I asked him, 'Was this hypnosis?' He replied that he didn't do hypnosis.

Someone grounded in the dynamics of clinical hypnosis might well have termed this 'success imagery' procedure an 'age progression' technique, an *experiential*, not only cognitive, orientation to the future that encouraged the client to develop an association between a specific set of thoughts, feelings and behaviors, and a particular context. Clinicians employing hypnosis routinely make use of age progression as well as 'post-hypnotic suggestions' for exactly this reason: to establish links (i.e., associations) between desired responses and specific contexts. Such goal-oriented suggestions are typically well-elaborated and carefully delivered with the intention of making the links as strong as possible.

There is something quite special about the experience of hypnosis. Hypnosis allows for an enhanced sense of personal control (i.e., a greater internal locus of control) and greater flexibility in responding in multi-dimensional ways. Particularly relevant, though, is how hypnosis encourages a greater *automaticity* in responding, meaning a quality of response that is therapeutically valuable that seems to arise quite effortlessly in the hypnotized person.

Well before they were called 'automatic thoughts' by cognitive therapists, such non-volitional and typically non-conscious responses were called ideocognitive responses. While identifying negative automatic thoughts has become a major focus in CBT, clinicians studying hypnosis were developing innovative ways to encourage *positive ideocognitions*. Is the goal of treatment to reduce negative or distorted thinking or increase positive or clear thinking? Should therapy be aimed at re-training the conscious mind to recognize and correct cognitive distortions, or aimed at unconscious processes that can help mobilize more effective information processing and reflexive positive responses? These are tantalizing questions to consider, and how one answers them no doubt shapes one's clinical style and methods.

The hypnosis literature is replete with examples of successfully integrated suggestions to change the quality and direction of one's thinking. Furthermore, the use of hypnosis to reduce anxiety and ease the learning process has made for easier – and better – therapy. In particular, there is a growing body of scientific literature attesting to the fact that hypnosis enhances CBT; in fact, much of this literature is referenced and critically reviewed in this substantive book.

Through this impressive volume, which introduces the reader to Dr. Assen Alladin's *Cognitive Hypnotherapy* (CH) model, we get a well-thought out answer to the question many of us ask: How might we enhance the merits of CBT? The essence of the answer is *integrate hypnosis into the treatment process*. Dr. Alladin takes on the challenge of presenting a theoretical foundation for integrating hypnosis with CBT, and he provides a structured means for doing so with his case-formulation guidelines. He offers detailed and illuminating examples of specific intervention strategies, and he even provides a flexible template for ways other models of psychotherapy may be combined with methods of clinical hypnosis.

Dr. Alladin is uncommon in his having one foot in the world of psychotherapy and the other foot in the world of research. His expertise in both domains comes shining through in these pages. He strives to not only solve problems, but teach problem-solving. He sees beyond the limitations of one-dimensional procedures and offers us a variety of hypnotic methods that reach beyond conscious minds and go into areas where more typical CBT techniques just don't usually go. He emphasizes the merits of hypnosis as a means of empowering people to use their minds in new and creative ways that can enhance their lives. And, Dr. Alladin provides us with the empirical evidence we need that there is good reason to absorb what he is teaching us.

It is my privilege to write the Foreword to this volume. I hope you will find it as instructive, intelligent, interesting and practical as I did.

Michael D. Yapko, Ph.D.
Fallbrook, CA
February 12, 2008
www.yapko.com

PREFACE

In writing this book, I have addressed three main concerns about hypnotherapy that have evolved in my 27-year career as a practitioner and teacher of clinical hypnosis. First, many writers advocate that hypnotherapy is very effective in the treatment of various disorders, but provide little or no empirical research to support their claims. Second, they describe numerous hypnotic techniques that can be utilized with a variety of medical and psychological conditions. However, it is not made clear how these techniques differ from other forms of psychotherapy, what are the empirical bases for using them, and how they modify the underlying pathology. The reader is often left with the impression that hypnotic techniques are utilized without giving much consideration to recent advances in etiology and treatments. Third, most books emphasize the adjunctive role of hypnotherapy, but they do not describe in detail the multimodal strategies within which hypnotic techniques are incorporated. Most often a single-modality hypnotic approach is described. Considering that most clinical disorders are complex and compounded by comorbid factors, it is surprising that some authors take a single-modality approach to treatment. On the other hand, some writers have made attempts to integrate hypnotic techniques with other forms of psychotherapy (e.g., cognitive behavior therapy or psychodynamic therapy), but they have not provided a theoretical or scientific rationale for integration.

This book takes a multimodal approach to understanding and treating emotional disorders. It is written to encourage evidence-based clinical practice and research in hypnotherapy. It provides directions on how to assimilate hypnosis with cognitive behavior therapy (CBT) in the management of various emotional disorders. It lays down a solid theoretical foundation for integrating hypnosis with CBT in the management of emotional disorders. Furthermore, cognitive hypnotherapy is conceptualized as an assimilative model of psychotherapy. The assimilative approach to psychotherapy is the latest integrative psychotherapy model described in the literature. It is considered to be the best model for integrating both theory and empirical findings to achieve maximum flexibility and effectiveness under a guiding theoretical framework. Evidently, cognitive hypnotherapy meets criteria for assimilative model of psychotherapy. Hypnotherapy can now be formally recognized as a valid adjunct to cognitive psychotherapy. This is an important recognition for the field of clinical hypnosis.

Unlike other books on hypnotherapy, this book advocates a case formulation approach to clinical practice. Such a model of practice allows the assimilation of techniques to be based on empirical findings rather than using techniques haphazardly in a hit and miss fashion. Evidence suggests that matching of treatment to particular patient characteristics increases outcome.

Each clinical chapter focuses on a particular emotional disorder and offers a detailed step-by-step treatment protocol. The treatment protocol, based on latest empirical evidence, provides an *additive design* for studying the additive effect of hypnosis. The treatment protocols are specifically designed in a structured way to allow validation of the clinical efficacy of adding a hypnotherapy component to CBT. An *addidtive design* involves a strategy in which the treatment to be tested is added to another treatment to determine whether the treatment added produces an incremental improvement over the first treatment.

Moreover, the book provides a template for integrating other forms of psychotherapy with hypnotherapy. Cognitive hypnotherapy, as an assimilative model of psychological intervention, chooses CBT as the host psychotherapy for integration because CBT meets criteria for scientific theory; it is empirically validated; and it constitutes a unifying theory of psychotherapy and psychopathology. Theory is essential to clinical practice; without theory, the practice of psychotherapy becomes a purely technical exercise, devoid of any scientific basis. Although cognitive hypnotherapy meets criteria for an assimilative model of psychotherapy, it is not to be seen as a finished product, but as an evolving process. It requires further empirical validation; without empirical validation it is not possible to establish whether the importation of the hypnotic techniques into CBT positively impact therapy, especially when the techniques are decontextualized and placed in a new framework. It is only through empirical validation that ineffective and idiosyncratic assimilation can be avoided. The book offers several structured and well-described cognitive hypnotherapy protocols that can be easily validated empirically.

Considering modern hypnosis has been around for over a quarter of a century, the relative empirical foundation of clinical hypnosis is not very solid and hypnotherapy is far from being recognized as mainstream psychotherapy. To increase credibility and utilization of clinical hypnosis, the empirical basis of hypnotherapy needs to be widely established. There is an immediate need for more research evaluating the efficacy of hypnotherapy with both medical and psychological conditions, either as a single treatment or part of a multi-treatment modality. Once this efficacy is established, the utilization of hypnotherapy will be increased and the demand for its services as a non-biologic treatment will be augmented. It is hoped that this book, by formally recognizing hypnotherapy as a valid adjunct to psychotherapy, will serve as a springboard for further additive studies of clinical hypnosis. It is also hoped that readers will find the assimilation of some of the treatment techniques described in the book both innovative and clinically enriching. For example,

Chapter 5, by integrating CBT, hypnotherapy and imagery rescripting therapy (IRT), provides a multifaceted, imagery-focused, evidence-based treatment for reducing PTSD symptoms, altering negative beliefs, and enhancing the trauma survivor's ability to self-calm and self-nurture. Chapter 6 dicusses the interface between psychiatry and dermatology and provides a framework for utilizing cognitive hypnotherapy within the new field of *psychocutaneous medicine*. Chapter 9 describes the application of cognitive hypnotherapy to erectile dysfunction in the context of the 'Viagra revolution' and discusses innovative ways of delivering treatment for erectile dysfunction within the context of sexual medicine.

Assen Alladin
Calgary, Alberta, Canada
February 2008

THE RATIONALE FOR INTEGRATING HYPNOSIS AND COGNITIVE BEHAVIOUR THERAPY IN THE MANAGEMENT OF EMOTIONAL DISORDERS

INTRODUCTION

This book adopts the position that there is an enhancement in treatment effect when cognitive behaviour therapy (CBT) is integrated with hypnosis in the management of emotional disorders. Although many clinicians have blended hypnosis with various psychotherapies, the approach to integration has ranged from being arbitrary and idiosyncratic to very systematic, rather than driven by a coherent integrated theory. As hypnosis is not a school of therapy and does not provide a theory of personality, psychopathology or behaviour change, hypnotherapists have combined their techniques with a variety of psychotherapies, for example CBT (e.g. Alladin, 1994, 2006, 2007a; Bryant et al., 2005; Golden, 2006), multimodal therapy (Lazarus, 1973), psychoanalysis (e.g. Fromm & Nash, 1996) and rational emotive behaviour therapy (e.g. Ellis, 1986, 1993, 1996). To my knowledge, none of the writers has developed a coherent integrative model of psychotherapy that assimilates hypnosis with CBT.

I developed a theoretical or working model called the *Cognitive Dissociative Model of Depression* (Alladin, 1994, 2006, 2007a), which provides the rationale for combining hypnosis with CBT in the management of depression. From this model evolved *Cognitive Hypnotherapy*, a multimodal approach for treating depression, mainly consisting of CBT and hypnotic techniques (Alladin, 1994, 2006, 2007a). The cognitive hypnotherapy approach to integration is similar to the psychodynamically based integrative therapy developed and described by Gold and Stricker (2001, 2006). Gold and Stricker (2001, 2006) have developed an assimilative model of psychotherapy that integrates standard psychodynamic methods with other therapies 'when called for' in order to 'advance certain psychodynamic goals as well as address the target concern effectively' (Gold & Stricker, 2006, p. 12). In this chapter cognitive hypnotherapy is conceptualised as an assimilative model of psychotherapy.

Cognitive hypnotherapy uses CBT as the base theory for integration because the cognitive theory provides a unifying theory of psychotherapy and psychopathology, and it effectively integrates theory and clinical practice. Absence of a good theory can be problematic as it is likely to lack conceptual coherence (Bergin & Garfield, 1994). Another distinguishing characteristic of CBT is that it is technically eclectic. Although most of the techniques utilised in CBT are 'behavioural' or 'cognitive', it routinely combines techniques from various psychotherapies. Alford and Beck (1997, p. 90) write: 'any clinical technique that is found to be useful in facilitating the empirical investigation of patients' maladaptive interpretations and conclusions may be incorporated into the clinical practice of cognitive therapy'. However, in CBT the techniques are not chosen haphazardly. They are selected in the context of cognitive case formulation that is used to guide the practice of CBT for each individual case (Needleman, 2003; Persons, 1989; Persons & Davidson, 2001; Persons, Davidson & Tompkins, 2001). Evidence suggests that matching of treatment to particular patient characteristics increases outcome (Beutler, Clarkin & Bongar, 2000). Alford and Beck (1997, p. 91) went on further to say;

> The technically eclectic nature of cognitive therapy has been described previously as follows: 'By working within the framework of the cognitive model, the therapist formulates his [sic] therapeutic approach according to the specific needs of a given patient at a particular time. Thus, the therapist may be conducting cognitive therapy even though he is utilizing predominantly behavioral or abreactive (emotion releasing) techniques' (Beck et al., 1979, p. 117). Techniques can be selected from other psychotherapeutic approaches, provided that the following criteria are met: (1) The methods are consistent with cognitive therapy principles and are logically related to the theory of therapeutic change; (2) the choice of techniques is based on a comprehensive case conceptualization that takes into account the patient's characteristics (introspective capacity, problem-solving abilities, etc.); (3) collaborative empiricism and guided discovery are employed; (4) the standard interview structure is followed, unless there are factors that argue strongly against the standard format (Beck, 1991a).

As CBT is technically eclectic and adopts multiple approaches to case formulation and treatment, it offers an excellent framework for integrating hypnotic and cognitive strategies with a variety of syndromes. It is hoped that the integrated approach described in this chapter will provide a clear understanding of how to use hypnotic techniques to enhance treatment effect and how to use hypnosis as an adjunct treatment in the context of CBT. Before discussing the rationale for integrating hypnosis with CBT in the management of emotional disorders, theories of psychotherapy integration are reviewed to provide readers with some background information on the psychotherapy integration movement.

PSYCHOTHERAPY INTEGRATION MOVEMENT

For decades the field of psychotherapy was marked by deep division and segregation of theories and methods. This sentiment is eloquently described by Gold and Stricker (2006, pp. 3–4):

> Psychotherapists of one orientation or another have been loath to learn from their colleagues. Our collective behavior seems to have been governed by a powerful xenophobic fear and loathing that caused immediate and reflexive dismissal of approaches to psychotherapy that were different than one's own. When psychotherapists of one orientation did in fact take notice of the work of another school of psychotherapy, they typically did so with disdain and hostility. The clinical and research literatures were compiled primarily with reports meant to demonstrate that the writer's preferred brand of psychotherapy clinically outperformed all others, or that the author's theory was the best in terms of theoretical accuracy and sophistication.

Fortunately, there have been some pioneers in the field who tried to integrate different forms of psychotherapy. For example, French (1933) attempted to synthesise ideas from classical conditioning within psychoanalytic theory. Dollard and Miller (1950) integrated the central ideas about unconscious motivation and conflict with the concepts drawn from learning theories; and Wachtel (1977) integrated psychoanalysis with behaviour therapy. During the last decade of the 20th century, interest in the psychotherapy integration movement was at its peak and it culminated in the formation of the Society for the Exploration of Psychotherapy Integration, the founding of the *Journal of Psychotherapy Integration* in 1991, and the publication of two handbooks on psychotherapy integration: *Handbook of Psychotherapy Integration* (Norcross & Goldfried, 1992) and *Comprehensive Handbook of Psychotherapy Integration* (Stricker & Gold, 1993). These handbooks covered most of the important integrative therapies available at that time and went beyond the exclusive focus on the synthesis of psychoanalytical and behavioural models. The current trend in integrative therapies is to 'combine cognitive, humanistic, experiential, and family systems models with each other and with sophisticated psychoanalytic, behavioural and humanistic components of treatment in ever more complex permutations' (Gold & Stricker, 2006, p. 8). This chapter blends hypnosis with CBT and proposes *cognitive hypnotherapy* as an assimilative model of psychotherapy for the management of emotional disorders.

Norcross and Newman (1992) have identified eight factors that have promoted psychotherapy integration in the past 20 years:

1. There has been a proliferation in the number of schools of psychotherapy.
2. Lack of unequivocal empirical support for the superiority of any single psychotherapy.
3. The inability of any psychotherapy theory to completely explain and predict psychopathology.
4. The exponential increases in short-term psychotherapies.
5. Increase in communication between clinicians and scholars.
6. Lack of support for long-term psychotherapy from third-party payers.
7. Recognition of common factors in all psychotherapies that are related to outcome.
8. Growth of journals, conferences and professional organizations dedicated to psychotherapy integration.

MODELS OF PSYCHOTHERAPY INTEGRATION

Psychotherapy integration can be defined as the 'search for, and study of, the ways in which the various schools or models of psychotherapy can inform, enrich, and ultimately be combined, rather than to a specific theory or method of psychotherapy' (Gold & Stricker, 2006, p. 8). From the current psychotherapy integration literature, four models of integration can be identified, including *technical eclecticism, common factors approach, theoretical integration* and *assimilative integration*. Each of these models of psychotherapy integration is briefly reviewed before describing Cognitive Hypnotherapy, an assimilative model that combines CBT with hypnotic techniques.

Technical Eclecticism Integration Model

Technical eclecticism, loosely referred to as eclectic psychotherapy, is an empirically based approach that advocates selectively combining the best techniques, regardless of their theoretical origin, and applies them in such a way as to maximise the therapeutic results for a specific client in as short a time as possible (Lampropoulos, 2001). Technical eclecticism can be approached haphazardly, arbitrarily, idiosyncratically or very systematically, where the techniques are chosen, based on clinical knowledge and research findings, to match the patient's needs. Multimodal therapy (Lazarus, 1992, 2002) and prescriptive psychotherapy (Beutler *et al.*, 2002) are the two well-known versions of technically eclectic psychotherapy. *Multimodal therapy* was developed by Lazarus, who became disenchanted with the limits of then traditional behaviour therapy, and hence decided to develop a broad-spectrum behaviour therapy, supplemented by cognitive, experiential and imagery-based interventions. *Prescriptive psychotherapy*, developed by Beutler et al. (2002), is a flexible and empirically driven system in which the therapist matches the patient's concern with the most efficacious interventions, drawn from a variety of therapeutic orientations. Although technical eclecticism allows the flexibility to draw techniques from different schools of therapy, the model presents some serious problems. First, since none of the integrative therapies is related to any theory of personality and psychopathology, a framework for explaining and predicting human behaviour and change is lacking. Secondly, eclecticism is often practised as if a therapeutic technique can be easily disembodied from its contextual framework and readily transported to another context without consideration of its new psychotherapeutic context (Lazarus & Messer, 1991). Thirdly, it is very problematic to evaluate technical eclecticism. Because of the myriad interactions involved in empirical eclecticism, it is very difficult to determine the relative effectiveness of each treatment component included.

Common Factors Approach Integration Model

The common factors approach to psychotherapy integration is based on Rosenzweig's (1936) seminal discovery that all therapies share certain change processes, irrespective of their theoretical orientation. Therapists who operate within the common principles of change across different therapies look for common factors that may be most important in the treatment of their patients. For example, a common principle in many forms of psychotherapy consists of helping clients to become aware of and challenge their self-criticism. The common factors approach to psychotherapy integration has generated considerable research, produced several lists of proposed common factors and facilitated a rapprochement between different therapies (Lampropoulos, 2001). However, due to many serious methodological issues, recently there has been no further development in research and practice on the common factors approach.

One of the main problems with this approach relates to the common principles themselves. Although a common factor may appear similar on the surface, on closer inspection important differences may be represented. For instance, the common factors related to clients' awareness of self-criticism mentioned above are understood and accomplished very differently in the context of diverse psychotherapies. Within the CBT context, self-criticism is seen as maladaptive thinking that needs to be recognised, controlled and eliminated via cognitive restructuring. By contrast, in gestalt therapy, self-criticism is considered to be an aspect of the self that must be recognised and then integrated with other parts of the self, which can be achieved by the 'empty chair' technique (Safran & Messer, 1997).

Theoretical Integration Model

In this form of integration, different theories are combined in an attempt to construct a new and superordinate theoretical framework that can meaningfully guide research and practice. The best example of this kind of integration is Wachtel's *cyclical psychodynamics* (Wachtel, 1977, 1997), which assimilates psychoanalytic and behavioural theories within an interpersonal psychodynamic framework. The model acknowledges and uses reinforcement and social learning principles, thus allowing the therapist to use behavioural, cognitive, systems and experiential interventions in the context of psychodynamic therapy.

Lampropoulos (2001) has articulated four weaknesses related to the theoretical integration model of psychotherapy:

weaknesses

(a) Although the goal of this model is to integrate as many theories as possible, the existing models have succeeded in combining only two or three theories.
(b) The focus of the existing theoretical integration models is on specific psychological disorders only, thus neglecting other diagnostic categories.
(c) Because of their inherent theoretical differences and contrasting worldviews, integration presents great difficulties.
(d) Theoretical integration lacks systematic empirical validation.

Assimilative Integration Model

Best

In this mode of psychotherapy integration the therapist maintains a central theoretical position but incorporates or assimilates techniques from other schools of psychotherapy (Gold & Stricker, 2006). It is the most recent model of psychotherapy integration described in the literature, drawing from both theoretical integration and technical eclecticism. This approach to integration is well illustrated by the psychodynamically based integrative therapy developed and described by Gold and Stricker (2001, 2006). In this approach, 'therapy proceeds according to standard psychodynamic guidelines, but methods from other therapies are used when called for, and they may indirectly advance certain psychodynamic goals as well as address the target concern effectively' (Gold & Stricker, 2006, p. 12).

Messer (Lazarus & Messer, 1991; Messer, 1992) argues that when techniques from different theories are incorporated into one's preferred theoretical orientation, both the host theory and the imported technique interact with each other to produce a new assimilative model. Assimilative integration is considered to be the best model for integrating both theory and empirical findings to achieve maximum flexibility and effectiveness under a guiding theoretical framework (Lampropoulos, 2001). The cognitive hypnotherapy approach to treating emotional disorders described in this book is conceptualised as an assimilative integration model of psychotherapy.

COGNITIVE HYPNOTHERAPY AS AN ASSIMILATIVE INTEGRATION MODEL OF PSYCHOTHERAPY

Traditionally the practice of hypnosis has embraced a psychoanalytic framework, although Freud abandoned hypnosis and went on to develop free association. Like other schools of therapy, 'classical' hypnotherapists have also been resistant to diluting hypnotherapy with behaviour therapy or CBT. Chapman (2006) has identified several barriers that have impeded the integration of CBT with hypnosis:

- CBT practitioners have tended to use relaxation training or imagery procedures rather than hypnosis. CBT therapists often wonder: 'How is relaxation and imagery training different from hypnosis?' or 'What can hypnosis offer beyond relaxation or imagery training?'
- Training programmes for CBT have not taught clinical hypnosis or emphasised the role of hypnosis in therapy.
- Practitioners from other theoretical models, for example psychodynamic therapists, have embraced hypnosis but have not endorsed formal CBT strategies, although they often employ techniques used by CBT therapists (Golden, 1994).
- Differing views of the concept of the unconscious exist among different schools of therapy. Behaviour therapy has traditionally rejected the role of the unconscious, while other therapies, such as psychodynamic therapy, have readily embraced the unconscious.
- Lack of agreement exists over the definition of hypnosis.
- Lack of agreement exists over the definition of CBT.

To this list we can also add:

- Hypnosis does not provide a theory of personality, psychopathology and behaviour change.
- Empirical validation of hypnosis techniques is in its infancy.

Nevertheless, some clinicians have attempted to combine hypnosis with behaviour therapy (e.g. Clarke & Jackson, 1983; Kroger & Fezler, 1976; Lazarus, 1973) and hypnosis with CBT (e.g. Alladin, 1994, 2006, 2007a; Ellis, 1986, 1993; Golden, 1986, 1994, 2006). To my knowledge, none of these writers has formally attempted to combine hypnosis with CBT within any of the four psychotherapy integration models described above. Previously, I described the *cognitive-dissociative* model of depression (Alladin, 1994, 2006), recently revised and renamed the *Circular Feedback Model of Depression* (Alladin, 2007a), to establish the theoretical rationale for utilising cognitive hypnotherapy, hypnosis combined with CBT, in the management of depression (Alladin, 1989, 1994, 2006, 2007a). In this chapter, cognitive hypnotherapy is formally conceptualised as an assimilative model of psychotherapy for emotional disorders.

It is only fitting to consider cognitive hypnotherapy as an assimilative integration model of psychotherapy since it meets the six criteria for assimilative integration laid down by Lampropoulos (2001), including (a) empirical validation of host theory; (b) evidence-based imported techniques; (c) empirically based assimilation; (d) sensitivity around assimilation; (e) coherent assimilation; and (f) empirical validation of assimilated therapy.

Empirically Validated Theory

Both CBT and hypnotherapy comprise several empirically validated components. One of the requirements for integrative assimilation is that some of the components of the host theory of therapy should be empirically validated, or at least empirically informed. A good scientific theory should meet a number of criteria, including internal consistency, parsimony of explanatory constructs, testability and scope of clinical application (Alford & Beck, 1997). CBT meets all these criteria and it provides an excellent paradigm for integrative clinical practice, as it constitutes a unifying theory of psychotherapy and psychopathology. Theory is essential to clinical practice; without theory the practice of psychotherapy becomes a purely technical exercise, devoid of any scientific basis.

The cognitive theory of psychopathology and psychotherapy views *cognition* to be the key to psychological disorders. Alford and Beck (1997, p. 14) define cognition as 'that function that involves inferences about one's experiences and about the occurrence and control of future events' and state that cognitive theory 'suggests the importance of phenomenological perception of relationships among processes of identifying and predicting complex relations among events, so as to facilitate adaptation to changing environments'. CBT is the application of the cognitive theory of psychopathology to the individual case. Cognitive theory relates the various psychiatric disorders to specific cognitive variables and it includes a formal, comprehensive set of principles or axioms, including:

1. The *schemas* or cognitive structures regulate our psychological functioning or adaptation and give meaning to contextual relationship.
2. Assignment of meaning, whether at conscious or unconscious levels, activates behavioural, emotional, attentional or memory strategies for adaptation.
3. There is an interactive relationship between cognitive systems and other systems.
4. Each category of meaning has *cognitive content specificity* or the potential to produce specific patterns of emotion, attention, memory and behaviour.
5. Meanings do not always represent pre-existing components of reality but construction of a given context or goal, and are therefore subject to *cognitive distortions* or *bias* (dysfunctional or unadaptive meanings). Cognitive distortions can produce errors in either cognitive content (meaning) or cognitive processing (meaning elaboration), or in both.
6. Some individuals are vulnerable (predisposition or diathesis) to specific cognitive distortions. Specific cognitive vulnerabilities predispose individuals to specific syndromes.

7. Psychopathology results from *cognitive triad* or cognitive distortions related to the self, the world (environmental context) and the future (goals). Each psychological disorder manifests specific cognitive distortions associated with the components of the cognitive triad.

8. Two levels of meaning – *public meaning* and *personal meaning* – can be attached to any event. The public meaning of an event has few major implications for the individual, whereas the personal or private meaning has significant implications as the person is likely to access the cognitive triad.

9. Cognitive processing involves three levels of processing, including (a) pre-conscious, unintentional or automatic processing; (b) conscious processing; and (c) metacognitive processing, which includes 'realistic' or 'rational' responses. The conscious level of processing is predominantly utilised in CBT.

10. Schemas are *teleonomic* structures; that is, they facilitate adaptation of the individual to the environment. A given psychological state is therefore neither adaptive nor maladaptive in itself, but only in relation to the larger social or environmental context of the person.

Moreover, CBT provides a common language for psychotherapy integration. A survey of 58 members of the Society for the Exploration of Psychotherapy Integration carried out by Norcross and Thomas (1988) found the absence of a common language to be rated as the most severe impediment to psychotherapy integration. CBT constructs are compatible with divergent schools of psychotherapy. CBT uses ordinary language and concepts from cognitive psychology that are widely used by therapists from different/varying orientations. While ordinary language is applicable across several generations, cognitive concepts such as 'schemas', 'scripts' and 'metacognition' describe therapeutic phenomena observed across differing psychotherapies. According to Kazdin (1984, p. 163), the concepts of cognitive psychology 'deal with meaning of events, underlying processes, and ways of structuring and interpreting experience. They can encompass affect, perception, and behaviour. Consequently, cognitive processes and their referents probably provide the place where the gap between psychodynamic and behavioural views is leas wide.'

Evidence-Based Imported Techniques

The second criterion for integrative assimilation requires the techniques to be synthesised into the host theory to be empirically supported, or at least empirically informed, within the research guidelines proposed by the American Psychological Association (APA) Task Force (Chambless & Hollon, 1998). Hypnosis has been used, in one form or another, to relieve pain and suffering since prehistoric times. Review of the well-controlled empirical studies of the role of hypnosis in the treatment of a variety of medical and psychiatric conditions provides convincing evidence for the clinical efficacy of hypnosis (Alladin, 2007b; Lynn *et al.*, 2000; Pinnell & Covino, 2000). The effectiveness of hypnosis in the management of pain has been even more remarkable. A meta-analysis of controlled trials of hypnotic analgesia demonstrates that hypnotherapy can provide relief for 75% of the patients studied (Montgomery, DuHammel & Redd, 2000). Other comprehensive reviews of the clinical trial literature indicate that hypnotherapy is effective with both acute and chronic pain (Elkins, Jensen & Patterson, 2007; Patterson & Jensen, 2003). The American Psychiatric Association recognises hypnosis as a legitimate therapeutic tool. It is therefore not surprising that hypnosis has been used as an adjunctive treatment with a variety of psychiatric conditions, including anxiety, depression, dissociative disorders, somatoform disorders, eating disorders, sleep disorders and sexual disorders.

Moreover, there is some empirical evidence for combining hypnosis with CBT. Schoenberger (2000), from her review of the empirical status of the use of hypnosis in conjunction with cognitive-behavioural treatment programmes, concluded that the existing studies demonstrate substantial benefits from the addition of hypnosis with cognitive-behavioural techniques. Similarly, Kirsch, Montgomery and Sapirstein (1995), from their meta-analysis of 18 studies comparing a cognitive-behavioural treatment with the same treatment supplemented by hypnosis, found that the mean effect size of the difference between hypnotic and non-hypnotic treatment was 0.87 standard deviations. The authors concluded that hypnotherapy was significantly superior to non-hypnotic treatment. Alladin and Alibhai (2007) demonstrated the additive effect of combining hypnosis with CBT in the management of chronic depression. The study also met criteria for *probably efficacious* treatment for depression as laid down by the American Psychological Association (APA) Task Force (Chambless & Hollon, 1998) and it provides empirical validation for integrating hypnosis with CBT in the management of depression. Similarly, Bryant *et al.* (2005) demonstrated hypnosis combined with CBT to be more effective than CBT and supportive counselling in the treatment of acute stress disorder.

Empirically Based Assimilation

The circumstances and rationale for selecting the techniques to be assimilated should be empirically guided. Alladin (2007a) has listed 19 strengths related to hypnosis that can be easily integrated with CBT. Those techniques that add strengths to hypnotherapy, and are empirically informed or supported, are listed below.

Hypnosis adds leverage to treatment

When used properly, hypnosis adds leverage to treatment and shortens treatment time (Dengrove, 1973). The rapid changes are attributed to the brisk and profound behavioural, emotional, cognitive and physiological changes brought on by hypnosis (De Piano & Salzberg, 1986). Hypnotherapists routinely observe such rapid changes in their patients, which is succinctly documented by Yapko (2003, p. 106):

> I have worked with many people who actually cried tears of joy or relief in a session for having had an opportunity to experience themselves as relaxed, comfortable, and positive when their usual experience of themselves was one of pain and despair.

Hypnosis serves as a strong placebo

For the majority of patients, hypnosis serves as a strong placebo. Lazarus (1973) and Spanos and Barber (1974, 1976) have provided evidence that hypnotic trance induction procedures are beneficial for those patients who believe in their efficacy. There is a considerable body of evidence that patients' positive attitudes and beliefs about a treatment can have a profound therapeutic effect in both medical and psychological conditions (Harrington, 1997). Such observations led Kirsch (1985, 2000) to develop the sociocognitive model of hypnosis, known as the *response set theory*. Kirsch provided considerable empirical evidence to support the hypothesis that the positive effect of hypnosis is due to the patients' positive expectancy. However, the studies on hypnotic induced analgesia conducted by Goldstein and Hilgard (1975) and Spiegel and Albert (1983) clearly indicate that hypnotic reduction of pain is not due to placebo, stress inoculation or changes in the level of endorphins. Moreover, there is a growing literature providing empirical evidence for the effectiveness of hypnotherapy with a variety of medical and psychological disorders (see Lynn *et al.*, 2000; Lynn & Kirsch, 2006; Yapko, 2003). Whether hypnosis works via a placebo effect or by influencing behavioural and physiological responses, the sensitive therapist can create the right atmosphere to capitalise on suggestibility and expectation effects to enhance therapeutic gains (Erickson & Rossi, 1979). Kirsch (1999, p. 216) stresses that the 'placebo effect is not something to be avoided, provided that it can be elicited without deception. Instead, therapists should attempt to maximize the impact of this powerful psychological mechanism.'

Hypnosis breaks resistance

Indirect hypnotic suggestions can be provided to break patients' resistance (Erickson & Rossi, 1979). For example, an oppositional (to suggestions) patient may be instructed (paradoxically) to continue to resist, as a strategy to obtain compliance.

Hypnosis fosters a strong therapeutic alliance

Repeated hypnotic experience fosters a strong therapeutic alliance (Brown & Fromm, 1986b). Skilful induction of positive experiences, especially when patients perceive them to be emerging from their own inner resources, gives patients greater confidence in their own abilities and help to foster trust in the therapeutic relationship.

Hypnosis facilitates rapid transference

Because of greater access to fantasies, memories and emotions during hypnotic induction, full-blown transference manifestations may occur very rapidly, often during the initial stage of hypnotherapy (Brown & Fromm, 1986a). Such transference reinforces the therapeutic alliance.

Hypnosis induces deep relaxation

Hypnosis induces relaxation, which is effective in reducing anxiety, making it easier for patients to think about and discuss materials that they were previously too anxious to confront. Sometimes anxious and agitated patients are also unable to pinpoint their maladaptive thoughts and emotions. But once they close their eyes and relax, many of these same individuals appear to become more aware of their thoughts and feelings. Through relaxation, hypnosis also reduces distraction and maximises the ability to concentrate, which enhances learning of new materials. The relaxation experience is particularly helpful to patients who have comorbid anxiety. For example, many depressives experience anxiety; approximately 50–76% of depressives have comorbid anxiety disorder (see Dozois & Westra, 2004).

Hypnosis strengthens the ego

Ego strengthening is an approach whereby positive suggestions are repeated to oneself with the belief that these suggestions will become embedded in the unconscious mind and exert an automatic influence on feelings, thoughts and behaviour. Ego strengthening is incorporated in hypnotherapy to enhance patients' self-confidence and self-worth (Heap & Aravind, 2002). Alladin (1992) has pointed out that depressives tend to engage in negative self-hypnosis (NSH) and Araoz (1981, 1985) considers NSH to be the common denominator of all psychogenic problems. More recently, Nolen-Hoeksema and her colleagues (see Nolen-Hoeksema, 2002 for review) have provided empirical evidence that individuals who ruminate a great deal in response to their sad or depressed moods have more negative and distorted memories of the past, the present and the future. These ruminators or moody brooders then become increasingly negative and hopeless in their thinking, resulting in protracted depressive symptoms.

Ego-strengthening suggestions are offered to counter the NSH. Alladin and Heap (1991, p. 58) consider ego strengthening to be 'a way of exploiting the positive experience of hypnosis and the therapist–patient relationship in order to develop feelings of confidence and optimism and an improved self-image'.

Hypnosis facilitates divergent thinking

Hypnosis facilitates divergent thinking by maximising awareness along several levels of brain functioning, maximising the focus of attention and concentration, and minimising distraction and interference from other sources of stimuli (Tosi & Baisden, 1984). In other words, through divergent operations the potential for learning alternatives is increased.

Hypnosis directs attention to wider experiences

Hypnosis provides a frame of mind where attention can be directed to wider experience, such as feelings of warmth, feeling happy and so on. Hypnosis provides a vehicle for exploring and expanding experience in the present, the past and the future. Such strategies can enhance divergent thinking and facilitate the reconstruction of dysfunctional 'realities'.

Hypnosis allows engagement of the non-dominant hemisphere

Hypnosis provides direct entry into the cognitive processing of the right cerebral hemisphere (in right-handers), which accesses and organises emotional and experiential information. Therefore hypnosis can be utilised to teach restructure cognitive and emotional processes influenced by the non-dominant cerebral hemisphere.

Hypnosis enables access to non-consciousness processes

Hypnosis allows access to psychological processes below the threshold of awareness, thus providing a means of restructuring non-conscious cognitions.

Hypnosis allows integration of cortical functioning

Hypnosis provides a vehicle whereby cortical and subcortical functioning can be accessed and integrated. Since the subcortex is the seat of emotions, access to it provides an entry to the organisation of primitive emotions.

Hypnosis facilitates imagery conditioning

Hypnosis provides a basis for imagery training/conditioning. When the patient is hypnotised the power of imagination is increased, possibly because hypnosis, imagery and affect are all mediated by the same right cerebral hemisphere (Ley & Freeman, 1984). Under hypnosis, imagery can be used for the following reasons:

(a) systematic desensitisation (in their imagination the patient rehearses coping with in vivo difficult situations)
(b) restructuring of cognitive processes at various levels of awareness or consciousness
(c) exploration of the remote past
(d) directing attention on positive experiences

According to Boutin (1978), the rationale for using hypnosis is that it intensifies imagery and cognitive restructuring. Lazarus (1999, p. 196) writes:

> Clinically speaking, the use of the word *hypnosis* and the application of various hypnotic techniques appear to enhance the impact of imagery methods on susceptible clients. They also appear to augment the power of most suggestions. There seems to be a greater veridical effect when suggestible clients picture various scenes 'under hypnosis.'

Hypnosis induces dreams

Hypnosis can induce dreams and increase dream recall and understanding (Golden, Dowd & Friedberg, 1987). Dream induction provides another vehicle for uncovering non-conscious maladaptive thoughts, fantasies, feelings and images.

Hypnosis induces positive moods

Negative or positive moods can be easily induced under hypnosis and therefore patients can be taught, through rehearsal, strategies for controlling negative or inappropriate affects. Mood induction can also facilitate recall. Bower (1981) has provided evidence that certain materials can only be recalled when experiencing the coincident mood (mood-state-dependent memory). Bower's research into mood-state-dependent memory led him to propose the associative network theory, which states:

(a) An emotion serves as a memory unit that can easily link up with coincident events.
(b) Activation of this emotion unit can aid retrieval of events associated with it.
(c) It primes emotional themata for use in free association, fantasies and perceptual categorisation.

Repeated hypnotic induction of positive mood can lead to the development of 'antidepressive' pathways (Alladin, 2007a; Schwartz, 1984). Goldapple *et al.* (2004) have provided functional neuroimaging evidence to show that CBT produces specific cortical regional changes in treatment responders.

Similarly, Kosslyn *et al*. (2000) have demonstrated that hypnosis can modulate colour perception. Their investigations showed that hypnotised subjects were able to produce changes in brain function (measured by PET scanning) similar to those that occur during visual perception. These findings support the claim that hypnotic suggestions can produce distinct neural changes correlated with real perception. Moreover, Schwartz *et al*. (1976) have provided electromyographic evidence that depressive pathways can be developed through conscious negative focusing. Schwartz's investigations led him to believe that if it is possible to produce depressive pathways through negative cognitive focusing, then it would be possible to develop antidepressive or happy pathways by focusing on positive imagery (Schwartz, 1984). From the foregoing evidence it would not be unreasonable to infer that the positive affect and images, coupled with ego-strengthening suggestions, produced by the hypnosis and Positive Mood Induction Technique might have exerted some cortical changes in the brains of the depressives subjected to repetitive positive hypnotic experience. To verify the extent and locus of changes, further studies involving hypnotherapy and brain imaging are required.

Post-hypnotic suggestions

Hypnosis provides post-hypnotic suggestions, which can be very powerful in altering problem behaviours, dysfunctional cognitions and negative emotions. Often post-hypnotic suggestions are used for shaping behaviour. Barrios (1973) regards post-hypnotic suggestion to be a form of 'higher-order conditioning', which functions as positive or negative reinforcement to increase or decrease the probability of desired or undesired behaviours, respectively. Clarke and Jackson (1983) have utilised post-hypnotic suggestions to enhance the effect of in vivo exposure among agoraphobics. Yapko (2003) regards post-hypnotic suggestions to be a very necessary part of the therapeutic process if the patient is to carry new possibilities into future experience. Hence many clinicians use post-hypnotic suggestions to shape behaviour.

Hypnosis enhances training in positive self-hypnosis

Self-hypnosis training can be enhanced by hetero-hypnotic induction and post-hypnotic suggestions. Most of the techniques mentioned above can be practised under self-hypnosis, thus fostering positive self-hypnosis by deflecting preoccupation away from negative self-suggestions. Patients with various emotional disorders have the tendency to ruminate negatively, which can be considered to be a form of self-hypnosis (Alladin, 1994, 2006, 2007a; Araoz, 1981, 1985). For example, Abramson and his colleagues (Abramson *et al.*, 2002) have examined the relationship between cognitive vulnerability and Beck's theory of depression. They found cognitive vulnerability to underlie the tendency to ruminate negatively and they posited that cognitively vulnerable individuals are at high risk of engaging in rumination. Depressive rumination involves the perpetual recycling of negative thoughts (Wenzlaff, 2004). Evidence indicates that negative rumination can lead to negative affect, depressive symptoms, negatively biased thinking, poor problem-solving, impaired motivation and inhibition of instrumental behaviour, impaired concentration and cognition, and increased stress and problems (for review, see Lyubomirsky & Tkach, 2004). Depressive ruminators, in particular, are caught in a vicious cycle. Due to their rumination they become keenly aware of the problems in their lives, but at the same time they are unable to generate good solutions to those problems and therefore they feel hopeless about being able to change their lives (Nolen-Hoeksema, 2002). Training in positive self-hypnosis provides a strategy for counteraction negative ruminations (Alladin, 2007a).

Hypnosis creates perceived self-efficacy

Bandura (1977) believes that expectation of self-efficacy is central to all forms of therapeutic change. The positive hypnotic experience, coupled with the belief that one has the ability to experience hypnosis and use it to ameliorate symptoms, give one an expectancy of self-efficacy. The perceived self-efficacy not only creates a sense of hope but also affects the treatment outcome (Lazarus, 1973).

Hypnotic techniques are easily exported

Hypnosis provides a broad range of short-term techniques, which can be easily integrated as an adjunct with many forms of therapy, e.g. with behaviour therapy, cognitive therapy, developmental therapy, psychodynamic therapy, supportive therapy and so on. Since hypnosis itself is not a therapy, the specific treatment effects will be contingent on the therapeutic approach with which it is integrated. Nevertheless, the hypnotic relationship can enhance the efficacy of therapy when hypnosis is used as an adjunct to a particular form of therapy (Brown & Fromm, 1986b).

Sensitivity Around Assimilation

The therapist should be sensitive to the assimilation process, as not all the techniques imported can be easily assimilated into one's theory without contradicting or opposing its central meaning and worldview (Messer, 1989). For example, the technique of regression commonly used in hypnotherapy contradicts one of the principal tenets of CBT. In hypnotherapy regression is often used to access unconscious experience (Alladin, 2007a, pp. 151–3) and it is readily accepted that one can have an affect without conscious cognition, which is contradictory to the cognitive theory which holds that cognition precedes affect. The therapist needs to be very sensitive to the patient, particularly to a patient who is well versed in CBT, when introducing hypnotic regression to access unconscious cognitions, otherwise the patient will be confused and may question the credibility of the therapy or the integrity of the therapist. One of the ways of approaching hypnotic regression is to inform the patient:

> Not always, but sometimes, it is possible for us to be upset in a situation without knowing why. This may sound contrary to what you learned from the CBT sessions. It is true that 99% of the time we are able to identify the cognitions related to the event or situation that upset us, but on rare occasions we can't identify the thoughts related to our feelings. Last Sunday is a good example – you indicated that you were upset at the wedding but don't know why, you could not identify your cognition. Hypnotic regression is an effective tool for accessing unconscious cognition related to an event or situation.

Coherent Assimilation

The assimilative integration process should be coherent or theoretically compatible with the major propositions and principles of the main guiding theory. This means that the final product of the assimilative integration is theoretically compatible with the host theory, without seriously altering it. Otherwise it might result in any of these three possibilities (Lampropoulos, 2001): a new theoretical integrative therapy is evolved; a multimodal or eclectic mode of therapy is produced; and a meaningless and contradictory hodgepodge of techniques is assembled. Hypnosis, not being therapy but a bunch of short-term strategies, is easily integrated with CBT without seriously altering the theoretical conceptualisation of CBT. Kirsch's (1993, p. 153) description of hypnosis in the context of CBT reinforces this point:

> The use of hypnosis in cognitive-behavioral therapy is as old as behavior therapy itself. Wolpe and Lazarus (1966), for example, reported using hypnotic inductions instead of progressive relaxation with about one third of their systematic desensitization patients. From a cognitive-behavioral perspective, hypnosis provides a context in which the effects of cognitive-behavioral interventions can be potentiated for some clients. Specifically, hypnosis is likely to enhance the effects of cognitive-behavioral therapy among clients with positive attitudes and expectancies toward hypnosis.

Empirical Validation of Assimilated Therapy

Without empirical validation it is not possible to establish whether the importation of a technique into a host therapy has a positive impact on therapy, especially when techniques are decontextualised and placed in a new framework. It is only through empirical validation that the creation and practice of ineffective and idiosyncratic assimilative integration can be avoided. Moreover, empirical validation may lead to re-evaluation of the assimilative model. Several studies (e.g. Alladin & Alibhai, 2007; Bryant *et al.*, 2005; Schoenberger *et al.*, 1997) and reviews (Flammer & Alladin, 2007; Kirsch, Montgomery & Sapirstein, 1995; Schoenberger, 2000) have demonstrated the effectiveness of combining hypnosis with CBT. However, all the studies have combined several hypnotic techniques with CBT. For example, Alladin and Alibhai (2007) utilised hypnotic relaxation, ego strengthening, expansion of awareness, positive mood induction, post-hypnotic suggestions and self-hypnosis with CBT in the treatment of depression. Without further studies using a dismantling design, there is no way of knowing which techniques were effective and which were superfluous.

COGNITIVE HYPNOTHERAPY AS AN ASSIMILATIVE INTEGRATION MODEL OF PSYCHOTHERAPY

From the reviews of the integrative models, it would appear that the assimilative model provides the best mode of psychotherapy integration. There are many reasons for assimilating hypnotic techniques with CBT.

1. CBT meets all the criteria for assimilative integration proposed by Lampropoulos (2001), including empirical evidence for the additive effect when CBT is combined with hypnotic techniques (Alladin & Alibhai, 2007; Bryant *et al.*, 2005; Kirsch, Montgomery & Sapirstein, 1995; Schoenberger, 2000; Scheonberger *et al.*, 1997).
2. Cognitive hypnotherapy allows CBT therapists to continue practising in the framework of their training, experience, investments and preferred theoretical orientations without losing the benefits of effective techniques generated from the area of clinical hypnosis. CBT therapists do not have to abandon their theoretical orientation nor do they have to change the beliefs around which they built their professional identity, self-esteem and professional credibility. Hypnosis provides a broad range of short-term techniques that can be easily integrated as an adjunct with CBT.
3. Cognitive hypnotherapy can equally be beneficial to therapists who practise clinical hypnosis within their own preferred theoretical orientations (e.g. psychodynamic approach). Since hypnosis does not provide a theory of personality, psychopathology and behaviour change, it seems logical to assimilate effective hypnotic techniques within an empirically based theory of psychotherapy such as CBT. Such an integrative approach is particularly suited when hypnosis is regarded as an adjunctive therapy.
4. In the assimilative integration of CBT and hypnosis, therapists faithful to each mode of therapy are able to transcend the limitations of their original theory by using highly effective but previously 'forbidden' techniques (Lampropoulos, 2001). Alladin (2007a) reviewed the strengths and limitations of CBT and hypnosis and concluded that the 'strengths of CBT and hypnotherapy can be combined to form a powerful treatment approach' (p. 54) for a variety of emotional disorders.

SUMMARY

After reviewing the well-known integrative theories of psychotherapy, the rest of the chapter focused on conceptualising cognitive hypnotherapy as an assimilated model of integrative psychotherapy. Cognitive hypnotherapy meets the criteria for an assimilative integrative model of psychotherapy. It is hoped that the application of the model with various clinical disorders will inform and guide clinicians on how to select treatment strategies, not haphazardly but based on case formulation of each individual case. However, the model should not be seen as a finished product, but an evolving process. Although it is important to evaluate and validate assimilative integrative therapies empirically, it is important to bear in mind that *psychotherapy integration* is synonymous with *psychotherapeutic creativity and originality*' and thus 'many advances occur in the consulting room of individual therapists who cannot submit their work to large-scale research investigations' (Gold & Stricker, 2006, p. 13). Moreover, beyond blending techniques, clinicians should attempt to integrate patients' insight and feedback into their assimilative therapies.

CHAPTER 2

COGNITIVE HYPNOTHERAPY CASE FORMULATION

INTRODUCTION

One of the most important clinical skills is the ability to formulate a case in terms of the most effective treatment plan. This chapter describes the cognitive hypnotherapy (CH) approach to case formulation, which guides the clinician in selecting the most effective and efficient treatment strategies for his or her patient. CH case conceptualisation stresses the role of cognitive distortions, negative self-instructions, irrational automatic thoughts and beliefs, schemas, and negative ruminations or negative self-hypnosis in the understanding of the patient's problem(s). Evidence suggests that matching of treatment to particular patient characteristics increases outcome (Beutler, Clarkin & Bongar, 2000). By formulating a case, the clinician develops a working hypothesis on how the patient's problems can be understood in terms of negative self-hypnosis and cognitive behavioural theories. This understanding provides a compass or a guide to understanding the treatment process.

Persons (1989) has posited that psychological disorders can occur at two levels: *overt difficulties* and *underlying psychological mechanisms*. Overt difficulties are signs and symptoms presented by the patient that can be described in terms of beliefs, behaviours and emotions. The manifestation and intensity of the cognitive, behavioural or emotional symptoms are determined by the dysfunction of the underlying biological and psychological mechanisms. As the focus of this book is on psychological treatment, the underlying psychological mechanism of each disorder described in the book will be examined in detail. But this is not meant to imply that biological factors are not important. Whenever possible, the psychobiological mechanism of a disorder will be examined. The chapter will also discuss how the clinician can translate and tailor the nomothetic (general) treatment protocol to the individual (idiographic) patient. Within this framework, clinical work becomes systematic and hypothesis-driven, rather than adopting a hit-and-miss approach to treatment.

RATIONALE FOR USING INDIVIDUALISED CASE FORMULATION IN PSYCHOTHERAPY

The main function of a case formulation is to devise an effective treatment plan. Needleman (2003) defines case formulation as the process of developing an explicit, parsimonious understanding of patients and their problems that effectively guides treatment. Although the effectiveness of CBT (e.g. with depression, see Chapter 3) and hypnotherapy (e.g. migraine, see Chapter 4) with various disorders has been empirically validated, the clinical significance levels were derived from *nomothetic* (general) or standardised treatment protocols studied in randomised controlled trials (RCTs). In the clinical setting there is no standard treatment protocol that can be applied systematically to all patients. The task of the clinician in such a setting is to translate the nomothetic findings from RCTs to an *idiographic* or individual patient basis in an evidence-based way. To accomplish this task, many writers (e.g. Persons, 1989; Persons & Davidson, 2001; Persons, Davidson & Tompkins, 2001) have recommended an evidence-based case-formulation approach to treatment. Persons, Davidson & Tompkins (2001) regard an evidence-based formulation-driven approach to the treatment of each individual patient as an experiment. Within this framework, treatment begins with an assessment, which generates a hypothesis about the mechanisms causing or maintaining the problem. The hypothesis is the individualised case formulation, which the therapist uses to develop an individualised treatment plan. As treatment proceeds, the therapist collects data via further assessment to evaluate the effects of the planned treatment. If it becomes evident that the treatment is not working, the therapist reformulates the case and develops a new treatment plan, which is also monitored and evaluated. Clinical work thus becomes more systematic and hypothesis-driven. Such an approach to treatment becomes principle-driven rather than delivering treatment in a hit-and-miss fashion.

The greatest advantage of a formulation-driven approach to clinical work is:

> when the therapist encounters setbacks during the treatment process, he or she can follow a systematic strategy to make a change in treatment (consider whether a reformulation of the case might suggest some new interventions) rather than simply making hit-or-miss changes in the treatment plan. (Persons, Davidson & Tompkins, 2001, p. 14)

Nevertheless, there are two important drawbacks to a formulation-driven approach to treatment. First, individualised formulation-driven treatments have not been widely subjected to evaluation in RCTs. Secondly, while monitoring treatment outcome systematically, a clinician may rely on idiosyncratic or non-evidence-based formulation and treatment. To minimise clinical judgement errors and to secure solid evidence-based individualised formulation-driven treatment, Persons, Davidson & Tomplins (2001) offer two suggestions:

- Base the initial idiographic formulation on a strong evidence-based nomothetic formulation.
- Base the initial idiographic treatment plan on nomothetic protocols that have been shown to be effective in RCTs.

The CH case formulation described in this book is based on Beck's (1976) cognitive theory and therapy of psychopathology, Persons and colleagues' (Persons, 1989; Persons & Davidson, 2001; Persons, Davidson & Tompkins, 2001) evidence-based formulation-driven treatment, and Alladin's (2007b) and Chapman's (2006) case-conceptualisation model of integration of CBT and hypnosis in the management of psychological disorders.

ASSUMPTIONS IN COGNITIVE HYPNOTHERAPY CASE FORMULATION

The CH case-formulation approach is recommended for three main reasons: it provides a systematic method for individualising treatment; it allows the therapist to take an empirical approach to treatment of each case; and it provides direction and evaluation during the treatment process. As CH case formulation make several assumptions about psychological disorders, it is important for the cognitive hypnotherapist to have a complete understanding of the patient's belief systems and thought processes, and how they relate to the assumptions listed below:

1. Emotions are not produced by external events, but by the perception of the events.
2. Maladaptive emotions are produced by cognitive distortions.
3. Cognitive distortions are mediated by underlying negative schemas.
4. Underlying negative schemas can be latent and unconscious from early life.
5. Symptoms are produced when certain life events activate negative schemas.
6. Negative rumination is considered to be a form of negative self-hypnosis (NSH).
7. NSH can lead to exacerbation of symptoms and loss of control.
8. NSH leads to negative kindling of the brain and may create negative pathways.
9. Psychological disorders are caused by biopsychosocial factors within the context of the diathesis-stress model.
10. Psychological disorders have many underlying risk factors and they can be comorbid with other medical and psychological disorders.

LEVELS OF COGNITIVE HYPNOTHERAPY CASE FORMULATION

The individualiaed case formulation should include an exhaustive list of the patient's problems and should describe the relationships among these problems. Exhaustive information is particularly necessary when treating severe cases with multiple psychiatric, medical and psychosocial problems. Patients with complex profiles are not usually included in RCTs. In the clinical settings it is the norm for therapists to treat these patients, and therefore it is important to obtain an exhaustive list of problems that will help the therapist develop a working hypothesis and prioritise treatment goals. CH case formulation can occur at three different levels:

- formulation at the case level
- formulation at the problem or syndrome level
- formulation at the situation level

The initial case-level formulation is developed after three or four sessions of therapy. At this level, the clinician develops a conceptualisation of the case as a whole. In the formulation at this level it is very important to explain the relationships among the patient's problems. Establishing the relationship among the problems helps the clinician to focus first on problems that may be causing other problems. For example, social anxiety may be caused or maintained by poor social skills and thus social skills training should be the focus of early intervention.

Formulation at the problem or syndrome level provides conceptualisation of a particular clinical problem or syndrome, such as major depression, anxiety disorder, migraine headache, insomnia, bingeing and purging, and so on. Since hypnosis does not provide a model of personality or psychopathology, we need to rely on other models of psychological disorders. Within the CH formulation, cognitive behavioural theories are used to explain the symptoms and the syndromes. However, some clinicians have attempted to integrate the hypnotic paradigm with cognitive behaviour theory to explain symptoms. For example, Alladin (2007b) uses the circular feedback model to explain depression (see Chapter 3). The clinician's treatment plan for the syndrome or problem depends on the formulation of the problem. For example, a patient's complaint of fatigue in response to a recent professional setback can be attributed to either abuse of hypnotics or negative thoughts ('There's no point in trying – I always fail'). Different formulations suggest different interventions. Moreover, the case formulation is determined by the theoretical orientation of the clinician.

The formulation at the situation level provides a 'mini-formulation' of the patient's reactions in a particular situation in terms of cognitions, ruminations, behaviours and affect that guides the clinician's intervention in that situation. Beck has provided the Thought Record format (see the CAB form in

Appendix A) to develop a situation-level formulation. The case-level formulation is derived from the information collected in the situation-level and the problem-level formulations.

As noted above, all levels of formulation provide directions for intervention. However, all formulations should be treated as hypotheses and the clinician should continually revise and sharpen the formulations as the therapy proceeds. Moreover, a complete case formulation should also contain many other relevant components that the therapist considers important, such as religious background, spirituality, cultural influence, minority group and so on.

COGNITIVE HYPNOTHERAPY CASE FORMULATION

In order to identify the mechanisms that underlie the patient's problem, the eight-step case formulation derived from the work of Persons, Davidson and Tompkins (2001), Ledley, Marx and Heimberg (2005) and Alladin (2007b) can be used. The eight components summarised in Table 2.1 are described in detail below. Appendix C provides a generic template for a CH case formulation and treatment plan. This template can be utilised with any specific psychobiological disorder the therapist wants to treat with CH. Appendix D provides a completed example of a CH case-formulation and treatment plan for Jackie (a depressed patient), while Chapter 3 describes some of the CH strategies utilised with Jackie.

Table 2.1   Eight-step cognitive hypnotherapy case formulation

1. List the major symptoms and problems in functioning.
2. Formulate a formal diagnosis.
3. Formulate a working hypothesis.
4. Identify the precipitants and activating situations.
5. Explore the origin of negative self-schemas.
6. Summarise the working hypothesis.
7. Outline the treatment plan.
8. Identify strengths and assets and predict obstacles to treatment.

Problem List

The problem list is derived from the assessment information, consisting of an exhaustive list of the patient's main presenting problems and other relevant psychosocial issues. Persons and Davidson (2001) recommend stating the patient's difficulties in concrete behavioural terms. The problem list should include any difficulties the patient is having in any of the following domains:

- psychological/psychiatric symptoms
- medical symptoms
- interpersonal difficulties
- occupational problems
- financial difficulties
- housing problems
- legal problems
- leisure activities

Making a comprehensive list of problems ensures that important problems are not missed and this exercise protects the therapist from becoming overwhelmed with the patient's multitudinous problems. Moreover, the list provides themes about causal relationships among problems and helps to develop working hypotheses. For example, a patient with chronic migraine headache, in an attempt to control an attack, may avoid social situations, prefers routine and may be finicky with food.

Diagnosis

An accurate diagnosis provides information for the initial formulation of the hypotheses and the treatment plan. It is recommended that a formal diagnostic nomenclature such as the DSM-IV-TR (American Psychiatric Association, 2000) is used to make a psychiatric diagnosis. Beck *et al.* (1987) have provided empirical evidence for his *content-specificity* hypothesis, which maintains that although negativity is common to all emotional disorders, each disorder has its own specific set of cognitive distortions. Therefore an accurate diagnosis provides schema hypotheses. For example, it is known that depressives hold typical negative schemas about themselves, others, the world and the future, and therefore a diagnosis of depression will guide the therapist to look for depressive schemas hypotheses. A psychiatric diagnosis also serves as a link to RCTs and empirically supported nomothetic treatment interventions (Persons, Davidson & Tompkins, 2001).

When dealing with a medical or neurological condition, it is important to obtain information and clearance from the attending physician. In such a case it may be important to combine CH with the medical treatment.

Working Hypotheses

The working hypothesis is central to case formulation and it can be subdivided into four headings: schema, activating events, origins and summary.

Schemas

Schemas or core beliefs are deep cognitive structures that people have held for much of their lives and they are activated across a wide range of situations. The schemas have a profound influence on how people feel, appraise situations, and see themselves and the world (Needleman, 2003). The therapist attempts to offer hypotheses about the core beliefs that may be causing or maintaining the difficulties identified in the problem list. For example, when formulating a case with depression, it will be important for the therapist to understand the patient's beliefs about self, others, world and future (cognitive triad); the extent to which the patient ruminates and indulges in negative self-hypnosis; and the capacity of the depressed patients to experience hypnotic trance. Therefore within the CH case formulation for depression, maladaptive cognitions, negative ruminations, negative self-hynosis and hypnotic suggestibility are routinely assessed.

Appendix D provides Jackie's negative views on several cognitive domains. Although patients with a particular condition may have multiple negative beliefs, they tend to ruminate with one or two core beliefs. According to Nolen-Hoeksema (1991) rumination represents a process of perseverative attention that is directed to specific, mainly internal content. For example, an anxious person may become focused on his or her anxious feeling, the causes of the anxious feeling and the consequences of the anxiety. In such a case the core beliefs may centre around: 'I am abnormal, there's something wrong with me and I will never be normal'. And the patient will ruminate with the negative self-suggestions that 'I am not normal' and thus 'I will be anxious for the rest of my life and I will never be able to achieve anything'. Such perseverative attention can be regarded as a form of negative self-hypnosis (NSH). Moreover, the negative schemas and the negative beliefs add more vitality to NSH, which serves to counter positive suggestions from self or others.

Patients who are highly suggestible to hypnosis are more likely to be experientially involved in their ruminations. For example, Bliss (1984) found that patients with conversion disorders scored an average of 9.7 on the Hypnotic Induction Profile (HIP) 12-point scale. This finding was corroborated by Maldonado (1996a,b), which led him to hypothesise that patients with conversion disorder may be using their own capacity to dissociate to displace uncomfortable emotional feeling on to a chosen body part, which then becomes dysfunctional. Therefore Maldonado and Spiegel (2003) argue that since the hypnotic phenomena may be involved in the etiology of some conversion symptoms, hypnosis can be used to control the symptoms. This is the reason for assessing negative self-hypnosis and hypnotic suggestibility within the CH case formulation. Although the concept of hypnotic suggestibility is controversial, it is my belief that patients who score low on standard hypnotic suggestibility scales may not derive maximum benefit from hypnotherapy. For such patients, relaxation or imagery training can be substituted for hypnosis. The standard tests not only indicate which patient is highly suggestible, but the assessment also serves as an experiment to discover what kinds of suggestions the patient would naturally respond to. Such information guides the therapist to craft and deliver congruent induction, and hypnotic and posthypnotic suggestions. For instance, if a patient obtained the highest score on 'arm heaviness' and a low score on 'arm levitation' on the Barber Suggestibility Scale (Barber & Wilson, 1978/79), then it would be more appropriate to use suggestions of heaviness for hypnotic induction, deepening and post-hypnotic suggestions regarding self-hypnosis.

Precipitants and activating situations

In this stage of case conceptualisation, the therapist specifies external events that activate schemas to produce symptoms and problems. External events can be categorised into two classes: *precipitating events* and *activating situations*. Precipitating events are large-scale, molar events that trigger the primary symptoms. For example, a depressive episode can be precipitated in a young adult who leaves home to go to university. Activating situations refer to smaller-scale events that precipitate negative affect or maladaptive behaviours. Often these smaller-scale activating situations can trigger the same schema activated by precipitating events. For example, the student who left home felt lonely while studying in his room at the university residence. In this example, both the precipitating event (leaving home) and the activating situation (alone in his room) triggered the same schema ('I'm weak, I can't cope').

There are several important reasons for assessing external events and situations. First, since the cognitive-behavioural theory of emotional disorders attributes symptoms to activation of underlying schema, and not to external events or intrapsychic events, there ought to be a match between the patient's schema and the external events that activated the schema. It is therefore important for the therapist to have a good understanding of the relationship between external events and core beliefs, as the focus of CBT is to change the schema. Secondly, there are times when a connection cannot be made between external events and core beliefs as the schema remains unconscious. CBT is not designed to explore deep unconscious cognitions. This limitation of CBT is compensated for by the inclusion of hypnotherapy in the CH approach to treatment. Hypnotherapy provides several effective techniques for eliciting and changing unconscious schemas. Thirdly, although the focus of CBT is on core beliefs and not on external events, external events can be problematic to some patients. For example, an abusive relationship may create situations where safety for a partner may be compromised. Identification of such problematic events can provide important information while formulating intervention strategies. Fourthly, at times it is beneficial for patients to change their situations rather than simply changing their reactions to the situations. For example, the young man who went to university can share his room with another student in order to avoid loneliness. The foregoing clearly illustrates that emotional disorders are complex disorders, involving multiple factors, and hence treatment should be broadened to deal with all the triggering, maintaining, and risk factors.

Origins

In this section of the case formulation, the therapist draws information from the patient's early history to understand how the patient might have learned the problematic schema. It is recommended that the therapist summarises this understanding with a simple statement or by providing a brief description of one or two poignant incidents that capture the patient's early experience. For example, as a child, Mary (who suffered recurrent depression during her early adulthood) was continually punished by her parents for playing outside her house, while her brother got away with doing the same. The parents pointed out to her that girls are not allowed to play outside the house as the girl's place is in the home. Consequently, Mary learned that 'I am not important, I am inferior'. Information about modelling experiences (e.g. Mary learned from her parents to treat boys and girls differently) and failure to learn certain important skills or behaviours (e.g. Mary was afraid to question her parents and did not learn to be assertive) can also be included in this section.

It is also important to obtain a history of mental illness in the family. Although emotional disorders are not hereditary illnesses, within the biopsychosocial (diathesis-stress) model biological factors serve as a diathesis to emotional problems. Because of the biological diathesis, a person may be predisposed to develop problematic schemas. Mary's mother had a long history of major depressive disorder and Mary had held a pessimistic view of life since childhood. Her negative self-schemas were shaped by the way she was treated by her father and by a traumatic experience (an incident where her father forced her out of the shower naked to switch off the television, which she had left on while having her shower) that she could not get out of her mind.

Summary of working hypothesis

This section forms the heart of the case formulation. Here the therapist describes how the components of the working hypothesis (schema, precipitants and activating situations, and origins) interact with each other to produce the symptoms and the problems listed on the patient's problem list. The summary of the working hypothesis can be described either verbally or in a diagram with arrows linking the components on the formulation (see Persons & Davidson, 2001). In the case of Mary, her negative schema, originating from her abusive father, is triggered by special social events such as engagements and weddings, leading to the triggering and maintenance of anxiety and depression.

[handwritten note: diathesis = constitutional predisposition or tendency, as to a particular disease of affection]

Strengths and Assets

Gathering information about the patient's strengths and assets (e.g. social support, good social skills, financial resources, a stable lifestyle, good physical health and so on) serves several purposes. It helps the therapist develop a working hypothesis, it enhances the treatment plan by integrating the patient's strengths and assets, and it can assist in the determination of realistic treatment goals. Mary's strengths and assets included over-average intelligence, a stable lifestyle, an excellent social life and having several close friends.

Treatment Plan

Although the treatment plan is not part of the case formulation, it is included here to stress the point that the treatment plan is based directly on the case formulation. One of the main reasons for CH case formulation is to guide the therapist in selecting effective and efficient interventions. As mentioned before, there is evidence that therapeutic success is increased when interventions are matched to particular patient characteristics (Beutler, Clarkin & Bongar, 2000). The treatment plan derived from the case formulation has six components: goals, modality, frequency, interventions, adjunct therapies and obstacles. Each of these components is described in detail below.

Goals

The therapist and the patient collaborate to develop treatment goals to deal with the symptoms and problems listed on the problem list. Most patients seek treatment to address one or two important or distressing problems, rather than trying to solve all their problems. It is therefore important for the therapist and the patient to have complete agreement on the treatment goals. It is unlikely that treatment will succeed if there is no agreement between the therapist and the patient regarding the treatment goals or the problem list.

Within the CH formulation, it is recommended that the treatment goals are stated concretely and the progress towards the goals is measured. Specifying treatment goals in clear, concrete statements facilitates therapeutic work. For example, a vague goal statement such as 'Jane will get better' is not concrete enough to provide guidance on setting specific goals for the treatment sessions. A concrete statement such as 'Jane will reduce her depressive symptoms' provides clear guidance on setting agendas for the treatment sessions. Moreover, setting concrete goals facilitates outcome measurement. Measurement of progress towards the treatment goal provides a tool for the therapist to track down progress. If the initial treatment plan does not work, it will be necessary to revise the case formulation and the treatment plan. For each formulated goal, it is advisable to use at least one measure to monitor treatment progress. Measures can range from simple counts (e.g. keeping a count of daily activities, number of panic attacks) to self-rating measures (e.g. Beck Depression Inventory). As recommended by Persons, Davidson and Tompkins (2001), I routinely ask my depressed patients to complete the revised Beck Depression Inventory (BDI-II; Beck, Steer & Brown, 1996), the Beck Anxiety Inventory (BAI; Beck & Steer, 1993a) and the Beck Hopelessness Scale (BHS; Beck & Steer, 1993b) prior to each therapy session to monitor the weekly progress. The scores from these three self-rating measures can be plotted on a graph to track the patient's progress with depressive and anxiety symptoms. The graph provides a visual representation of the patient's progress. Idiographic measures such as self-monitoring (e.g. Daily Activity Schedule, Headache Intensity Scale) can also be tailored to assess the patient's problems.

Changes in dysfunctional thinking can also be monitored by utilising any of the three self-rating assessment tools suggested by Nezu, Nezu and Lombardo (2004): the Automatic Thought Questionnaire – Revised (Kendall, Howard & Hays, 1989), the Cognitive Triad Inventory (Beckham et al., 1986) and the Dysfunctional Attitude Scale (Weissman & Beck, 1978).

Modality

Specify the treatment approach to be utilised, for example individual cognitive hypnotherapy.

Frequency

State the frequency of treatment sessions required, for example once a week.

Interventions

The interventions proposed in the treatment plan are based directly on CH formulation, but most importantly they are related to the deficits described in the working hypothesis. The interventions are designed specifically to address some of the problems identified on the problem list in order to accomplish of the goals (Persons, Davidson & Tompkins, 2001). For example, activity scheduling will be a logical intervention for a depressed man who is passive and inactive and spends most of his time staying in bed in his apartment. A socially anxious person, who is lacking social skills because of social inhibition based on the belief that he or she is criticised by everyone, will benefit from social skills training. McKnight et al. (1984), from a series of single-case studies, have provided evidence that interventions tailored to address patients' deficits are most beneficial in reducing primary symptoms. They found depressed patients with social skills deficits to benefit most from social skills training, while those with cognitive distortions benefited most from cognitive restructuring. It is therefore recommended that therapists use evidence-based interventions within the context of CH formulation.

Adjunct therapies

The majority of the patients seen in clinical practice have multitudinous problems and comorbid conditions. Very often adjunctive interventions such as pharmacotherapy, family therapy or substance abuse counselling may be required. It is recommended that the therapist is alert to the patient's complex needs and facilitates adjunctive interventions as necessary.

Obstacles

The final component of the treatment plan uses the information from the case formulation to predict difficulties that might arise in the therapeutic relationship or in the course of the therapy. Certain items from the problem list, such as interpersonal difficulties, financial problems, medical problems and occupational difficulties, can alert the therapist to the factors that may interfere with therapeutic progress. Early awareness of these potential obstacles helps the patient and the therapist cope more effectively with the problems when they arise.

SUMMARY

The CH case formulation provides a model for selecting effective treatment strategies for the individual (idiographic) patient from the available nomothetic research literature. This model stresses the role of multiple risk factors in the onset, exacerbation and maintenance of the disorder. By formulating a case, the therapist develops a working hypothesis on how the patient's problems can be understood in terms of the CH conceptualisation. This understanding provides a framework for comprehending the treatment process. Within this model, treatment begins with an assessment, which generates a hypothesis about the mechanisms causing or maintaining the problem. The hypothesis is the individualised case formulation, which the therapist uses to develop individualised treatment plan. As treatment proceeds, the therapist collects data via further assessment to evaluate the effects of the planned treatment.

Chapters 3 to 10 describe a number of treatment strategies within the CH framework for treating various conditions. If it becomes evident that the treatment is not working, the therapist reformulates the case and develops a new treatment plan, which is also monitored and evaluated. Within this framework, clinical work becomes systematic and hypothesis-driven driven rather than delivering treatment strategies randomly or in a predetermined order.

CHAPTER 3

COGNITIVE HYPNOTHERAPY IN THE MANAGEMENT OF DEPRESSION

INTRODUCTION

This chapter describes in detail how hypnotherapy can be integrated with cognitive behaviour therapy (CBT) in the management of major depressive disorder (MDD). MDD is one of the most common psychiatric disorders treated by psychiatrists and psychotherapists. Although MDD can be treated successfully with anti-depressant medication and psychotherapy (Moore & Bona, 2001), a significant number of depressives do not respond to either medication or the existing psychotherapy approach. It is thus important for clinicians to continue to develop more effective treatments for depression. Clinical depression also poses special problems to therapists as it is a complex disorder and it 'takes over the whole person – emotions, bodily functions, behaviors, and thoughts' (Nolen-Hoeksema, 2004, p. 280).

This chapter will describe *cognitive hypnotherapy* (CH), an evidence-based multi-modal treatment for depression, which can be applied to a wide range of patients with depression. CH represents the most comprehensive version of hypnotherapy for depression. Although the efficacy of the therapy has been examined in a controlled trial (Alladin & Alibhai, 2007), CH for depression is a work in progress as we continue to learn more about the etiology and treatment of depression.

DESCRIPTION OF DEPRESSION

MDD is characterised by feelings of sadness, lack of interest in formerly enjoyable pursuits, sleep and appetite disturbance, feelings of worthlessness, and thoughts of death and dying (Alladin, 2007b). The diagnosis of a major depressive episode is made when a person has been depressed or has lost interest or pleasure in nearly all activities for at least two weeks, and has experienced at least four of these additional categories of symptoms: changes in appetite or weight, sleep and psychomotor activity; decreased energy; feelings of worthlessness or guilt: difficulty thinking, concentrating or making decisions; and recurrent thoughts of death or suicidal ideation, plans or attempts (American Psychiatric Association, 2000, p. 349). MDD is extremely disabling in terms of poor quality of life and disability (Pincus & Pettit, 2001) and 15% of people with MDD commit suicide (Satcher, 2000).

MDD is on the increase (World Health Organization, 1998) and it is estimated that out of every 100 people, approximately 13 men and 21 women are likely to develop the disorder at some point in life (Kessler *et al.* (1994) and approximately one-third of the population may suffer from mild depression at some point in their lives (Paykel & Priest, 1992). The rate of major depression is so high that the World Health Organization (WHO) Global Burden of Disease Study ranked depression as the single most burdensome disease in the world in terms of total disability-adjusted life years among people in the middle years of life (Murray & Lopez, 1996). According to the WHO (1998), by the year 2020 clinical depression is likely to be second only to chronic heart disease as an international health burden, as measured by cause of death, disability, incapacity to work and medical resources used. Moreover, major depression is a very costly disorder in terms of lost productivity at work, industrial accidents, bed occupancy in hospitals, treatment, state benefits and personal suffering. The illness also adversely affects interpersonal relationships with spouses and children (Gotlib & Hammen, 2002), the rate of divorce is higher among depressives than among non-depressed individuals (e.g. Wade & Cairney, 2000) and the children of depressed parents are found to be at elevated risk of psychopathology (Gotlib & Goodman, 1999).

Approximately 60% of people who have a major depressive episode will have a second episode. Among those who have experienced two episodes, 70% will have a third; and among those who have had three episodes, 90% will have a fourth (American Psychiatric Association, 2000). Recurrence is very important in predicting the future course of the disorder as well as in choosing appropriate treatments. As many as 85% of single-episode cases later experience a second episode and the median lifetime number of major depressive episodes is four, with 25% of depressives experiencing six or more episodes (Angst & Preizig, 1996). Depression is therefore considered to be a chronic condition that waxes and wanes over time but seldom disappears (Solomon *et al.*, 2000).

MDD also co-occurs with other disorders, both medical and psychiatric. Kessler (2002), from his review of the epidemiology of depression, concludes that 'comorbidity is the norm among people with depression' (Kessler, 2002, p. 29). For example, the Epidemiologic Catchment Area Study (Robins &

Regier, 1991) found that 75% of respondents with lifetime depressive disorders also met the criteria for at least one of the other DSM-III disorders assessed in that survey. The most frequent comorbid condition with depression is anxiety. In fact, there is considerable symptom overlap between these two conditions. The presence of poor concentration, irritability, hypervigilance, fatigue, guilt, memory loss, sleep difficulties and worry may suggest a diagnosis of either disorder. The symptom overlap between the two conditions may be indicative of similar neurobiological correlates. At a psychological level, it seems reasonable to assume that depression can result from the demoralisation caused by anxiety, for example in a case of an agoraphobic who becomes withdrawn because of the fear of going out. Conversely, a person with depression may become anxious due to worry about being unable to hold gainful employment. Although there is an apparent overlap between anxiety and depression, it is common clinical practice to focus on treating one disorder at a time. The lack of an integrated approach to treatment means that a patient is treated only for depression while the patient is still suffering from anxiety. One of the rationales for combining hypnosis with CBT, as described in this chapter, is to address symptoms of anxiety.

TREATMENT OF DEPRESSION

In the past 20 years there have been significant developments and innovations in the pharmacological and psychological treatments of depression. The pharmacological, psychotherapeutic and hypnotherapeutic approaches to treatment are briefly reviewed.

Pharmacotherapy

Over the past 20 years tricyclics and monoamine oxidase inhibitors (MAOIs) have been replaced by a second generation of anti-depressants known as selective serotonin reuptake inhibitors (SSRIs). SSRIs have become extremely popular in the treatment of depression. Although these drugs are similar in structure to tricyclics, they work more selectively to affect the serotonin, thus the side effects are less severe and they produce improvement within a couple of weeks. Moreover, these drugs are not fatal in overdose and they appear to help with a range of disorders, including anxiety, binge eating and premenstrual symptoms (Pearlstein et al., 1997). A number of other drugs such as Remeron, Serzone, Effexor and Wellbutrin have also been introduced during the past decade. They share some similarities with SSRIs, but they cannot be classified in any one of the previously mentioned categories. Sometimes these drugs are used in conjunction with SSRIs. While there are a variety of anti-depressants available, but there are no consistent rules for determining which anti-depressant to use first. In clinical practice several anti-depressants are used before finding one drug that works well and has tolerable side effects.

Anti-depressant medication has relieved severe depression and undoubtedly prevented suicide in tens of thousands of patients around the world. Although this kind of medication is readily available, many people refuse or are not eligible to take it, however. Some are wary of long-term side effects. Women of child-bearing age must protect themselves against the possibility of conceiving while taking anti-depressants, because they can damage the foetus. In addition, 40–50% of patients do not respond adequately to these drugs, and a substantial number of the remainder are left with residual symptoms of depression (Barlow & Durand, 2005, p. 238).

Psychotherapy

Although anti-depressant medication works well for many depressed patients, it obviously does not alleviate the problems that might have caused the depression in the first place. The bad marriage, unhappy work situation or family conflict that precedes depression cannot be fixed by pills. Therefore, many depressed people benefit from psychotherapy designed to help them cope with the difficult life circumstances or personality vulnerabilities that put them at risk for depression. Psychotherapy is also indicated for people who have medical conditions (such as pregnancy and some heart problems) that preclude the use of medication.

Cognitive behaviour therapy (CBT), which is the most popular psychosocial treatment for depression, has been studied in over 80 controlled trials (American Psychiatric Association, 2000). It has been found to be effective in the reduction of acute symptoms and it compares favourably with pharmacological treatment in all but the most severely depressed patients. CBT also reduces relapse (Hollon & Shelton, 2001) and it can prevent the initial onset of the first episode or the emergence of symptoms in people at risk who have never been depressed (Gillham, Shatte & Freres, 2000). CBT is predicated on the notion that teaching patients to recognise and examine their negative beliefs and information-processing proclivities can produce relief from their symptoms and enable them to cope more effectively with life's challenges (Beck *et al.*, 1979). The primary goal of the CBT therapist is to educate patients in the use of various techniques that allow them to examine their thoughts and modify maladaptive beliefs and behaviours. The main role of CBT is to help the patient learn to use these tools independently. Such skills are not only important for symptom relief, but may also minimise the chances of future recurrence of symptoms. The goals of CBT are achieved through a structured collaborative process consisting of three inter-related components consisting of exploration, examination and experimentation (Hollon, Haman & Brown, 2002).

Hypnotherapy

Hypnosis has not been widely used in the management of clinical depression. The little published literature that exists can be categorised into case studies and adjunctive techniques. Alladin (2006a, 2007b) attributes the lack of progress in the application of hypnosis to depression to the myth created by some well-known writers (e.g. Hartland, 1971) that hypnosis can exacerbate suicidal behaviour in depressives. Alladin and Heap (1991) and Yapko (1992, 2001) have argued that hypnosis, especially when it forms part of a multi-modal treatment approach, is not contra-indicated with depression.

The bulk of the published literature on the clinical application of hypnosis to depression consists of case reports. These reports consist of a variety of hypnotherapeutic techniques, but are lacking in clarity on what therapists do with hypnosis in the management of depression (Burrows & Boughton, 2001). Nevertheless, several clinicians have used hypnosis as an adjunct to other forms of psychotherapy. For example, Golden, Dowd and Friedberg (1987), Tosi and Baisden (1984), Yapko (2001) and Zarren and Eimer (2001) have reported effective integration of CBT with hypnotherapy with depression in their clinical practice. However, with the exception of Alladin (1992a,b, 1994; Alladin & Heap, 1991), these writers have not provided a scientific rationale or a theoretical model for combining CBT with hypnosis in the management of clinical depression. Alladin has described a working model of non-endogenous depression that provides a theoretical framework for integrating cognitive and hypnotic techniques with depression. More recently, (Alladin, 2007b) he has revised the model and called it the circular feedback model of depression (CFMD).

CFMD stresses the biopsychosocial nature of depression and emphasises the role of multiple factors that can trigger, exacerbate or maintain the depressive affect. The model is not a new theory of depression or an attempt to explain the causes of depression. It is an extension of Beck's (1967) circular feedback model of depression, which was later elaborated on by Schultz (1978, 1984, 2003) and expanded by Alladin (1994). In combining the cognitive and hypnotic paradigms, CFMD incorporates ideas and concepts from information processing, selective attention, brain functioning, adverse life experiences, and the neodissociation theory of hypnosis (Hilgard, 1977). The initial model was referred to as the cognitive dissociative model of depression, because it encompassed the dissociative theory of hypnosis and proposed that non-endogenous depression was akin to a form of dissociation produced by negative cognitive rumination, which can be regarded as a form of negative self-hypnosis (NSH). CFMD consists of 12 interrelated components that form a circular feedback loop. These 12 components (see Alladin, 2007b) represent some of the major factors identified from the literature that may influence the course and outcome of depression. Any of these factors, such as negative affect, can trigger, exacerbate or maintain the depressive symptoms. The model also provides the theoretical underpinnings for using cognitive hypnotherapy (CH) with depression, which is described in the rest of this chapter. The conceptualisation of the model also highlights how hypnosis can be used as a useful construct to study and understand certain aspects of the depressive phenomenology.

CFMD states three pragmatic reasons for combining cognitive and hypnotic paradigms in the treatment and understanding of depression. First, since hypnosis can produce cognitive, somatic, perceptual, physiological and kinaesthetic changes under controlled conditions, the combination of the two paradigms may provide a conceptual framework for studying the psychological processes by which cognitive distortions produce the concomitant psychobiological changes underlying clinical depression. Secondly, hypnosis provides insight into the phenomenology of depression (Yapko, 1992). Like depression, hypnosis is a highly subjective experience. It allows remarkable insights into the subjective realm of human experience, thus providing a paradigm for understanding how experience, normal or abnormal, is moulded and patterned. Thirdly, after reviewing the strengths and limitations of CBT and hypnotherapy with depression, Alladin (1989) concluded that each treatment approach has marked limitations. For example, CBT does not allow access to unconscious cognitive restructuring, while hypnosis provides such access. On the other hand, hypnosis does not focus on systematic cognitive restructuring, while CBT's main focus is on cognitive restructuring via reasoning and Socratic dialogue. Alladin (1989) argued that some of the shortcomings of each treatment approach could be compensated for by integrating both treatment approaches.

Moreover, there is some empirical evidence for combining hypnosis with CBT. Schoenberger (2000), from her review of the empirical status of the use of hypnosis in conjunction with cognitive-behavioural treatment programmes, concluded that the existing studies demonstrate substantial benefits from the addition of hypnosis to cognitive-behavioural techniques. Similarly, Kirsch, Montgomery and Sapirstein (1995), from their meta-analysis of 18 studies comparing a cognitive-behavioural treatment with the same treatment supplemented by hypnosis, found the mean effect size of the hypnotic treatment to be larger than the non-hypnotic intervention. The authors concluded that hypnotherapy was significantly superior to non-hypnotic treatment. Alladin (Alladin & Alibhai, 2007) has conducted a study comparing the effects of CBT with cognitive hypnotherapy in 84 chronic depressives. The results showed an additive effect of combining hypnosis with CBT. The study also met criteria for *probably efficacious* treatment for depression as laid down by the American Psychological Association (APA) Task Force (Chambless & Hollon, 1998) and it provides empirical validation for integrating hypnosis with CBT in the management of depression.

STAGES OF COGNITIVE HYPNOTHERAPY

Cognitive hypnotherapy (CH) generally consists of 16 weekly sessions, which can be expanded or modified according to the patient's clinical needs, areas of concern and presenting symptoms. The stages of CH are briefly described below and, wherever relevant, the strategies used for treating Jackie during each stage of the treatment will be illustrated. The sequence of the stages of treatment can be altered to suit the clinical needs of each patient.

Session 1: Clinical Assessments

Before initiating CH it is important for the therapist to take a detailed clinical history to formulate the diagnosis and identify the essential psychological, physiological and social aspects of the patient's behaviours. The most efficient way to obtain all this information is to take the case-formulation approach described in Chapter 2. The case-formulation approach allows the clinician to translate and tailor nomothetic (general) treatment protocol to the individual (idiographic) patient (see Appendix C). Jackie's case formulation (Appendix D) clearly indicates her diagnosis, the role of cognitive distortions in the triggering and maintenance of her negative affect, and the treatment goals.

Sessions 2–5: Cognitive Behaviour Therapy

Cognitive behaviour therapy (CBT) is utilised to help depressed patients recognise and modify their idiosyncratic style of thinking through the application of evidence and logic. The main objects of the CBT sessions are to help the patients identify and restructure their dysfunctional beliefs that may be triggering and maintaining their depressive affect. CBT uses some very well-known and tested reason-based models such as Socratic logic-based dialogues and Aristotle's method of collecting and categorising information about the world (Leahy, 2003). CBT therapists engage their patients in scientific and rational thinking by guiding them to examine the presupposition, validity and meaning of their beliefs that lead to their depressive affect. As CBT techniques are fully described in several excellent books (e.g. Beck, 1995), they are not described in detail here. For a detailed description of the sequential progression of CBT within the CH framework, see Alladin (2007b). Whether hypnotherapy or CBT is introduced first is also determined by the clinical needs of the depressed patient. Introducing CBT first is recommended if the patient is overly preoccupied with dysfunctional cognitions and depressive rumination. In the case of a depressed patient who is overly preoccupied with anxious or depressive affect, hypnotherapy is recommended first.

The CBT component of CH can be extended over four to six sessions. However, the number of CBT sessions is determined by the needs of the patient and the severity of the presenting symptoms. Within the CH framework, Alladin (2006a) finds the following sequential presentation of the CBT components to be beneficial to depressed patients:

- The patient is given a simple but practical explanation of the cognitive model of depression. At least four sessions are devoted to CBT. The object of the CBT sessions is to help the patients identify and restructure their dysfunctional beliefs that may be triggering and maintaining their depressive affect. While explaining the model, the therapist writes the salient points on a piece of paper or on a board. Writing provides a visual representation of the model and both the patient and therapist can refer to the notes to check on a point.
- As part of the homework, the patient is advised to read the first three chapters of *Feeling Good: The New Mood Therapy* (Burns, 1999).
- Patients are encouraged to identify the cognitive distortions they ruminate with from the list of 10 cognitive distortions described by Burns (1999). This exercise helps patients identify and label their cognitive distortions.
- Patients are advised to log the CAB form (a form with three columns: A = Event; B = Automatic Thoughts; C = Emotional Responses; Figure 3.1). This homework helps patients identify their dysfunctional thoughts and discover the link between their distorted thoughts and negative feelings. This preparatory work sets the stage for evaluating and challenging the negative thoughts in the future.
- The patient is introduced to disputation (D) or how to challenge cognitive distortions after the patient has had the opportunity to log the ABC form for a week.

DATE	C = EMOTIONS	A = FACTS OR EVENTS	B = AUTOMATIC THOUGHTS ABOUT A
	1. Specify sad/anxious/ angry, etc. 2. Rate degree of emotion 0–100	Describe: 1. Actual event that activated unpleasant emotion/reaction 2. Images, daydreams, recollections leading to unpleasant emotion	1. Write automatic thoughts that preceded emotions/reactions 2. Rate belief in automatic thoughts 0–100%
Nov.06/04	Scared (100) Anxious (100) Depressed (85) Miserable (90)	Thinking of going to Christmas party organised by husband's office	I won't enjoy it (100) I will lose control (100) Everyone will hate me (90) I will spoil it for everyone (90) I can never go out and enjoy myself (100)

Figure 3.1   CAB form for monitoring irrational beliefs/thoughts/images/daydreams related to events/situations

- The Cognitive Restructuring (ABCDE) form is introduced to log disputation and the effects of disputation over negative affect. This form is an expanded version of the ABC form, by including two more columns (D = Disputation; E = Consequences of Disputation; see Figure 3.2 for a completed sample from Jackie).
- In order to get a better grasp of how to complete this form, patients are given a completed version of the Cognitive Restructuring form (with disputation of cognitive distortions in column D and the modification of emotional and behavioural responses in column E as a consequence of cognitive disputation). This homework provides patients with the opportunity to identify and restructure their cognitive distortions. It should be reminded that CBT does not advocate the 'power of positive thinking', but rather the 'power of identifying whatever is being thought' (Leahy, 2003). CBT takes a constructivist approach to therapy by recognising that individuals' construction and interpretation of reality are based on unique information, personal categories and biases in perception or cognition.
- Patients are coached to differentiate between surface or automatic cognitive distortions ('I can't do this') and deeper or enduring ('I'm a failure') negative cognitive structures (self-schemas) and therapists use different strategies to restructure the deeper self-schemas. The term 'schema' refers to enduring, deep cognitive structures or 'templates' that are particularly important in structuring perceptions and building up 'rule-giving' behaviours (Sanders & Wills, 2005).
- For uncovering core beliefs the Downward Arrow Method can be used and the Circle of Life Technique is used for restructuring core beliefs (see below).
- The patient is advised to constantly monitor and restructure negative cognitions until it becomes a habit.

Downward Arrow Method

The Downward Arrow Method is the most common CBT technique used for uncovering core beliefs. This excerpt from one of the CBT sessions in which Jackie stated 'I hate going to parties' (her surface cognition) demonstrates how the therapist can use the Downward Arrow Method to get to core beliefs:

Th = Therapist; *J* = Jackie
Th: Jackie, what do you mean by 'I hate going to parties'?
J: I don't like being around people.
Th: What do you mean?
J: Well, I feel nervous.
Th: What makes you feel uneasy?
J: Well, people will notice that I am not confident.
Th: What do you mean?
J: Well, I'm not as calm or relaxed as others.
Th: What do you mean?
J: I'm no good.
Th: What do you mean?
J: Well, I am a failure, I am useless, I can never do anything right.

DATE	A ACTIVATING EVENT	B IRRATIONAL BELIEFS	C CONSEQUENCES	D DISPUTATION	E EFFECT OF DISPUTATION
	Describe actual event, stream of thoughts, daydream etc. leading to unpleasant feelings	Write automatic thoughts and images that came in your mind. Rate beliefs or images 0–100%	1. **Emotion**: specify sad, anxious or angry. Rate feelings 1–100% 2. **Physiological**: Palpitations, pain, dizzy, sweat etc. 3. **Behavioural**: Avoidance, in bed 4. **Conclusion**: Reaching conclusions, self-affirmation	Challenge the automatic thoughts and images. Rate belief in rational response/image 0–100%	1. **Emotion**: Re-rate your emotion 1–100% 2. **Physiological**: Changes in bodily reactions (i.e. less shaking, less tense, etc.) 3. **Behavioural**: Action taken after disputation 4. **Conclusion**: Reappraise your conclusion and initial decision. Future beliefs in similar situation
Nov 06/04	*A worked example: Thinking of going to Christmas party organised by husband's office*	1. *I won't enjoy it (100)* 2. *I will lose control (100)* 3. *Everyone will hate me (90)* 3. *I will spoil it for everyone (90)*	1. *Scared (100), anxious (100), depressed (85), miserable (90)* 2. *Weak, tired, shaky* 3. *Don't want to go, prefer staying at home*	1. *How do I know I won't enjoy it, I haven't been there yet? The chances are I may like being with others (60)*	1. *Less scared (10), less anxious (20), less depressed (20), no longer feeling miserable (0)* 2. *Still feeling tired and weak but feel more relaxed*

Figure 3.2 Completed cognitive restructuring (ABCDE) form

DATE	A ACTIVATING EVENT	B IRRATIONAL BELIEFS	C CONSEQUENCES	D DISPUTATION	E EFFECT OF DISPUTATION
		4. I can never go out and enjoy myself (100)	4. I will never be able to go out and enjoy myself	2. I may feel anxious; it may be uncomfortable but I will not lose control, I have never lost control (80) 3. No one hates you because of your looks. I am conscious of my looks, but my friends don't even focus on my looks (80) 4. I may be nervous or depressed, but how I feel has no bearing on the party (90) 5. This is not true; there are many situations where I enjoyed myself, although initially I did not want to go (100)	3. Out of bed, looking for the dress I can wear 4. Even if I feel anxious or depressed, I can make myself feel better by going out to social functions

Figure 3.2 (Continued)

Circle of Life Technique

Once the core beliefs (in this case 'I am useless; I am a failure') are uncovered, several CBT techniques can be used to restructure them. I find the Circle of Life Technique very effective in dealing with such core beliefs.

The next part of the transcript illustrates how the Circle of Life Technique was utilised to help Jackie restructure her core beliefs: 'I am a failure' and 'I am useless'.

Th: Let's see how we can help you with these deep beliefs that you have that you are 'useless' and you are a 'failure'. Would you believe it if I say to you that a person can't be good or bad? (The therapist writes down on the top of a blank sheet of paper: Good/Bad; Success/Failure.)

J: Of course not! Some people are good and some people are bad.

Th: Would you believe me if I say to you a person can't be a success or a failure?

J: No.

Th: Let me show you why it's inaccurate to believe a person is either good or bad, or a success or a failure. Let's imagine this circle (the therapist draws a large circle on the blank sheet of paper just below where earlier he wrote Good/Bad; Success/Failure) represents life; of course, this is an oversimplification. We say we exist because we participate in hundreds of activities daily (the therapist fills the inner circle with about 20 large dots). Let's imagine each dot represents one activity and as you can imagine we participate in hundreds of activities every day. We go to school, we walk, we talk, we work, and so on. Do you agree?

J: Yes. You are right, we do many things every day.

Th: That's right, we do many things in a day. Do you know of anyone who does everything very well?

J: No.

Th: Do you know of anyone who does everything badly?

J: No. I see what you mean. Not everyone does everything well or badly.

Th: That's right! No one does everything badly or very well. It's more accurate to say that we all do some things well and we do some things badly.

J: You are right. I never thought about it this way.

Th: Let's suppose I do some things badly (the therapist crosses three dots inside the circle). Does this make me a bad person?

J: No. You are still good at doing other things.

Th: That's right. I am still good at other things although I mess up some of the things I do. Because I am not good with these things (therapist pointing to the three crossed-out dots), it does not mean all the other activities that I am good at (the therapist pointing to the uncrossed dots) are totally wiped out.

J: It's so amazing, I never thought about it this way. Because I feel nervous in the presence of people, it doesn't mean I am no good at anything. I thought because I feel nervous I can't be a good person, I thought I must be a failure.

Th: I'm happy that you can relate to this and you realise that you were thinking the wrong way.

Sessions 6–7: Hypnotherapy

The hypnotherapy component of CH is introduced to provide leverage to the psychological treatment of depression (Alladin, 2006a, 2007b) and to prevent relapses (Alladin, 2006b; Alladin & Alibhai, 2007). Hypnotherapy is specifically utilised to induce relaxation (as 50–75% of depressives have comorbid anxiety; see Dozois & Westra, 2004); reduce distraction; maximise concentration; facilitate divergent thinking; amplify and expand experiences; acquire sense of control; and provide access to non-conscious psychological processes.

Cognitive hypnotherapy (CH) devotes four to six sessions to hypnotherapy. The first two or three sessions focus on inducing relaxation; producing somatosensory changes; demonstrating the power of the mind; expansion of awareness; ego strengthening; teaching self-hypnosis; and offering post-hypnotic suggestions. The other two to three hypnotherapy sessions concentrate on cognitive restructuring under hypnosis and unconscious exploration that are described under Sessions 8–10.

Relaxation training

One of the important goals for using hypnosis within the CH context is to induce relaxation. Most depressed patients experience high levels of anxiety either due to comorbid anxiety (Dozois & Westra, 2004) or due to their negative view of the future and their low level of confidence in their abilities to handle life challenges. For these reasons depressed patients benefit greatly from learning relaxation techniques. Various hypnotic induction techniques can be utilised to induce relaxation. I use the *relaxation with counting method* adapted from Gibbons (1979; see Alladin, 2007b) for inducing and deepening the hypnotic trance. I have chosen this technique as it is easily adapted for self-hypnosis training. The majority of the patients treated with CH in the study reported by Alladin and Alibhai (2007) indicated that the relaxation experience was empowering and it boosted their confidence to interrupt anxious sequences in their lives. The hypnotherapeutic script in Appendix E provides some examples of the types of hypnotic suggestions that can be utilised to induce a feeling of deep relaxation.

Producing somatosensory changes

Hypnosis is a powerful therapeutic tool for producing *syncretic cognition* (Alladin, 2006a), which consists of a variety of cognitive, somatic, perceptual, physiological, visceral and kinaesthetic changes. Hypnotic induction and modulation of these changes provide depressed patients with dramatic proof that they can change their feeling and experience. Such an experience provides hope that they can control their depressive affect. DePiano and Salzberg (1981) believe that such a positive experience in patients is partly related to the rapid and profound behavioural, emotional, cognitive and physiological changes brought on by the induction of the hypnotic experience.

Demonstration of the power of mind

Eye and body catalepsies are hypnotically induced to demonstrate the power of the mind over the body. These demonstrations reduce scepticism over hypnosis, foster positive expectancy and instil confidence in depressed patients that they can produce significant emotional and behavioural changes.

Expansion of Awareness

Hypnosis provides a powerful vehicle for expanding awareness and amplifying experience. I find Brown and Fromm's (in Hammond, 1990, pp. 322–4) technique of *enhancing affective experience and its expression* very effective in bringing underlying emotions into awareness; creating awareness of various feelings; intensifying positive affect; enhancing 'discovered' affect; inducing positive moods; and increasing motivation. The object of this procedure is to help depressed patients create, amplify and express a variety of negative and positive feelings and experience. Moreover, the technique further reinforces the view that the depressive affect can be modified and controlled.

To help Jackie bring on her underlying emotion into awareness while she is showering, under hypnosis it was suggested to her: 'When I count from ONE to FIVE . . . by the time you hear me say FIVE . . . you will begin to feel whatever emotion is associated with your body when you notice your body while showering.' Then Jackie was helped to amplify the affect associated with her body: 'When I count slowly from ONE to FIVE . . . as I count you will begin to experience the upsetting feelings more and more intensely . . . so that when I reach the count of FIVE . . . at the count of FIVE you will feel the experience in your body as strongly as you can bear it . . . Now notice what you feel and you will be able to describe it to me.' This technique can also induce happy or pleasant feelings and the procedure can be expanded to access and frame past or future experiences by integrating time (past or future) projection methods.

Ego strengthening

Ego-strengthening suggestions are offered to depressives to increase self-esteem and self-efficacy. Bandura (1977) has provided experimental evidence that *self efficacy*, the expectation and confidence of being able to cope successfully with various situations, is one of the key elements in the effective treatment of phobic disorders. Individuals with a sense of high self-efficacy tend to perceive themselves as being in control. If depressives can be helped to view themselves as self-efficacious, they will perceive the future as hopeful. The most popular method for increasing self-efficacy within the hypnotherapeutic context is to provide ego-strengthening suggestions. The principles behind ego strengthening are to remove anxiety, tension and apprehension, and gradually to restore patients' confidence in themselves and their ability to cope with their problems (Hartland, 1971). Hence, the ego-strengthening suggestions consist of generalised supportive suggestions to increase the patient's confidence, coping abilities, positive self-image and interpersonal skills. Hartland (1971) believes that patients need to feel confident and strong enough to let go of their symptoms.

The hypnosis script in Appendix E provides a list of generalised ego-strengthening suggestions that can be routinely used in hypnotherapy with a variety of medical and psychological conditions. However, when working with depressives it is important to craft the ego-strengthening suggestions in such a way that they appear credible and logical to the patients. For example, rather than stating: 'Every day you will feel better', it is advisable to suggest: 'As a result of this treatment and as a result of you listening to your self-hypnosis tape/CD every day, you will begin to feel better'. This set of suggestions not only sounds logical, but improvement becomes contingent on continuing with the therapy and listening to the self-hypnosis tape daily (Alladin, 2006a,b, 2007b).

Post-hypnotic suggestions

Before terminating the hypnotic session, post-hypnotic suggestions are given to counter problem behaviours, negative emotions and dysfunctional cognitions (NSH) or negative self-affirmations. Depressives tend to ruminate with negative self-suggestions, particularly after experiencing a negative affect (e.g. 'I will not be able to cope'). This can be regarded as a form of post-hypnotic suggestion (PHS), which can become part of the depressive cycle. To break the depressive cycle it is very important to counter the NSH. Here are some examples of PHS provided by Alladin (2006a, p. 162) for countering NSH:

- While you are in an upsetting situation, you will become more aware of how to deal with it rather than focusing on your depressed feeling.
- When you plan and take action to improve your future, you will feel more optimistic about the future.
- As you feel involved in doing things, you will be motivated to do more things.

Yapko (2003) regards post-hypnotic suggestions as a very necessary part of the therapeutic process if the patient is to carry new possibilities into future experience. Hence, many clinicians use post-hypnotic suggestions to shape their patients' behaviour. For example, Clarke and Jackson (1983) regard post-hypnotic suggestion to be a form of 'higher-order-conditioning', which functions as positive or negative reinforcement to increase or decrease the probability of desired or undesired behaviours, respectively. They have successfully utilised post-hypnotic suggestions to enhance the effect of in vivo exposure among agoraphobics.

Self-hypnosis training

The self-hypnosis component of CH is designed to create positive affect and counter NSH via ego strengthening and post-hypnotic suggestions. At the end of the first hypnotherapy session, the patient is provided with an audiotape/CD of self-hypnosis (consisting of the full script from Appendix E) designed to create a good frame of mind; offer ego-strengthening suggestions; and provide post-hypnotic suggestions. The homework assignment provides continuity of treatment between sessions and offers patients the opportunity to learn self-hypnosis. The ultimate goal of psychotherapy is to help the depressed patient establish self-reliance and independence. Alman (2001) believes that patients can achieve self-reliance and personal power by learning self-hypnosis. Yapko (2003) contends that the teaching of self-hypnosis and problem-solving strategies to patients allows them to develop self-correcting mechanisms that give them control over their lives. These observations were confirmed by the study reported by Alladin and Alibhai (2007).

Sessions 8–10: Cognitive Restructuring under Hypnosis

Once the depressed patient becomes familiar with CBT and hypnosis, the next three sessions integrate cognitive and hypnotic strategies in the treatment. Very often in the course of CBT, a patient is unable to access cognitions preceding certain negative emotions. As hypnosis provides access to unconscious cognitive processing, non-conscious cognitive distortions and self-schemas can be easily retrieved and restructured under hypnosis. This is achieved by directing the patient's attention to the psychological content of an experience or situation. The patient is guided to focus attention on a specific area of concern (e.g. Jackie's fear of attending social functions) and to establish the link between cognition and affect. Once the negative cognitions are identified, the patient is instructed to restructure the maladaptive cognitions and then to attend to the resulting (desirable) syncretic responses. Hypnosis also provides a vehicle whereby cognitive distortions below the level of awareness can be explored and expanded. I use four hypnotic strategies for restructuring cognitive distortions under hypnosis: regression to the event that triggered the negative affect; regression to the original traumatic event; editing and deleting the unconscious file; and symbolic imagery techniques for dealing with a variety of emotional problems such as guilt, anger, fears, doubts and anxieties.

Regression to the activating event

While in a deep hypnotic trance state, it is suggested that the patient imagines a situation that normally causes upset. Then the patient is instructed to focus on the emotional, physiological and behavioural responses and then to become aware of the associated dysfunctional cognitions. Encouragement is given to identify or 'freeze' (frame by frame, like a movie) the faulty cognitions in terms of thoughts, beliefs, images, fantasies and daydreams. Once a particular set of faulty cognitions is frozen, the patient is coached to replace it with more appropriate thinking or imagination, and then to attend to the resulting (desirable) syncretic response. This process is repeated until the set of faulty cognitions related to a specific situation is considered to be successfully restructured. For example, when Jackie reported 'I don't know why I felt depressed at the party last week', she was hypnotically regressed back to the party and encouraged to identify and restructure the faulty cognitions, and to continue with the process until she could think of the party without being upset.

Regression to the trauma

This strategy is used when in therapy it becomes important to identify the origin of a core belief. Alladin (2006a) described the case of Rita, a 39-year-old housewife with a 10-year history of recurrent major depressive disorder who responded well to CH but continued to have symptoms of sexual dysfunction, which often served as a trigger for her depression. Whenever her husband showed an interest in her, including non-sexual scenarios, she would freeze and withdraw. Rita was 'convinced there was something wrong with her at an unconscious level that might be affecting her sexual desire and sexual activity' (Alladin, 2006a, pp. 176–7). Hypnotic regression helped to bridge the link between her affect and her cognition. From the hypnotic regression, Rita was able to remember an incident when she was molested by her uncle when she was 7 years old. She had so much love and respect for her uncle that she became confused after the incident and concluded, 'Men are bad; I will never let them come near me'. Once these core dysfunctional cognitions were identified, the Circle of Life Technique was used for her to come to the understanding that not all men are bad. She was also encouraged under hypnosis to give herself the permission to break the promise that she will never let a man touch her, as this promise was made while she was a child and totally confused.

Editing and deleting the unconscious file

A contemporary method of cognitive restructuring under hypnosis uses the metaphor of editing or deleting old computer files. This method is particularly appealing to children and adolescents. When the patient is in a fairly deep state of hypnotic trance, the patient is instructed to become aware of the 'good feelings' (after ego strengthening and amplification of positive feelings) and then directed to focus on personal achievements and successes (adult ego state). Here attempts are made to get the patient to focus on adult ego faculties of cognition, judgement and reality testing. Once this is achieved, the patient is ready to work on modification of old learning and experiences. The patient is instructed to imagine opening an old computer file that requires editing or deletion. At the outset of the session, it is usually decided which file the patient would be working on. Once the patient is able to access the specific file, the patient is instructed to edit or delete it, paying particular attention to dysfunctional cognitions, maladaptive behaviours and negative feelings. By metaphorically deleting and editing the file, the patient is able to mitigate cognitive distortions, magical thinking, self-blaming and other self-defeating mental scripts (NSH). Other hypnotic uncovering or restructuring procedures such as affect bridge, age regression, age progression and dream induction can also be used to explore and restructure negative self-schemas.

Symbolic imagery techniques

Depression can often be maintained by conscious or unconscious feelings of guilt and self-blame (old garbage). Various hypnotherapeutic techniques can be used to reframe the patient's past experiences that cause guilt or self-regret. Hammond (1990) describes several symbolic imagery techniques for dealing with guilt and self-blame. Four symbolic imagery techniques for dealing with guilt and self-blame are briefly described below. These techniques are normally used with depressed patients in the late phase of treatment, after the patient is sufficiently versed in both CBT and hypnotherapy. It is advisable to use these techniques when the patient is in a fairly deep trance state.

- *The Door of Forgiveness* (Watkins, 1990). This technique was devised by Helen Watkins to help patients find their own self-forgiveness. The patient is asked to imagine walking down a corridor, at the end of which is the Door of Forgiveness. While walking down the corridor, the patient notices several doors on either side of the corridor that he or she has to pass before reaching the Door of Forgiveness. Some of these doors may appear familiar or meaningful to the patient. The patient is encouraged to open each meaningful door in turn and describe to the therapist what he or she observes inside the door in the room. The idea is for the patient to resolve any experience or relationship from the past that causes guilt before reaching the Door of Forgiveness. Very often when a patient enters through a door, an emotional abreaction may occur. The therapist does not provide any interpretation and does not act as forgiver. The therapist's role is to provide direction and support.
- *Dumping the rubbish* (Stanton, 1990b). Stanton uses the image of laundry for helping patients wash away their unwanted rubbish, such as fears, doubt, anxieties and guilt. The patient is asked to imagine going into an old-fashioned laundry room, consisting of a sink. Then to imagine filling the sink with water, opening a trap door from the head and dumping the rubbish into the water, which becomes blacker and

blacker. Finally, the patient imagines pulling out the plug from the sink and letting the inky water drain down the sink.

- *Room and fire* (Stanton, 1990b). Here the image of a fireplace is used for burning unwanted garbage. The patient is asked to imagine going down in the elevator from the tenth floor of a hotel to the basement. In the basement there is a very cosy room with a large stone fireplace and a fire burning. The patient is asked to imagine throwing into the fire 'Things you may not wish to keep in your life, such as fears, doubts, anxieties, hostilities, resentments, and guilts . . . one at a time, feeling a sense of release as they are transformed into ashes' (Stanton, 1990b, p. 313).
- *The red balloon technique* (Hammond, 1990). Hammond uses the hot air balloon as a metaphor for getting rid of unwanted negative emotions such as guilt and anger. The patient is asked to imagine walking up the hill with a large backpack. As the patient imagines climbing up the hill, the backpack gets heavier and heavier. Then the patient imagines coming across a moored hot air balloon with a gondola underneath, containing a large basket. The patient imagines throwing the burdensome, heavy, large backpack on the ground next to the gondola. Then the patient opens the backpack and tosses all the excessive and unwanted objects from the backpack into the large basket in the gondola. Finally, the patient releases the balloon and as the balloon flies away, the patient feels relieved for having unloaded all the unwanted garbage.

Sessions 11–12: Attention Switching and Positive Mood Induction

Depressives have the tendency to become preoccupied with catastrophic thoughts and negative images. Such ruminations can easily become obsessional in nature and may also kindle the brain to develop depressive pathways, thus impeding therapeutic progress. To counter the development of depressive pathways, the Positive Mood Induction technique is used and attention-switching exercises are introduced to break the negative ruminative cycle.

Positive Mood Induction

Just as the brain can be kindled to produce depressive pathways through conscious negative focusing (Schwartz *et al.*, 1976), the brain can also be kindled to develop anti-depressive or happy pathways by focusing on positive imagery (Schwartz, 1984). There is extensive empirical evidence that directed cognition can produce neuronal changes in the brain and that positive affect can enhance adaptive behaviour and cognitive flexibility (see Alladin, 2007b). Within this theoretical and empirical context, Alladin (1994, 2006a, 2007b) has devised the Positive Mood Induction technique to counter depressive pathways and to develop anti-depressive pathways. Apart from providing a systematic approach for developing anti-depressive pathways, the technique also fortifies the brain to withstand depressive symptoms, thus preventing relapse and recurrence of future depressive episodes.

The Positive Mood Induction technique consists of five steps: education; making a list of positive experiences; positive mood induction; post-hypnotic suggestions; and home practice. To educate the patient, the therapist provides a scientific rationale for developing anti-depressive pathways. Then the patient is advised to make a list of 10 to 15 pleasant or positive experiences. When in deep trance, the patient is instructed to focus on a positive experience from the list of positive experiences, which is then amplified with assistance from the therapist. The technique is very similar to enhancing affective experience and its expression, described earlier. However, to develop anti-depressive pathways, more emphasis is placed on producing somatosensory changes in order to induce more pervasive concomitant physiological changes. The procedure is repeated with at least three positive experiences from the list of pleasant experiences. Post-hypnotic suggestions are provided so that the patient, with practice, will be able regress completely when practising at home with the list.

Attention switching

The patient is encouraged to practise with the list four or five times a day and to switch off from negative or 'undesirable' experiences; whenever the patient becomes aware of dwelling on these, they are instructed to 'put them out of your mind and replace them with one of the pleasant items from your list'. This procedure provides another technique for weakening the depressive pathways and strengthening the 'happy pathways'. In other words, the patient learns to substitute NSH with positive self-hypnosis. Yapko (1992) argues that since depressives utilise NSH to create the experience of depressive reality, they can equally learn to use positive self-hypnosis to create an experience of anti-depressive reality.

Session 13: Active Interactive Training

This technique helps to break 'dissociative' habits and encourages 'association' with the relevant environment. When interacting with their internal or external environment, depressives tend automatically to dissociate rather than actively interact with the relevant external information. Active interaction requires being alert and 'in tune' with the incoming information (conceptual reality), whereas automatic dissociation is the tendency to anchor to 'inner reality' (negative schemas and associated syncretic feelings), which inhibits reality testing or appraisal of conceptual reality.

To prevent automatic dissociation a person must become aware of such a process occurring; actively attempt to inhibit it by switching attention away from 'bad anchors'; and actively attend to relevant cues or conceptual reality. In other words, the patient learns to engage the left hemisphere actively by becoming analytical, logical, realistic and syntactical. Edgette and Edgette

(1995, pp. 145–58) have also discussed several techniques for developing adaptive dissociation. For example, a patient with habitual maladaptive dissociation can be trained to embrace adaptive dissociation, which helps to counter maladaptive dissociation, halt the sense of pessimism and the sense of helplessness, and detach from toxic self-talk.

Session 14: Social Skills Training

Youngren and Lewinshon (1980) have provided evidence that lack of social skills may cause and maintain depression in some patients. A session (or more sessions if required) is therefore devoted to teaching social skills and the patient is advised to read the appropriate bibliography. The social skills training can be enhanced by hypnosis via imagery training and imaginal rehearsal.

Session 15: Behavioural Activation

Lewinshon and Gotlib (1995) have proposed the behavioural theory of depression, which suggests that life stress can lead to depression by reducing positive reinforcers in a person's life. As a result, the depressed person begins to withdraw, causing further reduction in positive reinforcers, leading to more withdrawal, and thus creating the self-perpetuating cycle of depression. Therefore, it is not surprising that depression is characterised by feeling of sadness, misery and a sense of apathy, resulting in pervasive impairment of the capacity to experience pleasure or to respond positively to the anticipation of pleasure. Such inhibitions of the mechanism of pleasure lead to diminished interest and investment in the environment. Consequently, the depressives are unable to enjoy or participate in once-pleasurable activities such as hobbies, eating, sex or social interaction. At least one session is devoted to help depressed patients learn to deal with avoidant behaviours and they are encouraged to get involved in physical exercise. Forward projection, imaginal rehearsal, ego strengthening and post-hypnotic suggestions can be used to increase motivation (see Alladin, 2007b, Chapter 13 for a full description of behavioural activation therapy).

Session 16: Mindfullness Training

Depression involves withdrawing or turning away from experience to avoid emotional pain (Germer, 2005). Such withdrawal can deprive the depressed person of the life that can only be found in direct experience. Germer believes that a successful therapy outcome results from changes in a patient's relationship with his or her particular form of suffering. For instance, if a depressed patient decides to be less upset by events, then his or her suffering is likely to decrease. Mindfulness training helps the depressed person becomes less upset by unpleasant experiences and hence less reactive to negative events in the present moment. Teasdale *et al.* (2000) have provided empirical evidence that mindfulness-based CBT reduce relapses in depression.

Mindfulness can be easily integrated with hypnotherapy in the management of depression. Lynn *et al.* (2006, p. 145) suggest that 'hypnosis and mindfulness-based approaches can be used in tandem to create adaptive response sets and ameliorate maladaptive response sets'. They recommend using hypnosis to catalyse mindfulness-based approaches. Mindfulness training is introduced to the depressed patient nearer to the end of CH sessions. I find the following sequential training of mindfulness helpful to depressed patients: education, training and hypnotherapy.

Education

The patient is given an account, citing experimental evidence, of the risk factors involved in the exacerbation, recurrence and relapse of depression, particularly after the acute-phase treatment or when the illness is in remission. Then different strategies for relapse prevention are discussed, emphasising the simplicity and effectiveness of mindfulness training. Once the patient agrees to mindfulness training, the complexity of the human being is discussed and within this context it is emphasised that feelings and thoughts are part of us and not our whole self. It is pointed out that feelings and thoughts are not objective reality, but transitory states that 'come and go just like a cloud, but the sky stays the same'.

Training

The training involves *informal* mindfulness training consisting of the Body Scan Meditation exercise adapted from Segal, Williams and Teasdale (2002, pp. 112–13). The patient is provided with the following script for learning Body Scan Meditation.

Body Scan Meditation

1. Lie down on your back on a mat on the floor or on your bed and assume a comfortable posture and allow your eyes to close gently.
2. Take a few moments to get in touch with your breathing and the feelings in your body. Become aware of the movement in your belly, feeling it rise or expand gently with every inbreath, and it falls or recede with every outbreath. On each outbreath allow yourself to let go or sink on the mat or the bed.

3. Become aware of the physical sensations in your body, noticing the sensation of touch or pressure in your body where it makes contact with the mat or bed.

4. Remind yourself of the reasons for this practice. Your intention is not to feel any different, but to become aware of any sensation you detect as you focus your attention on each part of your body in turn. You may or you may not feel calm or relaxed.

5. Now bring your attention to your lower abdomen. Become aware of the physical sensations in your abdominal wall as you breathe in and breathe out. Stay connected with your abdominal wall for a few minutes, attending to the sensations and feelings as you breathe in and out.

6. Now move your focus or 'spotlight' of your awareness from your abdomen down to your left leg, into your left foot and all the way down to the toes of your left foot. Become aware of the sensations in the toes, maybe noticing the sense of contact between the toes, a sense of tingling or warmth, or no particular sensation.

7. Now you can move the spotlight to the breathing itself. Every time you breathe in, imagine the breath entering your lungs, travelling down into your left leg and left foot, all the way into the toes of your left foot. Every time you breathe out, you notice the outbreath leaving your toes, moving up your left foot and leg, into the abdomen and through your chest, all the way up, out through your nose. Continue breathing down into and out of your toes. This may appear difficult, but do the best you can and approach it playfully.

8. The next step is to let go of the awareness in the toes and to focus on the bottom of your left foot, becoming aware of the sensations in the sole of your foot, the instep and the heel, perhaps noticing the sensation in your heel where it makes contact with the mat or bed.

9. With the breath in the background, now allow your awareness to expand into the rest of your foot – into the ankle, the top of your foot, and right into the bones and joints. As you take a slightly deep breath, allow your awareness to move to the lower part of your left leg – into your calf, shin, knee and so on in turn.

10. Now continue to bring your awareness to the physical sensations in each part of the rest of your body in turn – to the right toes, right foot, right leg, pelvic area, back, abdomen, chest, fingers, hands, arms, shoulders, neck, head and face. It's not important how well you do, simply do your best. Just continue to bring the same detailed level of awareness to the bodily sensation present. As you leave each area, 'breathe in' to it on the inbreath and let go of the region on the outbreath.

11. When you become aware of any tension or intense sensations in any part of your body, just 'breathe in' to them. Use your inbreath gently to bring your awareness right into the sensations and have a sense of release or let go on your outbreath.

12. From time to time your mind will wander away from your breath and your body. This is normal. This is what the mind does. So when you notice your mind wandering, just notice it, gently acknowledge it, notice where it has gone off to, and gently return your awareness to the part of the body you intended to focus on.

(Continued)

13. After scanning your whole body in this way, spend a few minutes being aware of a sense of your body as a whole and your breath flowing in and out of your body.
14. While practising, if you find yourself falling asleep, you may prop up your head by using a pillow, or you may practise sitting up.

Hypnotherapy

Lynn *et al.* (2006) argue that basic instructions to practise mindfulness can be offered as hypnotic suggestions, just as other imaginative or attention-altering suggestions can. These scripts from Lynn *et al.* (2006, p. 155) illustrate how hypnotic suggestions and images can facilitate mindfulness training.

> Imagine that your thoughts are written on signs carried by parading soldiers (Hayes, 1987), or thoughts continually dissolve like a parade of characters marching across a stage (Rinpoche, 1981, p. 53). Observe the parade of thoughts without becoming absorbed in any of them.

> The mind is the sky, and thoughts, feelings, and sensations are clouds that pass by, just watch them (Linehan, 1993).

> Imagine that each thought is a ripple on water or light on leaves. They naturally dissolve (Rinpoche, 1981, p. 44).

Lynn *et al.* (2006) also recommend using hypnotic and post-hypnotic suggestions to encourage patients to practise mindfulness on a regular basis; not to be discouraged when attention wanders off during training; learn to accept what cannot be changed; not to identify personally with feelings as they arise; learn to tolerate troublesome feelings; and appreciate that troublesome feelings and thoughts are not permanent.

Booster and Follow-up Sessions

CH as outlined above normally requires 16 weekly sessions. Some patients may, however, require fewer or more sessions. After these sessions, further booster or follow-up sessions may be provided as required.

SUMMARY

Following a brief review of the clinical description and current treatments of depression, the stages of cognitive hypnotherapy (CH) were described. CH provides a variety of treatment interventions for depression from which a therapist can choose the best-fit strategies for a particular depressed client. CH, which is based on the circular feedback model of depression (CFMD), embraces the rationale for combining cognitive behaviour therapy (CBT) with hypnotherapy in the management of depression, and the case-formulation approach adopted in the chapter guides the clinician in selecting the most effective and efficient treatment strategies for the particular patient. However, the number of sessions and the sequence of the stages of CH are determined by the clinical needs of each patient. CH also offers innovative techniques for treating depression, such as developing anti-depressive pathways and mindfulness hypnotherapy.

Although there is some empirical evidence for the effectiveness of CH, further studies are required before it can achieve the APA status of well-established treatment for depression. Conducting this kind of research can facilitate clinical hypnosis become recognised as a respectable and valid form of psychotherapy.

CHAPTER 4

COGNITIVE HYPNOTHERAPY IN THE MANAGEMENT OF MIGRAINE HEADACHES

INTRODUCTION

Although migraine headache is one of the most common disorders encountered by family physicians, it is under-recognised, under-diagnosed and under-treated in clinical practice (Taylor & Martin, 2004). It is estimated that approximately 18% of women and 6% of men in the United States suffer from migraine as defined by the International Headache Society (Stewart *et al.*, 1991). It is also more disabling and painful and longer in duration than other types of headache. Migraine is a public health problem that has an enormous impact on both the individual sufferer and on society. Nearly one in four US households have someone with migraine and 25% of these sufferers experience four or more severe attacks per month, 35% experience one to four severe attacks a month, and 38% experience at least one severe attack per month (Lipton *et al.*, 2005). About half of migraine sufferers are severely disabled or require bed rest during an attack (Lipton *et al.*, 2001) and many of them have psychiatric comorbidity such as anxiety and depression, and experience stress-related headache exacerbations (Lake, 2001).

Migraine reduces health-related quality of life and many migraineurs live in fear that at any time an attack could disrupt their ability to work, care for their families or meet social obligations (Lipton & Bigal, 2006); these concerns in their turn serve as a trigger for a migraine attack. Headache is reported by the US workforce to be the most common pain condition for lost productive time (Stewart *et al.*, 2003). It is estimated that approximately $23.7 billion is lost per year in the United States due to loss of productivity time (in terms of absenteeism and reduced productivity while at work) and utilisation of healthcare due to migraine headaches (Stewart *et al.*, 2002).

Despite its commonality and public health concern, the exact cause of migraine is not known and there is no medical or psychological cure for it. Ironically medication over-use for migraine may be an aggravating or causal factor for the headache progression, and may be a marker of headache intractability (Scher, 2006). Chronic headaches are predominantly 'primary' in origin; that is, only in rare instances are headaches found to be secondary to significant underlying pathology (Cady *et al.*, 2002). For these reasons, there is an urgent need to search for alternative treatment and methods of management.

This chapter describes a comprehensive approach, cognitive hypnotherapy, to the psychological management of migraine. Although the focus is on migraine, the treatment strategies can be adapted for other types of headache. After briefly reviewing the current theories and treatment of migraine, the chapter describes the cognitive hypnotherapy approach that can be easily incorporated in the management of migraine.

DESCRIPTION OF MIGRAINE HEADACHE

Migraine is a neurovascular disorder with heterogeneous clinical features, characterised by recurrent attacks of pain that vary widely in frequency, intensity and duration. As there is no available biochemical marker of migraine, the diagnosis is based on the patient's history.

Classification of Migraine

The Headache Classification Committee of the International Headache Society: Second Edition (ICHD-II; 2004) divides primary headaches into four major categories. Migraine is one of the major categories of headaches, subdivided into six subcategories consisting of migraine without aura; migraine with aura; childhood periodic syndromes that are commonly precursors of migraine; retinal migraine; complications of migraine; and probable migraine. Migraine without aura, migraine with aura and chronic migraine (a form of complicated migraine) are more often seen in clinical practice. Migraine attacks are associated with loss of appetite, nausea, vomiting and exaggerated sensitivity to light and sound, and often involve sensory, motor or mood disturbances. The diagnosis of migraine is usually made when a patient has a combination of these features:

1. Severe headache, often unilateral and located over the temple.
2. The pain is described as throbbing, pounding or pulsating.
3. Presence of nausea, vomiting and other gastrointestinal disturbances.
4. Aversion to strong sensory stimuli such as bright light, loud sounds or strong smell.
5. The pain is aggravated by movement or physical activity.

Migraine with aura is characterised by identifiable sensory disturbances that precede the head pain, whereas migraine without aura has a sudden onset and an intense throbbing, usually unilateral. Chronic migraine is diagnosed in patients having migraine on 15 days per month or more (in about 4% of the adult population) in the absence of medication over-use (Olesen & Lipton, 2006).

The Spectrum of Headaches

Some clinicians have questioned the validity of the categorical classification of headaches because, in clinical practice, many individuals with different subtypes of headache present similar symptoms. For example, the Spectrum Study (Lipton et al., 2000), which explored the relationship among different primary headaches in patients with migraine, found many migraineurs with or without aura fulfilling the criteria for probable migraine and tension-type headache. Thus, there was an observed spectrum of primary headaches in the population with migraine. Moreover, the study found that patients with different headache diagnoses showed a similar response rate to sumatriptan. Based on these findings, the investigators concluded that there may be a common underlying pathophysiological mechanism shared by phenotypically different primary headaches in the migraine population.

A subsequent study (Cady & Schreiber, 2004) found that 98% of sinus headache sufferers met criteria for migraine with or without aura (70%) or migrainous headache (28%) and their response to 50 mg of sumatriptan was comparable to the response of the migraine patients. These findings were further confirmed by a large placebo-controlled study of over 3000 subjects (Cady et al., 2002). It would therefore appear that sinus headaches are part of the spectrum of primary headache presentations observed in the migraine population. These results have also been observed in other cultures. A recent Turkish study (Turkdogan et al., 2006) with a large sample of 2504 schoolchildren aged 10 to 17 years also demonstrated the overlap between migraine and tension-type headache. They also concluded that the frequent co-occurrence of migraine and tension-type headache symptoms suggests the presence of a common pathogenesis.

Similarly, Bakal (1982) views chronic headache sufferers as falling along a continuum, so that the differences between different types of headaches are quantitative rather then qualitative. This view holds that there are no separate categories of headache as such (e.g. migraine, tension-type headache and so on); instead, there is chronic headache, which varies among individuals in terms of its intensity and frequency. A key component of this model is that chronic experience of headache is itself a stressor for the patient, which may help to perpetuate the headache disorder. The chronic pain and distress associated with the headache thus add to the total psychological and physiological stress with which the patient must cope. Having chronic headaches thus renders the sufferer more susceptible to new headaches. Cady *et al.* (2002) proposed the convergence hypothesis to explain the common pathophysiology underlying migraine and other types of common primary headaches (further discussed later in this chapter).

Clinical Anatomy of Migraine

It is critical to recognise that migraine involves a complex neurological process and that headache or pain is only one of its potential symptoms. Cady *et al.* (2002) describe three phases of migraine – pre-headache, headache and post-headache – to explain the progression from a well-functioning nervous system to a disabling migraine.

Pre-headache phase

The pre-headache phase is subdivided into the premonitory phase and the aura. The *premonitory phase* manifests signs and symptoms that are considered to be harbingers of an impending attack of migraine. About 70% of migraineurs with or without aura experience premonitory symptoms, which include a variety of mood alterations, muscle pain, food cravings, cognitive changes, fluid retension and yawning. However, only 50% of migraineurs who experience the premonitory symptoms have a migraine attack (Giffin *et al.*, 2003). Although this result supports the existence of the premonitory phase in migraine, it also demonstrates that the nervous system often recovers from the physiological process of migraine before the onset of headache. In contrast to the premonitory phase, the *aura* manifests focal, fully reversible, neurological symptoms that often precede the headache. The aura symptoms are estimated to precede about 15% of migraine attacks and they are supposed to be caused by an electrical phenomenon called *cortical spreading depression*. The fact that the prodrome can occur independently of the headache also demonstrates that in some instances the nervous system can escape the migraine process prior to the development of head pain.

Headache phase

The headache phase is subdivided according to the intensity of the headache: mild, moderate and severe. The duration of the mild phase can be quite variable, lasting minutes to days, and it can resolve itself spontaneously. During the moderate to severe phases the headache is often localised, aggravated by activity and associated with gastrointestinal symptoms, photophobia and phonophobia. These phases generally last for 4 to 72 hours.

Post-headache phase

The post-headache phase can be divided into the *resolution* and the *postdrome*. The postdrome phase is a period during which some migraine symptoms persist despite the resolution of the headache. This phase usually lasts for one to two days.

PATHOPHYSIOLOGY OF MIGRAINE

The pathogenesis of migraine is unknown (Rothner, 2001). Although several hypotheses have been advanced to explain the pathogenesis of migraine, none of the theories provides an over-arching explanation to account for the variety of symptoms presented by migraine patients. The dominant pathophysiological theory described in most textbooks is the neurovascular hypothesis (e.g. Rothner, 2001). The neurovascular hypothesis, which is based on biochemical, neurotransmitter and regional cerebral blood-flow studies, considers migraine to be an inherited sensitivity of the trigeminal vascular system. In response to internal or external stimuli, cortical, thalamic or hypothalamic mechanisms trigger migraine attack in genetically predisposed individuals. The generated impulses then spread to the cranial vasculature, producing a cascade of neurogenic inflammation and secondary vascular reactivity. This releases vasoactive neuropeptides that activate endothelial cells, mast cells and platelets, leading to an increase in extracellular amines, peptides and other metabolites. The end result is the sterile inflammation, causing pain, which is transmitted centrally via the trigeminal nerve. The sequential process involved in the pathogenesis of a migraine attack (see Hargreaves & Shepheard, 1999; Taylor & Martin, 2004) is summarised below:

- Endogenous (genetic predisposition) and exogenous factors (stress, diet, environment, lifestyle) coincide to precipitate an attack.
- The aura or pre-headache neurologic symptoms are secondary to vasospasm of cerebral arteries. The aura is primarily a neurological event caused by a mismatch of hypoperfusion and hyperfusion of cerebral blood flow and the cortical spreading depression.
- The vasospasm vasodilates the cerebral arteries and the trigeminal nerve becomes activated.
- Neuropeptides such as calcitonin gene-related peptide are released from the trigeminal nerve, leading to further vasodilation of the blood vessels. The vasodilation is perceived as a painful stimulus by the trigeminal nerve.
- The painful stimulus is transmitted from the peripheral trigeminal nerve to second-order neurons in the brainstem.
- The second-order neurons in the brainstem are activated and sensitised, leading to a relay of the painful stimulus to third-order neurons in the thalamus and later to the cerebral cortex, where the pain is perceived.

AETIOLOGY OF MIGRAINE

In discussing the aetiology of migraine, Feuerstein and Gainer (1982) have emphasised the delineation of those factors that predispose an individual to headache from those that exacerbate and maintain it. These factors, they argue, may be quite different from each other, and therefore their specification may help to clarify the controversies surrounding the various theories of migraine. Moreover, the identification of predisposing, exacerbating and maintaining factors may assist in the formulation of appropriate treatment protocols.

Some of the factors that are assumed to predispose, maintain and/or worsen headaches include diet, weather, sleep, hormonal change, psychosocial stress and various medical disorders. These factors, however, account for a small proportion of recurring headaches, as their removal often affords only modest benefits. Little research has been directed at the consequences of migraine, therefore less attention has been paid to factors that maintain chronic headache. Similarly, there has been virtually no research on the relationship between efforts to manage or cope with stress in a naturalistic environment and the frequency and intensity of headache symptoms. However, a large body of research suggests that the way an individual copes with stress can influence not only physiological stress responses, but also the onset and course of symptoms (e.g. Holroyd & Andrasik, 1982). But at this point it is not known what coping styles render individuals vulnerable to headache attacks.

Bakal (1982) has suggested an alternative approach to the study of the relationship between stress and headaches. Rather than studying the processes that mediate between the person and his or her environment, Bakal emphasises exploration of the relationship between the patient and his or her symptoms. Therefore the critical processes that mediate the chronic headache syndrome are found in the relationship among the symptoms experienced, the physiological mechanisms that mediate these symptoms and the cognitive evaluation of the condition, as the disorder develops across time. Chronic headache, Bakal suggests, should be viewed as a migraine pain disorder that is heavily influenced by the patient's cognitive actions and reactions in dealing with the symptoms themselves. At the behavioural level, a number of social learning factors such as pain behaviours, attention (secondary gain) for symptoms, pain medication and use of symptoms to avoid unpleasant environmental demands can prolong the occurrence of migraine (e.g. Philips, 1978).

The mechanisms that are considered of primary importance in the aetiology of migraine are biological, psychological and psychophysiological in nature. The biological theories focus on cerebro-vascular mechanisms and emphasise the role of biochemical agents (e.g. serotonin, histamine and catecholamine) as links in the chain of events that lead to head pain. The psychological theories concentrate on the relationship between psychological variables (e.g. emotional specificity, psychodynamic factors, personality, stress, psychiatric conditions and reinforcements) and the predisposition to migraine. The psychophysiological theories emphasise the potential role of 'stress' in the aetiology of migraine and attempt to elucidate the specific mechanisms by which stress could trigger a headache. While no single theory has been able to explain why certain individuals develop migraines and others do not, or even why headaches develop in certain situations and not in others, recently Cady and his colleagues (Cady *et al.*, 2002; Sheftell & Cady, 2006) have proposed the convergence hypothesis.

The Convergence Hypothesis

The convergence hypothesis takes a continuum view of primary headaches and attempts to connect common primary headaches with the pathophysiology of migraine. It proposes that an episode of migraine is initiated when a vulnerable nervous system is exposed to an environment (internal or external) that puts it at risk for migraine. Once placed in this migraine-risk environment, the nervous system undergoes changes in its normal homeostatic mechanism, producing premonitory symptoms. These changes start a chain of events, causing disruption of the nervous system, unique to each individual, resulting in different premonitory symptoms. This may lead to cortical spreading depression (CSD), thus starting the pre-headache phase. CSD is used to explain the physiological mechanism associated with the aura. However, the aura is associated with only 20% of migraine attacks and it is not known whether CSD occurs in migraine without aura (Bolay *et al.*, 2002).

The mild headache phase of the migraine results from a net loss of central inhibitory modulation of peripherally generated sensory inputs arising from trigeminal afferents and/or sensory input from the C-2-3 dermatomes. The early perception of headache is usually secondary to patients experiencing muscle tension and pain, skin sensitivity, or sinus pressure or congestion. According to Cady and his colleagues, these symptoms are erroneously interpreted as evidence for sinus headache or muscle tension headache. The symptoms are worsened primarily due to neurovascular activation of the trigeminal afferents. Once the moderate-to-severe headache phase sets in, the underlying migraine pathophysiology evolves and progresses, and the second-order neurons become sensitised. At this stage, physical activities that increase intracranial pressure such as coughing or bending forward can aggravate the pain. Sensory inputs are perceived as unpleasant or painful as the higher orders of the nervous system become sensitised and during some attacks patients may develop cutaneous allodynia (abnormal experience of pain in response to non-painful stimuli). As noted when describing the clinical anatomy of migraine, the moderate-to-severe headache can be arrested or terminated at any point in its evolution.

The convergence hypothesis has both diagnostic and clinical implications. The diagnostic implication is that the convergence hypothesis defines the experience of common primary headaches in terms of the extent of the activation and the disruption of the nervous system. Moreover, the model proposes that the entire spectrum of primary headaches can be understood as arising from the same pathophysiological process. Clinical management of primary headaches should therefore be shifted to understanding the pattern of headache rather than diagnosing each individual headache. Although the convergence hypothesis is controversial and is not accepted by all headache specialists (e.g. Olesen & Goadsby, 2006), the model is very applicable to psychological approaches to management of headaches, as the focus is on prevention and disruption of the headache patterns. Moreover, the model accounts for most of the psychological, physiological and environmental factors known to be associated with migraine.

MANAGEMENT OF MIGRAINE

Although migraine has existed for centuries, to date there is no cure for chronic migraine headache. Therefore it would be more accurate to speak of the management of migraine rather than its treatment. A variety of management techniques have been attempted with chronic migraine, ranging from surgery to psychotherapy. The next sections briefly review the pharmacological and psychological management of migraine.

Pharmacological Management of Migraine

Not all migraine sufferers benefit from pharmacotherapy. Pharmacological migraine management can either be *acute* (abortive) or *preventive* (prophylactic). Acute management can be further subdivided into *specific* and *non-specific* categories. Migraine-specific medications, such as triptans and ergotamine, relieve migraine but are generally ineffective with non-cephalic pain (Krymchantowski & Tepper, 2006). Acute treatment attempts to reverse or stop the progression of a headache once it has started by administering drugs with anti-migraine actions but no general anti-pain actions. Triptans have been successful in aborting migraine headache in about 20–68% of migraine patients (Taylor & Martin, 2004, p. 59). Non-specific medications are effective across a broad range of pain disorders not linked to migraine and they include such agents as aspirin, acetaminophen and other simple analgesics, non-steroidal anti-inflammatory drugs, neuroleptics, opioids and combination analgesics. In addition, some drugs can be used to target non-pain symptoms such as nausea and vomiting. Triptans provide vastly superior efficacy in comparison with non-specific agents (Lipton *et al.*, 2004). However, ergotamine and triptans are only effective with migraine attacks and not with the migraine pain. Therefore the clinician is faced with the decision whether to begin treatment with a triptan or a combination of non-specific treatments first. The choice of the treatment is usually determined by the characteristics of the migraine, the individual needs of the patient and the best outcome. In order to adopt an evidence-based approach to pharmacological management of migraine, physicians are encouraged to adopt the stepped-care approach (i.e. starting with the most simple and straightforward treatment and progressing to more intensive treatment as needed) described by Lipton and colleagues (Lipton *et al.*, 2000).

Preventive treatment is designed to reduce attack frequency and severity. Prophylactic medications for migraine are effective in reducing the frequency of attacks in fewer than 50% of patients (Adelman, Adelman & VonSeggern, 2002) and therefore Taylor and Martin (2004, p. 64) recommend that 'patients need to be told that a complete cure for headache is not possible with current migraine preventives and that it may take some time to see an improvement'. Mathew and Tfelt-Hansen (2006, p. 433) state:

> Physicians should encourage the patient to develop realistic expectations of the treatment of chronic migraine. It is important to explain that migraine is a recurrent disorder and that there is no total cure; the best that can be done is to keep the headaches under some control with abortive as well as preventive medications.

Moreover, some of the medications that are effective in some respects have adverse side effects and contra-indications (Mathew & Tfelt-Hansen, 2006). For these reasons, there is a need for alternative treatments.

Psychological Management of Migraine

Psychological or non-pharmacological interventions also do not provide a cure for migraine. The focus of psychological interventions, mainly consisting of biofeedback, relaxation training and cognitive behaviour therapy, is to prevent migraine, although psychological management skills may also be used to abort an attack or to cope with the occurrence of a migraine. Specifically, the goals of psychological interventions are to increase personal control over migraine; modify any behaviours that may trigger attacks, increase pain or prolong disability; reduce the frequency and severity of migraine; reduce migraine-related disability and affective distress; and limit reliance on poorly tolerated or unwanted pharmacotherapy (Holroyd, 2006).

Psychological procedures such as thermal and extracranial biofeedback, relaxation training, behaviour therapy, cognitive therapy and a combination of these procedures have been found to be generally effective in the management of migraine. Recently, a number of meta-analytic reviews indicated that relaxation training, temperature biofeedback training, temperature biofeedback plus relaxation training, EMG biofeedback training, cognitive-behavioural therapy (CBT), and CBT plus temperature biofeedback are more effective than wait-list and other controls (McGrath, Penzien & Rains, 2006). These behavioural interventions yielded 32–49% reductions in migraine versus a 5% reduction for no-treatment controls. Moreover, the follow-up data (e.g. Blanchard *et al.*, 1987) showed that 91% of migraine headache sufferers remained significantly improved five years after completing behavioural headache treatment.

Moreover, the effects of behavioural therapies are found to be comparable to the effects of pharmacotherapy. Recent meta-analyses (see review by McGrath, Penzien & Rains, 2006) demonstrated virtually identical improvement in migraine when treated either with propranolol and flunarizine or with a combination of relaxation with biofeedback training. These findings suggest that the 'best of the prophylactic medications and behavioural therapies may be equally viable treatment options' (McGrath, Penzien & Rains, 2006, p. 445) for migraine.

Hypnotherapy in the Management of Migraine

Hypnotherapy is another psychological approach for migraine management, although it is less widely used than cognitive behavioural interventions. A variety of hypnotic techniques has been used in the treatment of migraine. Hypnosis most often involves some form of relaxation in conjunction with hypnotic procedures, designed to modify pain perception and/or the emotional state of the patient. Bakal (1982) views hypnosis as a cognitive tool for teaching patients how to minimise the pain during attacks and to become aware of psychological events that lead to headache attacks. Spanos *et al.* (1979) assert that the effectiveness or ineffectiveness of hypnosis and suggestion procedures in the control of pain is largely determined by the patient's ability or inability to generate pain-control cognitions. Post-hypnotic suggestions have also been implemented. The general approach is ultimately directed at self-hypnosis, where the patient is able to implement specific strategies to reduce autonomic arousal, modify pain and enhance 'self-perception'. Specific techniques used with migraine include relaxation, glove anaesthesia, and symptom transformation via imagery and ego strengthening (Anderson, Basker & Dalton, 1975; Andreychuk & Skriver, 1975).

Finer (1974) has suggested that hypnosis should be used as the first, rather than the last, line of treatment for migraine. More recently, Hammond (2007), from his review of the effectiveness of hypnotherapy with migraine, concludes:

> not only has hypnosis been shown to be efficacious with headache and migraine, but it is also a treatment that is relatively brief and cost effective. At the same time it has been found to be virtually free of the side effects, risks of adverse reactions, and the ongoing expense associated with the widely used medication

treatments. Hypnosis should be recognized by the scientific, health care, and medical insurance communities as being an efficient evidence-based practice.

The National Institute of Health Technology Assessment Panel on Integration of Behavioural and Relaxation Approaches into the Treatment of Chronic Pain and Insomnia (National Institute of Health, 1996) also concluded, from a review of outcome studies on hypnosis with pain, that hypnosis is effective with chronic pain, including headaches. Similarly, a meta-analytic review of contemporary research on hypnosis and pain management (Montgomery, DuHamel & Redd, 2000) documented that hypnosis meets the American Psychological Association criteria (Chambless & Hollon, 1998) for being an efficacious and specific treatment for pain, showing superiority to medication, psychological placebos and other treatments. Moreover, Hammond's (2007) review of the literature on the effectiveness of hypnosis in the treatment of headaches and migraines concluded that hypnotherapy meets the clinical psychology research criteria for being a well-established and efficacious treatment for tension and migraine headaches.

Principles of Migraine Management

Based on our current understanding of the epidemiology, aetiology and management of migraine, the US Headache Consortium (Silberstein, 2000), the Canadian Headache Society (Pryse-Philips *et al.*, 1997) and the UK Migraine in Primary Care Advisors Migraine Guidelines Development Group (Dowson *et al.*, 2002) have all developed evidence-based guidelines for the management of migraine. These treatment guidelines can be summarised into seven principles (see Husid & Rapoport, 2006, p. 242):

- Establishment of a diagnosis.
- Assessment of disability and other factors.
- Education of patients about their conditions and their treatment.
- Establishment of realistic expectations.
- Encouragement of patients to become more active in their own care.
- Development of an appropriate, individualised treatment plan.
- Scheduling of regular follow-up visits to reassess and modify treatment.

COGNITIVE HYPNOTHERAPY FOR MIGRAINE

The seven treatment principles can be easily integrated within the cognitive hypnotherapy (CH) framework of the management of migraine. CH combines cognitive behavioural techniques with hypnotic strategies in order to maximise the treatment outcome. Although to my current knowledge there is no formal report in the literature of a study examining the additive effect of hypnotherapy and CBT in the management of migraine, there is evidence for such an effect with acute stress disorder (Bryant *et al.*, 2005) and depression (Alladin & Alibhai, 2007). Schoenberger (2000), from her review of the empirical status of the use of hypnosis in conjunction with cognitive-behavioural therapy in the treatment of a variety of emotional disorders, concludes that the existing studies demonstrate substantial benefits from the addition of hypnosis to cognitive-behavioural techniques. Similarly, Kirsch, Montgomery and Sapirstein (1995), from their meta-analysis of 18 studies comparing a cognitive-behavioural treatment with the same treatment supplemented by hypnosis for various emotional problems, found the mean effect size of the hypnotic treatment to be larger than the non-hypnotic intervention. However, it should be pointed out that CH should be used with migraine as an adjunctive treatment within a team approach, consisting of other health professionals, to maximise the effectiveness of the treatment. CH strategies for the management of migraine within the context of the seven treatment principles are described in detail in the rest of the chapter.

Establishing a Diagnosis

Before starting treatment it is important for the therapist to take a detailed clinical history and identify the essential psychological, physiological and social aspects of the patient's headache. In over 90% of cases, the diagnosis of migraine is established by history taking. Good history taking also enhances mutual respect and trust between the patient and clinician, which can make the difference between success and failure of treatment. When the migraine patient is treated by a non-physician, it is important to obtain medical clearance and diagnostic and other medical information, including pharmacological intervention, from the patient's attending physician. In addition it is crucial to rule out or identify organic aetiology that may require medical intervention.

Assessment of Disability

The disability caused by the migraine has the greatest impact on the patient and therefore a crucial part of headache management is to assess the disability status of the migraine patient (Husid & Rapoport, 2006). The MIDAS (migraine disability assessment) questionnaire can be used to assess the disability of migraine patients (Stewart *et al.*, 1999). However, it is recommended that the clinical assessment of the migraine patient is conducted within the context of the case-formulation model. As discussed in Chapter 2, the main function of a case formulation is to devise an effective treatment plan (see Appendices B and C). In order to identify the mechanisms that underlie the patient's migraine headache within the context of hypnotherapy, the eight-step case formulation (see Alladin, 2007b) can be used. Table 4.1 summarises the eight steps required to formulate the migraine case.

Table 4.1   Eight-step case formulation with migraine

---

1. List the major signs and symptoms of the migraine and indicate how they affect the functioning of the patient.
2. Formulate a formal diagnosis of the migraine and rule out organic causes.
3. Formulate a working hypothesis, e.g. whether the migraine is stress related, due to over-arousal or related to the patient's attitudes and beliefs.
4. Identify what triggers, exacerbates and maintains the migraine. Also identify the medication the patient may be on, noting the response to medication and the patient's 'pill-taking' behaviour.
5. Explore the origin of the migraine and how it has affected the patient.
6. Summarise the working hypothesis.
7. Outline the treatment plan, integrating the pharmacological or other treatment the patient may be having.
8. Identify strengths and assets and predict obstacles to treatment.

Educating Migraine Patients

The more understanding a patient has about his or her migraine and the treatment prescribed, the more collaborative the patient will be with the treatment. The education should particularly focus on:

- Understanding the role of triggering and aggravating factors.
- The importance of leading a reasonable life, with a predictable rhythm.
- The beneficial role of relaxation and self-hypnosis in mitigating headache.
- Understanding the relationship between certain activities (e.g. skipping meals, not getting enough sleep) and the triggering of a migraine attack.
- The importance of monitoring headaches to track 'trigger' behaviours.
- Providing information about the dangers of excessive pain medication.
- The rationale and outcome for using a particular treatment.
- The benefits and adverse effects of medication.
- The importance of active collaboration from the patient.

Establishing Realistic Expectations

In order to ensure a good outcome, it is fundamental to address the patient's expectations. The establishment of 'realistic expectations by setting appropriate goals and discussing the expected benefits of therapy and how long it will take to achieve them goes a long way in ensuring patient compliance' (Husid & Rapoport, 2006, p. 254). It is important to inform the patient that there are no magic remedies for curing the headaches. The realistic and practical goal of migraine treatment is to control pain, alleviate other associated symptoms and reduce disability, rather than eliminating the migraine completely. It is also important not to make assumptions about the patient's motive for seeking treatment. Each patient has his or her own concerns, fears, expectations and questions. In a survey of 100 headache patients attending a general neurology clinic, Packard (1987) found that while two-thirds of physicians believed that patients primarily sought pain relief, the patients themselves reported that they were more interested in having the causes of the pain explained to them.

Encouraging Patients to Become Active in Their Own Care

If a migraine patient is not willing to do most of the work and insists on looking for a magic pill, symptom relief may not be achieved. It is, therefore, very important to encourage patients to become active in their own care and assume control of their own migraine management, because without their active participation the treatment will fail. Husid and Rapoport (2006, p. 255) draw the analogy with diabetes mellitus to make this point: 'Just as diabetics must take responsibility for monitoring blood sugar and maintaining an appropriate diet, so must headache patients take appropriate beneficial measures.' Headache calendars can be used to get the patient involved in effective migraine management. As headache calendars require self-monitoring of symptoms and medication intake, the patients become automatically involved as active participants in their treatment.

Developing an Appropriate Individualised Treatment Plan

As each patient is unique, the treatment plan should be individualised. The case-formulation approach utilised in this book facilitates individualised treatment plans and translates nomothetic findings into an idiographic perspective in an evidence-based way. The next section describes cognitive hypnotherapy (CH), a multi-modal approach to the psychological management of migraine.

COGNITIVE HYPNOTHERAPY FOR MIGRAINE

CH for migraine is provided within the context of the general treatment principles described above. The CH treatment prototype described below represents the routine hypnotic procedure I have been using over the past 20 years with migraine patients. Although the focus is on hypnotherapy, the treatment usually involves a multi-modal approach consisting of medication, cognitive behaviour therapy (CBT), stress inoculation and pain management. It should also be borne in mind that migraine sufferers do not form a homogenous group. The treatment should be adapted to each individual patient's clinical needs. CH prototype for migraine consists of hypnotic induction and deepening; relaxation and induction of well-being; mind over body training; ego strengthening; pain management via relaxation and transfer of warmth; imagery training for healing; post-hypnotic suggestions; cognitive behaviour therapy; problem-solving skills; and self-hypnosis training. Some strategies for dealing with complex cases will also be outlined.

Hypnotic Induction and Deepening

The hypnotic procedure is targeted at the three main components of migraine: physiological changes (usually blood vessel dilation); the subjective experience of pain (aching, distress, fatigue etc.); and the behaviour motivated by the pain (e.g. pill taking, withdrawal from family and social activities, absence from work). Any formal or informal method of hypnotic induction and deepening can be used. However, it is advisable to consider a few points before choosing an induction and deepening method. A patient with migraine may often have blurred vision or difficulty focusing, or may feel very anxious and irritable and may be hypersensitive to various stimuli. A therapist should be aware of these factors and should therefore choose a hypnotic induction or deepening technique that may not require eye fixation or hyper-attentiveness, or any approach that is likely to strain the patient further. Moreover, if the initial hypnotic induction is recorded for making an audiocassette or CD to assist the patient in self-hypnosis training, the induction technique needs to be simple and effective. I have adopted the *relaxation with counting method* from Gibbons (1979), which is easily adapted for self-hypnosis training (see Appendix D for the complete script for induction and deepening).

Relaxation and Induction of Well-Being

One of the main objectives of using hypnosis is to induce a deep sense of relaxation. By learning to relax, migraine sufferers are able to reduce sympathetic arousal, manage the physiological responses associated with migraine, reduce stress and enhance feelings of self-efficacy and control (Bernstein, Borkovec & Hazlett-Stevens, 2000). Moreover, by inducing relaxation, hypnosis reduces anxiety and creates a feeling of well-being, thus providing migraineurs with the evidence that they can relax, calm down, modify their symptoms and feel different. These experiences create a sense of control and promote positive expectancy and a strong therapeutic alliance.

Mind over Body Training

Hypnosis provides a commanding tool for demonstrating the credibility of psychological therapy for migraine. The more credible and powerful the treatment is perceived to be by the patient, the better the treatment outcome (DePiano & Salzberg, 1981). When the patient is in a fairly deep hypnotic trance, eye and body catalepsies (associated with the challenge to open eyes and get out of the chair or couch) are induced to demonstrate the power of the mind over the body. These demonstrations reduce scepticism over hypnosis and instil confidence in the migraine patients that they can produce significant emotional, behavioural and physiological changes.

This approach is exemplified by the case of Michael. Michael, a 40-year-old geologist with a 10-year history of chronic classical (with aura) migraine, was referred to me for hypnotherapy by his neurologist. Michael was very sceptical of psychological treatment, especially hypnosis, for his migraine, which he considered to be a vascular disorder. Not only did the demonstration of the power of mind over body via eye and body catalepsies reduce his scepticism about hypnosis, he also became a model patient and the frequency of his migraine attacks (from one per week to one attack every six to eight weeks) significantly decreased after 12 sessions of hypnotherapy.

Ego Strengthening

When experiencing hypnosis, ego-strengthening suggestions are offered to the migraine patient to increase self-confidence, boost self-esteem and optimise treatment effect. The enhancement of feelings of self-confidence and self-esteem produces positive expectancy and perceived self-efficacy. Bandura (1977) has provided experimental evidence that *self-efficacy*, the expectation and confidence of being able to cope successfully with various situations, is one of the key elements in the effective treatment of phobic disorders. Individuals with a sense of high self-efficacy tend to perceive themselves as being in control. If migraine patients can be helped to view themselves as having the ability to control their symptoms, they will perceive the future as hopeful. The most popular method for increasing self-efficacy within the hypnotherapeutic context is to provide ego-strengthening suggestions. According to Hartland (1971), ego-strengthening suggestions 'remove tension, anxiety and apprehension, and . . . gradually restore the patient's confidence in himself and his ability to cope with his problems'. Hence his ego-strengthening suggestions (see Appendix B) consist of generalised supportive suggestions to increase the patient's confidence, coping abilities, positive self-image and interpersonal skills.

However, to ensure credibility and acceptance of the ego-strengthening suggestions, it is of paramount importance that they are crafted in such a way that they appear credible and logical to the migraine patient. For example, rather than stating 'Your migraine will disappear', it is advisable to suggest:

> As a result of this treatment and as a result of you listening to your self-hypnosis tape every day, you will begin to relax and learn to let go. And every day as you listen to your tape, you will begin to feel more and more deeply relaxed, less tense, less anxious and less upset, so that every day your mind, your body and your nerves will become more and more relaxed. As a result of this deep relaxation, every day, your mind, your body and your nerves will become stronger and healthier. As a result of this, your migraine will become less frequent, less severe, until they will disappear completely.

This set of ego-strengthening suggestions sounds logical, and improvement becomes contingent on continuing with the therapy and listening to the self-hypnosis tape daily.

Pain Management via Relaxation and Transfer of Warmth

Hypnotherapy provides a powerful tool for producing a variety of cognitive, somatic, perceptual, physiological, visceral and kinaesthetic changes under controlled conditions. Hypnotic production and modulation of these changes provide migraine patients with dramatic proof that they can change their feelings and experience, thus providing hope that they can alter their migraine symptoms. After two or three sessions of hypnosis and ego strengthening, I begin to introduce relaxation and 'warming' techniques for symptom management. Here's an example of the kind of relaxation suggestions that can be given to the patient to gradually reduce the head pain:

> You have now become so deeply relaxed and you are in such a deep trance that your mind and your body feel so relaxed, so comfortable, that you can let yourself go completely. You begin to feel a sensation of peace and tranquillity, relaxation and calm flowing all over your mind and body, giving you such a pleasant and such a soothing sensation all over your mind and body that you begin to feel all the tension, all the pressure easing away from your head. As you become more and more relaxed, you feel all the tension, all the pressure, all the discomfort easing away from your head. Soon you will feel so relaxed and so calm that your head will feel clear and comfortable.

The above suggestions can be repeated, modulated and expanded to produce the desired effects. When using this technique, if the patient has a headache it is important to assess and monitor the pain via a 10-point self-report scale (0 = no pain; 10 = worst pain) throughout the procedure. It is useful to rate the pain before starting the hypnotherapy and then to monitor the level by regularly asking the rating from the patient. This monitoring of pain provides feedback both to the therapist and to the patient. In the event that the pain has aborted during the course of the session, the therapist can use future tense when making suggestions of pain control (e.g. 'In the future whenever you have a headache, you will be able to control it by relaxing your forehead'). With chronic and severe migraine, relaxation suggestions may not be sufficient to ease away the pain. Very often, the relaxation suggestions have to be substantiated with the warming technique to bring about the desired changes:

> You have now become so deeply relaxed and you are in such a deep trance that your mind has become so powerful, so sensitive to my suggestions, that you will be able to feel, imagine and experience everything I ask you to imagine, feel and experience. Now I want you to imagine yourself sitting in front of a bucket full of warm water. You know the water is warm because you can see the steam

rising. (*It is advisable to monitor the patient's experience by regularly checking via an established ideomotor signal.*)

Become aware of the warm water surrounding your hand, dipped in the warm water. You feel the warmth from the water penetrating your hand and soon you will feel your hand feeling warm. When you experience your hand feeling warm, let me know by nodding your head (*I normally use a head nod for 'yes' and head shake for 'no'*). As you focus on your hand, you begin to feel the warmth increasing, and soon you will feel a very warm feeling in your hand. You may begin to feel a tingling sensation in your hand. (*The therapist needs to wait until these changes occur; that is, they are reported by the patient.*)

Now I want you to take your hand out of the warm water and gently rest it against your forehead. Gently massage your forehead, and as you do that you begin to feel the warmth from your hand spreading over your forehead. As you feel this warmth spreading over your forehead, you begin to feel your forehead becoming more and more relaxed, more and more comfortable. You will soon begin to feel the warmth spreading inside your head (*suggestions repeated until the patient can feel the warmth inside the head*). As the warmth spreads inside your head, you feel your head becoming more and more relaxed, more and more comfortable, drifting into a deeper and deeper hypnotic trance. Soon you will feel so relaxed, so comfortable, that your head will feel relaxed and comfortable, and as your head becomes more and more relaxed you feel all the tension, all the pressure, all the discomfort easing away from your head, and soon your head will feel clear and comfortable.

As a result of this hypnotic procedure, many migraine patients report a dramatic reduction in their symptoms. DePiano and Salzberg (1981) maintain that the rapid positive changes experienced by migraine patients are partly due to the profound behavioural, emotional, cognitive and physiological changes brought on by hypnotic induction.

Imagery Training for Healing

Imagery training is used within the context of warming the head to promote healing inside the brain. Once the migraine patient is able to induce the warm feeling inside the head, the therapist capitalises on this experience to promote healing and modification of the perceived underlying pathophysiology of migraine. The suggestions are worded to associate warmth inside the head with increased blood circulation, which appears logical to the patient:

Just continue to experience this warm feeling inside your head. The warm feeling inside your head is due to the fact that the blood circulation inside your head has increased. Imagine the blood flow is increasing inside your head (*wait for the affirmative before proceeding further*). Imagine the extra blood flow is bringing in more oxygen and more nutrition to the areas where you need them most. As a result of this extra blood, the tissues, the nerves, the blood vessels will become stronger and healthier, and as a result of this your migraines will become less frequent, less severe, until they will disappear completely.

Post-hypnotic Suggestions

Post-hypnotic suggestions are provided to ratify the hypnotic experience, to promote self-hypnosis and to counter problem behaviours, negative emotions and dysfunctional cognitions that may trigger or exacerbate the migraine symptoms. Post-hypnotic suggestions are regarded as a very necessary part of the therapeutic process if the patient is to carry new possibilities into future experience (Yapko, 2003). Hence many clinicians use post-hypnotic suggestions to shape behaviour. Clarke and Jackson (1983) regard post-hypnotic suggestion as a form of 'higher-order conditioning', which functions as positive or negative reinforcement to increase or decrease the probability of desired or undesired behaviours, respectively. They have successfully utilised post-hypnotic suggestions to enhance the effect of in vivo exposure among agoraphobics.

The following post-hypnotic suggestions can be used with migraine patients. These post-hypnotic suggestions not only sound logical to patients, they also convey the contingent relationship between their behaviour (e.g. listening to the self-hypnosis tape) and improvement.

> As a result of this treatment, and as a result of you listening to your self-hypnosis tape every day, you will become less preoccupied with yourself, less preoccupied with your migraine and less preoccupied with what you think other people think about you. As a result of this, every day you will become more and more interested in what you are doing and what is going on around you.

> And every day as you listen to the tape, you will learn how to relax, how to let go, so that even when you have a headache, you will be able to relax . . . You will be able to unwind, relax and let go even when you have a headache. As a result of this, every day you will have more and more confidence in controlling your headache, and you will become more and more confident in coping with your migraine.

> As a result of this treatment, you will also learn to warm your hand easily and quickly . . . so that when you have a headache you will be able to transfer the warmth to your head and the warmth will replace any discomfort you may have in your head. And also as you imagine the blood flow increasing inside your head, the nerves, the tissues and the blood vessels inside your head will become stronger and healthier. As a result of this your migraines will become less frequent, less severe, until they will disappear completely.

Cognitive Behaviour Therapy

The rationale for using cognitive behaviour therapy (CBT) with migraine is derived from the observation that the way in which individuals cope with everyday stresses can precipitate, exacerbate or maintain migraines and increase migraine-related disability and distress (Holroyd & Andrasik, 1982). CBT directs patients' attention to the role that their thoughts and behaviours play in generating stress and stress-related headaches, and in increasing headache-related disability (Holroyd, 2006). Three to five sessions may be spent with CBT and this component is particularly useful when migraine patients have comorbid anxiety or depression.

The CBT approach used with migraine patients is similar to the sequential format of CBT described with depression in Chapter 3. More specifically, migraine patients use the Cognitive Restructuring (ABCDE) form to monitor the circumstances (events) in which their headaches occur, including their automatic thoughts, feelings, bodily sensations and behaviours prior to the onset of the headaches. Once the migraine-related stressful situations are identified, the patient is coached to identify and restructure the dysfunctional cognitions (see Chapter 3). Cognitive targets may be stress-generating *thoughts* (e.g. 'I can't cope with this') or an underlying *belief* or *assumption* (e.g. 'I'm weak; there's something wrong with me') that distils the meaning or theme from many stress-generating thoughts (Holroyd, 2006). The goal of CBT is to train the patients to 'catch' their stress-generating thoughts, 'thereby controlling stress and other negative effects, and to render the patient less vulnerable to stress-related negative effect' (Holroyd, 2006, p. 262).

Problem-Solving Skills

As mentioned above, migraine can be triggered, exacerbated and maintained by stress. Patients are encouraged to identify physical (e.g. noise) and psychosocial (e.g. lack of assertiveness at work) problems or situations that can trigger, maintain or worsen their migraine symptoms. Once the patient has been able identify a stressor (e.g. a lack of social skills), the patient and the therapist can work collaboratively to find a solution to the problem. In this example, it will be important for the therapist to coach the patient to acquire appropriate social skills. Hypnosis can be used to make the cognitive-behavioural strategies more experiential, and therefore more meaningful.

Self-Hypnosis Training

Alman (2001) believes that patients can achieve self-reliance and personal power by learning self-hypnosis' and Yapko (2003) contends that the teaching of self-hypnosis and problem-solving strategies to patients allow them to develop self-correcting mechanisms that give them control over their lives. Therefore it is of paramount importance to teach self-hypnosis to patients with chronic pain. At the end of the first hypnotherapy session, the

patient is provided with an audiocassette or CD of self-hypnosis to practise at home. The homework assignment provides continuity of treatment
between sessions and offers patients the opportunity to learn self-hypnosis.
The self-hypnosis component of the hypnotherapy is devised to induce
relaxation, promote parasympathetic dominance and provide tools for controlling the migraine symptoms. The self-hypnosis also helps to counter
negative emotions, attitudes and behaviours.

Complex cases

Insight-orientad or exploratory hypnotic techniques can be used when the
patient does not respond to the usual treatment protocol. This approach allows
the therapist and the patient to explore intrapersonal dynamics and the unconscious origin or purposes of the migraine. There are many insight-oriented
hypnotic methods (e.g. Brown & Fromm, 1986a). The simplest and the most
widely used one is ideomotor signalling. Hammond (1998, p. 114) introduces
ideomotor signalling to his hypnotised patient in the following manner:

> We all have a conscious mind, and an unconscious mind; like a front of the
> mind, and a back of the mind. Your unconscious mind has tremendous capacity
> and power to help you. Your unconscious mind also knows a great deal about
> you, and sometimes it may be aware of things that we're are not fully aware
> of consciously. And your unconscious mind can establish a method of signaling
> and communicating with us. Now I don't want you to consciously or voluntarily
> try to move or lift any of your fingers. But simply allow your unconscious mind,
> that it wishes to use as a signal for a response of 'yes.' And all by itself, entirely
> on its own, you'll simply discover one of those fingers developing a feeling of
> lightness, as if a helium balloon is attached with a string to the fingertip, and
> it will float up into the air all by itself. And just notice which finger begins to
> develop that light, floaty sensation, and then begins floating up, all by itself. Your
> unconscious mind will select one of the fingers on your right/left hand, that it
> wishes to use as a signal for 'yes.' And you'll notice a tendency to movement in
> one of those fingers. And you can just think over and over in your mind, 'yes, yes,
> yes,' and a finger will begin getting lighter, and lighter, and begins floating up.

Seven key areas can be explored with migraine patients using the ideomotor
signalling technique:

- Adaptive function or secondary gain for the symptoms.
- Self-punishment by having the migraine.
- Inner conflict causing the migraine.
- Imprints or commands transformed into migraine.
- Migraine symbolic of past experiences.
- Migraine adopted as a form of identification.
- Migraine symbolic of inner pain.

Once the underlying cause of the migraine is established, the therapist can help the patient deal with the issue in a satisfactory manner. Migraine can also be compounded by comorbid psychiatric and/or medical problems. With these a comprehensive psychiatric and/or medical treatment will be required.

Scheduling of Regular Follow-up Visits

As migraine is a chronic condition and not yet curable, regular follow-up visits are essential for successful long-term care.

SUMMARY

This chapter briefly reviewed the theories and the psychological treatment of migraine headache. The main focus of the chapter was on the description of the cognitive hypnotherapy prototype for migraine. The techniques described can be easily adapted to a variety of headache patients. Clinicians are encouraged to standardise these procedures and to validate the relative effectiveness of these procedures in the management of migraine.

CHAPTER 5

COGNITIVE HYPNOTHERAPY WITH POST-TRAUMATIC STRESS DISORDER

INTRODUCTION

Stress is an inevitable fact of everyday life and in some cases stress can be desirable. However, some stressors can be so catastrophic and horrifying that they can cause serious psychological harm such as anxiety, depression, dissociative symptoms, substance abuse, acute stress disorder (ASD) and post-traumatic stress disorder (PTSD; Cardeña, Butler & Spiegel, 2003; Van Ommeren et al., 2002; Yehuda *et al.*, 1993). This chapter will focus on PTSD, which is characterised by re-experiencing of the traumatic event accompanied by symptoms of increased arousal, numbing of emotional responses and avoidance of stimuli associated with the trauma. The causes and the treatments of PTSD are briefly reviewed before providing a detailed description of cognitive hypnotherapy (CH) for PTSD. CH is an evidence-based multi-modal treatment that can be applied to a wide range of traumatised patients. To provide an empirical and conceptual basis for utilising hypnosis with PTSD, the hypnotherapy techniques are integrated with imagery rescripting therapy (IRT), a multi-faceted, imagery-focused, evidence-based treatment designed to alleviate PTSD symptoms, alter negative beliefs and schemas, and enhance the trauma survivor's ability to self-calm and self-nurture (Grunert *et al.*, 2003; Smucker, 1997). The implications for using hypnosis within the context of IRT are highlighted.

CLINICAL DESCRIPTION OF POST-TRAUMATIC STRESS DISORDER

The diagnosis of PTSD is based on a history of exposure to a traumatic event. This makes it a unique disorder over other psychiatric diagnoses classified in the fourth, text revised edition of the *Diagnostic and Statistical Manual of Mental Disorders* (DSM-IV-TR; American Psychiatric Association, 2000) because of the great importance attached to the traumatic stressor in the diagnostic criteria of the disorder. In fact, one cannot make a diagnosis of PTSD unless the 'stressor criterion' is met by the patient. DSM-IV-TR defines an event as traumatic:

1. When a person experienced, witnessed or was confronted with an event or events that involved actual or threatened death or serious injury, or a threat to the physical integrity of self or others; and
2. The response involved intense fear, helplessness, or horror (in children this may be expressed as disorganised or agitated behaviour).

Examples of traumatic events include combat experiences, assault, rape, prolonged abuse, or observing the serious injury or violent death of another person. To meet the diagnostic criteria for PTSD, the traumatised person should also present symptoms from these three major categories of symptoms: re-experiencing; avoidance/numbing; and hyperarousal. Moreover, the symptoms should last more than one month and they should cause clinically significant distress or impairment in social, occupational or other important areas of functioning. When the duration of the symptoms has been less than one month, the diagnosis of Acute Stress Disorder (ASD) should be made. The three categories of symptoms are described below.

1. *Re-experiencing the traumatic event.* The patient frequently recalls the event or has flashbacks of the event and has nightmares about it. Intense emotional upset is produced by the stimuli that symbolise the event (e.g. screeching of tyres may remind one of a serious motor vehicle accident) or anniversaries of some specific experience. The re-experiencing of the trauma is considered to be a central feature of the disorder as it triggers other categories of symptoms. Moreover, it interferes with the process of integrating the traumatic experience into an existing schema or the person's general beliefs about the world (e.g. Foa, Zinbarg & Rothbaum, 1992). Re-experiencing can be associated with chronic somatic distress, anxiety, depression, dissociation, avoidance of situations linked with their emergence, paranoid thinking and sleep disturbance (see Lynn & Cardeña, 2007).
2. *Avoidance of stimuli associated with the event or emotional numbing.* As a defense against intrusive thoughts, the patient tries to avoid thinking about the trauma, avoids anything that might remind him or her of the event, or withdraws emotionally. Emotional numbing refers to decreased interest in others, a sense of estrangement and an inability to feel positive emotions. Emotional numbing appears to contradict the symptoms related to re-experiencing; that is, a person cannot be emotionally numb while experiencing intense emotions. This paradox makes sense when the fluctuation of the symptoms is considered – PTSD patients go back and forth between re-experiencing and numbing. Nonetheless, recent research suggests that avoidance and numbing may have to be divided into different clusters of symptoms in the DSM-V (Asmundson, Stapleton & Taylor, 2004) as they (a) differ in their clinical correlates (numbing is more strongly correlated with depression while re-experiencing is more anxiety related); (b) differ in their prognostic significance (numbing predicts poor outcome); and (c) differ in their response to treatment (CBT has greater impact on avoidance than on numbing).

3. *Heightened autonomic arousal*. The symptoms of heightened arousal include difficulties falling or staying sleep, difficulty concentrating, hypervigilance, an exaggerated startle response, and loss of control over aggression. Laboratory studies have confirmed the presence of these clinical symptoms in PTSD patients (Morgan *et al.*, 1996, 1997; Orr *et al.*, 1995).

PREVALENCE OF POST-TRAUMATIC STRESS DISORDER

The lifetime prevalence rate of PTSD in community samples in North America is approximately 8% (APA, 2000), but it is higher in some subgroups such as the armed forces, emergency service workers, law enforcement officers, and among survivors of rape. For example, lifetime prevalence rate of PTSD among combat veterans is 22–31% (Prigerson, Maciejewski & Rosenheck, 2002) and for rape victims it is 75.8% (Kilpatrick *et al.*, 1989). Approximately 50% of people with PTSD recover and approximately 50% develop a persistent, chronic form of the illness (First & Tasman, 2004). The prevalence of PTSD is also higher in countries in which there is widespread persecution of ethnic groups or ongoing armed conflicts. A recent epidemiological survey found the lifetime prevalence of PTSD to be 16% in Gaza, 28% in Cambodia and 37% in Algeria (De Jong *et al.*, 2001).

There are significant gender differences in the prevalence rate of PTSD, women having higher lifetime prevalence of PTSD than men (10% vs 5%; Kessler *et al.*, 1995). This is mainly due to the nature of the trauma that men and women experience. Men are more often subjected to physical assault, while women more often experience sexual assault. Sexual assault such as rape may involve various stressful sequelae such as sexually transmitted disease, unwanted pregnancy and aversive experiences when reporting the incident to the police or when testifying in court (Taylor, 2006) that may cause double trauma. Once a person is traumatised, the risk of re-experiencing a second trauma is as high as 50% (Resnick *et al.*, 1993).

Although 40–60% of community adults are exposed to trauma, only a fraction (8%) develops PTSD (APA, 2000; Kessler *et al.*, 1995; Yehuda & Wong, 2002). This suggests that the trauma alone is insufficient to cause PTSD. Many studies have identified several risk factors that may make an individual vulnerable to developing the disorder. From his review of the studies of PTSD risk factors, Taylor (2006) has synthesised the findings into four classes of risk factors:

1. Historical features such as family psychiatric history, low intelligence, family instability and personal history of PTSD or trauma exposure.
2. Severity of the trauma.
3. Threat-relevant psychological processes, such as dissociation or perception of threat, occurring during and immediately after the trauma.
4. Life stressors and low social support after the trauma.

Similarly, the severity and the chronicity of PTSD depend on the interaction of a number of variables, including the characteristics of trauma and individual differences (Lynn & Kirsch, 2006). Although not officially recognised in the Diagnostic and Statistical Manual (DSM) taxonomy, some authors have advocated the creation of a diagnosis of 'complex PTSD' or 'disorder of extreme stress not otherwise specified (DESNOS)' for traumas that disrupt affect, character structure and major areas of functioning above and beyond ASD and PTSD symptoms (see Cardeña, Butler & Spiegel, 2003, for a review). This chapter focuses on 'simple' PTSD rather than on a complex symptomatology profile that may require considerable character restructuring and relearning of basic psychological skills (Gold, 2000).

CAUSES OF POST-TRAUMATIC STRESS DISORDER

By definition, the cause of PTSD is known; that is, an individual develops the disorder after experiencing a trauma. What is not known is how some individuals develop the disorder while others are unaffected. Complex issues comprising of biological, psychological and social factors are involved in the development of the disorder (Barlow, Durand & Stewart, 2006). A wide range of social, psychological and biological theoretical explanations have been proposed to explain the causality of the disorder. Each theory attempts to explain why some individuals develop PTSD in response to a traumatic event while others do not. However, none of the explanations provides a unitary biopsychosocial theory of PTSD. Thus, a summary of the various psychological and biological processes implicated in the etiology of PTSD is given here.

Biological Theories of PTSD

Biological theories of PTSD are derived from the observation of various biological changes that occur in PTSD patients. It has been observed that patients with chronic PTSD have increased circulating levels of norepinephrine and increased reactivity of the alpha-2-adrenergic receptors (Yehuda, 2002). These changes have been hypothesised to account possibly for some of the somatic symptoms that occur in patients with PTSD. Evidence from neuroanatomical studies of PTSD patients indicates alterations in the amygdala and the hippocampus (Rauch et al., 2000). Moreover, functional magnetic resonance imaging (fMRI) and positron-emission tomography (PET) studies of exposure to trauma-related stimuli have shown increased reactivity of the amygdala and the anterior paralimbic region (Lieberzon et al., 1999) and decreased reactivity of the anterior cingulated and orbitofrontal areas in PTSD patients (Shin et al., 1999). These biological alternations suggest that there may be a neuroanatomical substrate for symptoms of thought intrusion and other cognitive problems that characterise PTSD (First & Tasman, 2004; Schnuff et al., 2001). Heightened sympathetic tone (Pitman, 1993) and higher resting heart rate (Yehuda, McFarlane & Shalev, 1998) have been found in individuals with a current diagnosis of PTSD. There is also evidence for brain dysfunction in individuals with PTSD, manifested in increased cortical inhibition to high-intensity stimuli, impairments in memory and concentration, auditory gating deficits and heightened selective attention to trauma-related stimuli (Pitman *et al.*, 1999). However, at this point it is not known whether these biological and processing changes result from PTSD or were pre-existent before the emergence of the disorder.

Changes in the neuroendocrine system of PTSD patients have also been investigated. The results of the hypothalamic–pituitary–adrenal (HPA) axis studies suggest that chronic PTSD is accompanied by supersuppression of the emergency HPA response to acute stress (Yehuda *et al.*, 1991). Yehuda and her colleagues contend that these changes may result from the organism's attempt to protect itself from the potentially toxic effect of high levels of corticosteroids that might occur with repeated exposure to stress or from reminders of the trauma.

Psychological Theories of PTSD

The most popular psychological models of PTSD are cognitive-behavioural conceptualisations. Cognitive-behavioural models of PTSD are based on two main assumptions (Zayfert & Becker, 2007):

1. PTSD is viewed as an anxiety disorder that is associated with non-anxiety symptoms. Anxiety and fear stem from three interrelated factors: cognition (e.g. fearful thoughts), behaviour (e.g. avoidance behaviour) and physiology (e.g. autonomic arousal). Each factor interacts and influences the others.
2. The same mechanisms that are involved in the development of adaptive fear also operate in the development of maladaptive fear. CBT practitioners assume that humans are born with few fears, such as loud noises and falling (O'Leary & Wilson, 1987), while the remaining fears, both adaptive and maladaptive, are learned. The function of realistic anxiety is to help us escape from dangerous situations.

The foundation of the CBT conceptualisation of PTSD is based on Mowrer's (1947) two-factor theory of anxiety. Mowrer proposed that there are two types of learning involved in the development of fears: classical and operant conditioning. He suggested that anxiety is initially developed via classical and maintained by operant conditioning. He also proposed that fear is maintained over time because extinction is prevented through escape and avoidance. The origin and maintenance of James's fear of dogs, described by Zayfert and Becker (2007, p. 11), illustrates the two-factor theory of anxiety:

> James developed a pronounced fear of large dogs after being bitten by a Labrador retriever. After the attack, James discovered that his anxiety rapidly diminished when he escaped because the dog's owner took it away, or because he himself

left the situation. As a result, his escape behavior was reinforced and therefore increased. He started by crossing the street whenever he saw a dog coming toward him and eventually limited his activity outside his home to avoid any possible contact with dogs. According to Mowrer, escape and avoidance behaviors, by limiting the time James spent with dogs without being harmed, prevented James' anxiety from diminishing naturally. Thus, James failed to learn that his anxiety was unnecessary around most dogs, because the presence of a dog does not reliably predict being bitten.

Some aspects of PTSD, particularly the fear and avoidance, can be explained by the two-factor conditioning theory, as Zayfert and Becker (2007, pp. 11–12) state:

> Mowrer's theory is directly applicable to patients with PTSD, who after experiencing a traumatic event, typically avoid objects or situations closely associated with the event, and report (like James) extreme anxiety if forced into contact with such situations or objects. In addition, many trauma survivors attempt to block trauma memories, which may produce an effect similar to that of behavioral avoidance of real-life stimuli (Keane, Fairbank, Caddell, Zimering, & Bender, 1985). In other words, trauma survivors may fail to extinguish conditioned fears because they avoid trauma reminders both behaviorally and cognitively. For example, Sandra, who was beaten with a baseball bat during a mugging, coped with the fear evoked by bats and her memories of the mugging by giving up softball (i.e., avoiding bats) and avoiding thoughts about the mugging. Thus, she failed to learn that neither bats nor her traumatic memory could hurt her.

Mowrer's theory, however, does not account for the full range of fears that trauma survivors experience. To account for the wide range of fears that PTSD patients develop, two fundamental principles of conditioning, higher-order conditioning and stimulus generalisation, are added to the two-factor model (Keane *et al.*, 1985). *Higher-order conditioning* occurs when a previously neutral stimulus triggers a conditioned response by being paired with a conditioned stimulus. For example, James became fearful of the streets in the neighbourhood where he encountered large dogs, although the streets were not paired with the unconditioned stimulus (dog). *Stimulus generalisation* occurs when a person responds to stimuli that resemble the conditioned stimulus, for instance James started to fear small dogs. Higher-order conditioning and stimulus generalisation explain why such a wide range of stimuli trigger traumatic memories and associated physiological and emotional arousal in PTSD patients (Brewin & Holmes, 2003).

Moreover, apart from explaining many core features of PTSD, the conditioning models also make sense to the patient. For example (Zayfert & Becker, 2007, p. 12):

> Elizabeth, who had been repeatedly raped by her mother's boyfriend, reported experiencing a panic attack whenever she saw a wall clock. A clock hung over

the bed in which she was raped and Elizabeth always stared at it while waiting for the rape to end. Using Mowrer's two-factor theory, we can hypothesize that Elizabeth's fear of wall clocks did not extinguish after the rapes stopped, because she avoided the room with the wall clock and averted her gaze whenever she encountered a wall clock. Elizabeth reported feeling "crazy," because she did not understand *why* something harmless that was associated with her rape would produce fear. The two-factor conceptualization helped her understand why and how she had come to fear wall clocks. She then reported that she no longer felt quite so crazy, because the model made sense and pointed to specific solutions.

Nevertheless, Mowrer's original theory has several limitations. First, studies have shown that pathological anxiety can occur without classical conditioning (Rachman, 1977). For example, fears can be acquired via information (e.g. after reading about a plane crash, John developed flying phobia). Therefore the model does not account for the role of dysfunctional beliefs in PTSD. Second, the theory does not easily account for non-anxiety symptoms associated with PTSD (e.g. guilt, shame, numbing etc.). Third, the theory does not account for pre-morbid factors such as childhood experiences that pre-date the traumatic experience that may influence the development of PTSD. Finally, the two-factor theory does not account for delayed-onset PTSD, in which the person may have few or no symptoms after the trauma and then, months or years later, develop full-blown PTSD. Keane and Barlow (2002) developed a more complex learning model of PTSD within the diathesis-stress (biopsychosocial) paradigm, in which they addressed the weaknesses of Mowrer's theory. They proposed that both genetic and psychological factors (diatheses) can predispose an individual to develop PTSD after a traumatic event. In addition, they contended that other factors such as the nature of the trauma and repeated traumatic experiences can increase the risk for the development of PTSD. They use the concepts of 'true alarms' and 'learned alarms' to explain the incubation of fear and avoidance behaviour in PTSD patients. When a person is exposed to a traumatic event, the 'true alarm', which has an evolutionary basis, is activated to mobilise the 'flight–fight–freeze' response (Beck, Emery & Greenberg, 1985). *True alarms* are fear reactions to actual dangerous situations (Barlow, 2002). Our natural reaction to dangerous situations is to flee or fight back. But there are situations where none of these options is available, as is often the case in sexual assaults, and therefore the person freezes. The fight–flight response produces a cascade of primary (e.g. increase in heart rate and breathing) and secondary (e.g. feeling dizzy or lightheaded) physiological responses that are commonly observed in patients with anxiety disorders.

Keane and Barlow (2002) contended that during a traumatic event, individuals associate a variety of stimuli (e.g. as in Elizabeth's case, the wall clock) with true alarm and consequently develop *learned alarms* (via classical conditioning). Learned alarms or false alarms are subsequently triggered by situations that resemble, symbolise (e.g. anniversaries) or contain features of the traumatic experience (Zayfert & Becker, 2007). Normally, early post-trauma learned alarms fade away over time. However, during the initial weeks after the traumatic event, in response to reminders of the event, false alarms cause sadness, shame, fear, anger, guilt and the reliving of the event in memories, dreams and flashbacks (e.g. Riggs, Rothbaum & Foa, 1995). These reactions cause anxiety and other associated emotional responses about encountering triggers. According to Keane and Barlow (2002), the anxiety motivates trauma survivors to avoid trauma-related stimuli. Moreover, the trauma survivors escape negative emotional reactions and distressing experience by numbing their feelings. However, the snowballing and the persistence of the symptoms depend on the trauma survivor's coping style, availability of resources and accessible social support. Like other psychological models of PTSD, Keane and Barlow (2002) consider avoidance as the critical factor in the development and maintenance of PTSD. It is well documented that trauma survivors who are exposed to triggers of learned alarms soon after the traumatic event are less likely to experience persistent distress (Wirtz & Harrell, 1987) compared to trauma survivors who avoid false alarms. Exposure therapy for PTSD is based partly on this finding.

Although Keane and Barlow (2002) have ameliorated and expanded on Mowrer's two-factor theory, their model does not fully explain the non-anxiety symptoms of PTSD. Cognitive behavioural models have, on the other hand, concentrated on explaining the emotional aspect of the disorder and, within this context, they have also examined the coping style of PTSD patients and their 'failure' to organise and process the traumatic experience successfully. Generally, individuals involved in stressful or emotional events deploy various strategies such as 'telling the story', 'making sense of the story' or discussion of traumatic experience to understand or 'process' the events. Studies suggest that people who mentally disconnect from traumatic events or inhibit their emotional reactions are at greater risk of developing PTSD (Ozer *et al.*, 2003). A variety of factors, such as the extreme nature of the traumatic event and the lack of predictability and control over the event, can interfere with adequate processing of the traumatic experience. Cognitive models assert that pathological fear develops when survivors of trauma incorrectly label benign stimuli as dangerous and fail to learn corrective information. In the case of Elizabeth, she labelled the 'clock' as dangerous, and due to avoiding clocks, she did not have the opportunity to learn that clocks are harmless.

According to cognitive models, trauma-related information is organised in the mind of the trauma survivor as a 'fear network' (e.g. Foa, Steketee & Rothbaum, 1989). *Fear networks* link together specific details of a dangerous or threatening event (including stimuli and memories) with the responses to the event (e.g. behaviours, thoughts and sensations) and the meanings or interpretations of the event. Fear networks serve as programs for survival when faced with life-threatening danger (Zayfert & Becker, 2007). Cognitive models of PTSD suggest that maladaptive conclusions (e.g. 'all clocks are dangerous') are reached because trauma survivors suspend information processing prior to the assimilation of corrective information that allows drawing of adaptive conclusions. Foa, Steketee and Rothbaum (1989) proposed that two conditions are necessary for complete processing and, hence, reducing maladaptive fears. First, the fear network must be activated to allow the individual to experience the fear elicited by the trauma cues and memories. Second, corrective information must be available at the same time to allow new learning to occur. Foa, Steketee and Rothbaum's (1989) proposal highlights the importance of exposure to fear networks in the adaptive processing of traumatic experience.

Non-anxiety-related symptoms such as anger, guilt and shame, which play an important role in many cases of PTSD, can be easily explained by the kinds of beliefs that survivors of traumatic events hold. Cognitive behavioural models assume that individuals who experience traumatic events hold pre-existing beliefs that are challenged by the event (Brewin, Dalgleish & Joseph, 1996). Thus after the traumatic event, individuals must resolve their conflicts between what they believed about the world and themselves prior to the event and what the traumatic experience tells them. This conflict is well illustrated by Elizabeth in the example provided by Zayfert & Becker (2007, p. 18):

> Elizabeth believed that she was generally safe in the world as long as she took certain precautions that she could control. Being assaulted in her home, an environment that she assumed was safe, provided experiential evidence that refuted her belief that she was 'safe unless proven otherwise.' According to Resick and Schicke (1992) there are three main cognitive solutions to this conflict. First, Elizabeth may alter her interpretation of the experience to fit with her belief system (e.g., *'I made him want to rape me by wearing sexy clothes, because I thought he was good looking; women don't get randomly raped in their own house by friends'* or *'It wasn't really rape, because I liked him and let him do it'*). Second, Elizabeth might radically alter her belief system in a maladaptive way (e.g., *'No place is safe anymore; I will never be safe'*). Third, she might alter, or accommodate, her belief system in a more moderate, productive manner (*'Although I liked him, I didn't ask him to rape me. Some men are dangerous, but many are not. I am still mostly safe as long as I am reasonably careful'*). PTSD is associated with the first two cognitive solutions. (Italics added for emphasis)

Conclusions such as 'no place is safe' and 'I will never be safe' are called 'stuck points' by Resick and Schnicke (1992). *Stuck points* are trauma-related thoughts that encourage focusing on danger and contribute to negative post-traumatic emotional reactions such as anger, fear, guilt, shame and lack of trust. Stuck points serve the purpose of reconciling previous beliefs with the traumatic event. According to Ehlers and Steil (1995) avoidance is motivated by emotional reactions invoked by the re-experiencing of the primary symptoms. The secondary emotional reactions, however, play a prominent role in perpetuating avoidance and thus maintaining the disorder. Moreover, by motivating further avoidance of processing the trauma, secondary emotional reactions also cause substantial suffering in the PTSD patient.

Although none of the biological or psychological models provided a comprehensive theory of the aetiology of PTSD, they provide valuable information in the management of the symptoms.

TREATMENT OF POST-TRAUMATIC STRESS DISORDER

Currently, there are a variety of effective pharmacological and psychological treatments, or a combination of the two, available for the treatment of PTSD. Irrespective of the treatment approach, the main goals are to help PTSD patients decrease intrusive thoughts, avoidance behaviour, hyperarousal, and numbing and withdrawal, and reduce psychotic symptoms and impulsive behaviour if they exist. Once these main symptoms are brought under control, the therapy should focus on (First & Tasman, 2004, p. 933):

- Developing the capacity to interpret perceived threat more realistically.
- Improving interpersonal and leisure functioning.
- Promoting self-esteem, trust and feelings of safety.
- Exploring and clarifying the meanings attributed to the event.
- Accessing and dealing with dissociated or repressed memories.
- Strengthening social support and social connections.
- Progressing from 'victim' to 'survivor' identification.

Four major treatment approaches – pharmacological, cognitive behavioural, psychodynamic and hypnotherapeutic – are briefly reviewed. None of the four approaches provides a comprehensive or integrated treatment for PTSD. Each treatment approach appears to emphasise different aspects of the problems. Following a brief review of each treatment approach, cognitive hypnotherapy, which integrates cognitive behaviour therapy and hypnosis, is described in the rest of the chapter.

Pharmacological Treatment of PTSD

As reviewed under biological causes, PTSD is associated with enduring neurochemical and psychophysiological changes that can lead to substantial impairment and distress. First and Tasman (2004) recommend the use of medication when the symptoms of PTSD are severe, rather than concentrating on 'trauma-focused psychotherapy' (p. 934). Although tricyclic anti-depressants and monoamine oxidase inhibitors (MAOIs) have been effective in the management of PTSD, because of the side effects the first-line medications nowadays are the selective serotonin reuptake inhibitors (SSRIs). First and Tasman (2004) suggest a sequencing approach to using medication with PTSD, as outlined in Table 5.1. Several placebo-controlled trials have shown the short- and long-term positive effects of SSRIs, including fluoxetine, sertraline (e.g. Davidson *et al.*, 2001) and paroxetine (e.g. Marshall *et al.*, 1998).

Each of these medications has broad-spectrum properties across the full symptom range of PTSD and they have been applicable with survivors of all the major classes of trauma, such as combat, sexual violence, non-sexual violence and accident. Moreover, they have been helpful to patients with or without comorbid depression (e.g. Davidson *et al.*, 2001).

Table 5.1   Sequential use of medications with PTSD

STEP 1

Selective serotonin reuptake inhibitor (SSRI)
Adjunctive medications:
  If prominent hyperarousal: benzodiazepine or buspirone
  If prominent mood liability or explosiveness: anticonvulsant or lithium
  If prominent dissociation: valproic acid
  If persistent insomnia: trazodone
  If psychotic: atypical antipsychotic

STEP 2

If no response or intolerance to SSRI:
  Dual action antidepressant, e.g. mirtazapine, venlafaxine
  Adjunctive medications as above

STEP 3

If no response to Step 1 or 2:
  Monoamine oxidase inhibitor
  Adjunctive medications as above

STEP 4

Other useful drugs:
Propranolol – hyperarousal
Clonidine – startle response
Neuroleptics – psychosis, poor impulse control

Source: Adapted from First, M. B. & Tasman, A. (2004) *DSM-IV-TR Mental Disorders: Diagnosis, Etiology, and Treatment*, Chichester: John Wiley & Sons Ltd, p. 936.

Presently, the role of anti-psychotic and mood-stabilising drugs with PTSD is not well understood, although they can be helpful in clinical practice. For example, anti-psychotic agents can be useful in patients with poor impulse control or with features of borderline personality disorder, and lithium and carbamazepine may benefit patients with mood swings and explosive outbursts (First & Tasman, 2004). Similarly, the validity of using benzodiazepines with PTSD is not well defined. While the anti-phobic and anti-arousal properties of benzodiapepines may be indicative with some PTSD patients, First and Tasman (2004, p. 936) caution the use of benzodiazepines as 'withdrawal from short-acting benzodiazepines may also introduce an additional set of problems with intense symptom rebound' and in 'individuals who have a propensity to abuse alcohol and other substances, benzodiazepines are not recommended'. Although medication, particularly SSRIs, is effective in reducing hyperarousal and the affective symptoms of PTSD, it does not address avoidance behaviour and interpersonal issues. The next section reviews the guidelines for the role of medication, as proposed by the expert consensus, in the management of PTSD.

Cognitive Behavioural Treatment of PTSD

As the cognitive behavioural approaches to the treatment of PTSD have gained most empirical support, CBT is reviewed here to assess the merits of CBT in relation to other treatments. Most CBT protocols involve a combination of imaginal exposure, situational exposure, anxiety-management techniques such as relaxation training and breathing retraining, and cognitive restructuring. Numerous carefully controlled randomised trials have shown CBT to be effective with PTSD and the gains are maintained at follow-ups of a year or more (Chard, 2005; Foa et al., 2005; Taylor, 2004). Meta-analytic studies comparing the effects of CBT with other treatments show CBT protocols, as a group, to have 'lower dropout rates than pharmacotherapies, and that CBT is equally effective in the short term as most potent pharmacotherapies, the selective serotonin reuptake inhibitors (SSRIs)' (see Taylor, 2006, p. 74). Moreover, the studies suggest that CBT is more effective than supportive counselling and short-term psychodynamic therapy, and equally effective as eye movement desensitisation and reprocessing (EMDR). More recent research with improved methodology, however, suggests that CBT is more effective and works faster than EMDR in reducing PTSD symptoms, and that the effect of EMDR is comparable to relaxation training (Taylor et al., 2003).

A group of internationally recognised PTSD experts has developed a consensus statement on the treatment of PTSD, based on research evidence and clinical experience (Ballenger et al., 2000; Foa, Davidson & Frances, 1999). The expert consensus recommends either SSRIs or psychosocial interventions using exposure therapy as the first-line interventions with PTSD. The group also concluded that exposure therapy is the fastest-acting and most effective psychotherapeutic technique and that 'the methods with the fewest negative side effects are anxiety management techniques, psychoeducation, and cognitive restructuring' (Taylor, 2006, p. 74). The expert consensus group also offers the following treatment guidelines (Foa, Davidson & Frances, 1999):

- Regardless of the patient's age, severity and duration of PTSD, the treatment should begin with either psychotherapy alone, e.g. CBT, or a combination of psychotherapy and medication.
- A combination of treatment should be used when PTSD is comorbid with major depression, bipolar disorder or anxiety disorders.
- When PTSD is comorbid with substance abuse or dependence, either treat the substance problem first or treat both problems simultaneously.

- Exposure therapy is recommended for avoidance and re-experiencing symptoms.
- Cognitive restructuring is recommended for numbing, irritability, anger, shame and guilt.
- Cognitive restructuring, with or without exposure therapy, is recommended for hyperarousal symptoms.
- Treatment for children and younger adolescents may include play therapy, psycho-education, anxiety-coping skills and cognitive restructuring.
- The treatment for older adolescents can be the same as cognitive behavioural interventions for young adults.
- If the patient fails to respond to psychosocial intervention, either add medication or switch to another psychotherapy.

From the review it would appear that CBT is recommended as a first-line treatment for PTSD. However, it should be used within the guidelines proposed by the expert panel; that is, the treatment approach should be comprehensive and when required, medication should be included.

Psychodynamic Psychotherapy for PTSD

The earliest psychological theories of PTSD were based on psychodynamic explanations. These theories postulated that symptoms of PTSD were manifested when the coping mechanisms failed to cope with overwhelming experience. This failure to cope led to avoidance or repression of the feeling, which interfered with the processing of the traumatic experience (Schwartz, 1990). The traumatic experiences themselves may produce the symptoms, or they may trigger painful memories of earlier unresolved unconscious conflicts, which may cause the anxiety to overflow (resulting from the inability to keep these memories repressed). For example, the experience of killing another person in battle may stimulate the emergence of previously aggressive impulses (Halgin & Whitbourne, 2006). Psychodynamic theories therefore consider the interpretation of the traumatic event to be critical in the determination of the symptoms.

From the clinical research and narrative-based literatures, two major psychodynamic approaches to psychotherapy with PTSD are identified (Ursano et al., 2006). The first approach focuses on the meaning of the trauma for the patient in terms of prior psychological conflicts, developmental experience, relationship issues and the developmental stage during which the trauma occurred. Within this approach, the therapist (a) assesses the patient's overall capacity to cope with the memories of the traumatic events; (b) examines the triggers of the traumatic memories; and (c) reviews the coping style the patient uses to manage these memories (Freud, 1967). The second approach concentrates on the effect of the traumatic experience on the patient's prior self-object experiences, overwhelmed self-esteem, altered experience of safety and loss of self-cohesiveness and self-observing functions, and helps the patient identify and maintain a functional sense of self in the face of the trauma

(Shaw, 1987). Both approaches appear to be useful in addressing the subject-ive and interpersonal sustaining factors of the disorder (e.g. issues of trust, shattered assumption of attachment), changing the patient's beliefs about the worldview, and altering the perception about safety. A mixture of supportive, insight-oriented and trauma-focused interventions are used to help the patient review personal values; examine how behaviour and experience were violated by the traumatic event; modify maladaptive defences and coping strategies; and fully process the traumatic experience (Yehuda *et al.*, 2002). The goal is the resolution of conscious and unconscious conflicts that were created by the traumatic event. In addition, the patient is helped to build self-esteem, self-control, reasonable personal accountability, sense of integrity and personal pride

Despite its widespread use with PTSD, psychodynamic psychotherapy has not been well studied by means of randomised, controlled trials. The little research that exists indicates that psychodynamic psychotherapy for PTSD lacks empirical validation (Freeman, 1989). For example, Brom, Kleber and Defare (1989) compared 18 sessions of brief psychodynamic psychotherapy (BPP) with systematic desensitisation, hypnotherapy and waiting-list control in a four-arm study. The result indicated that BPP was only marginally better than waiting-list control. Clinical consensus, however, maintains that psycho-dynamic psychotherapy is useful in reducing the core symptoms of PTSD by helping patients integrate past traumatic experience into a more adaptive schema of risk, safety, prevention and protection (Plakun & Shapiro, 2000).

Hypnotherapy for PTSD

Hypnosis has been used for treating traumatic experiences related to combat, sexual assaults, anaesthesia failure and accidents for over 200 years (Vijselaar & Van der Hart, 1992). However, with the rejection of hypnosis by Freud and the emerging popularity of psychodynamic psychotherapy during the first half of the 20th century, hypnosis lost its appeal. It was during and after the Second World War that hypnosis claimed its reputation again as a valid form of psychotherapeutic procedure. Hypnotic techniques were found to be efficient and effective in treating soldiers with 'traumatic neuroses', which nowadays will be described as PTSD. In those days, the hypnotherapy for PTSD was used as a single-modality treatment and it was very much influenced by psycho-analytic theories of ego defence and repression, and the hypnotic procedures were limited to abreaction and uncovering (Kardiner & Spiegel, 1947). The wide acceptance of the formal diagnosis of PTSD in the 1980s provided further impetus to hypnosis.

Consequently, hypnotherapy was used as an adjunctive psychotherapy (Spiegel, 1993) with a variety of traumatised patients, including survivors of war, crime, sexual assault, accidents and natural disasters. The formal recognition of the diagnosis and symptomatology of PTSD also led to intens-ive research in the aetiology and treatment of the disorder. This flurry of interest in PTSD led to the development of effective psychological and phar-macological treatment, and to the realisation that PTSD can be a complex disorder, especially when associated with comobid disorders. In recognition of these developments many hypnotherapists expanded the range of hyp-notic procedures with PTSD and acknowledged the limitation of hypnosis as a single-modality therapy by emphasising the adjunctive, albeit useful, role of hypnotherapy in the management of post-traumatic stress disorders. Therefore the focus of the hypnotic procedures shifted from uncovering and catharsis to reducing hyperarousal, restructuring dysfunctional beliefs and perception, and processing traumatic memories. Spiegel (1993, pp. 496-7) summarised the fundamental principles involved in the hypnotherapy of PTSD at that time:

> The fundamental principles involved in using hypnosis in the treatment of PTSD involve inducing controlled access to traumatic memories and helping patients to control the intense affect and strong physiological responses that may accom-pany memories of trauma. Hypnotic concentration can then be applied to help patients work through and grieve aspects of the traumatic experience and place the memories into a new perspective, a form of cognitive restructuring.

However, in practice, hypnotherapy for PTSD was still conducted in the tra-ditional psychoanalytic principle of remembering, repeating and working through (Spiegel, 1993). For instance, Spiegel (1993) described a fairly compre-hensive approach to treating PTSD with hypnosis, which can be summarised in eight principles (8Cs): confrontation, confession, consolation, condensa-tion, consciousness, concentration, control and congruence. Although Spiegel stresses the adjunctive nature of hypnosis and the multi-modal approach to treating PTSD, he did not provide a coherent description of how hyp-nosis is integrated with a particular type of psychotherapy. However, the work of Spiegel has pioneered the use of hypnosis with PTSD (Maldonado & Spiegel, 2003). Moreover, it is not clear how hypnosis affects change when it is combined with other forms of psychotherapy for PTSD.

Nonetheless, hypnotherapy was well established as a useful adjunct to cognit-ive, exposure and psychodynamic therapies. A randomised controlled study by Brom, Kleber and Defare (1989) demonstrated that hypnosis in the con-text of behaviour therapy, systematic desensitisation and psychodynamic psychotherapy was more effective than a waiting-list control group. Hyp-nosis and systematic desensitisation were found to be more effective with intrusion symptoms (e.g. flashbacks), whereas avoidance responded best to psychodynamic therapy. Nonetheless, there have been almost no system-atic studies on the efficacy of hypnosis for PTSD (Cardeña, 2000), although a comprehensive review of the literature (Cardeña et al., 2000) on the use of hypnosis with PTSD indicated that there are compelling reasons to use hypnosis as an adjunct for the treatment of the disorder. Similarly, a more recent review (Lynn & Cardeña, 2007) of empirically supported principles and practices of hypnosis with PTSD suggested that hypnosis can be a useful adjunctive procedure in the treatment of the disorder, but it is yet to be established as a 'proven' technique for ameliorating post-traumatic symptoms.

More recently, among some clinicians, there has also been a trend to integrate research into clinical practice. Historically, hypnotherapeutic approaches to PTSD have occurred in the absence of definitive knowledge concerning aetiology and new advances in treatment. This approach to intervention in the face of limited knowledge has resulted in the application of treatment approaches that were derived from speculation or theoretical construct based on post-hoc analyses of successful cases. The diversity of hypnotherapeutic procedures with PTSD and the fairly modest success rate produced by these, mainly single-treatment modality, attests to this attitude. In contrast, Lynn and his colleagues (Lynn & Cardeña, 2007; Lynn & Kirsch, 2006) have reviewed the literature on the aetiology and treatment of PTSD and identified the salient features that might be relevant to hypnosis. For example, they were impressed by:

> The fact that exposure therapy has been found to be effective in all 12 studies of the treatment of PTSD in which it was employed (see Rothbaum, Meadows, Resnick, & Foy, 2000), and that cognitive-behavioral treatments for PTSD are also highly effective (Deacon & Abormowitz, 2004; Van Etten & Taylor, 1998), make hypnosis a promising adjunctive intervention for ameliorating the suffering of victims of trauma. This impression is reinforced by the fact that patients with posttraumatic conditions seem to be more hypnotically suggestible than most other patient populations (Bryant, Guthrie, & Moulds, 2001; Spiegel, Hunt, & Dondershine, 1988; Stutman, & Bliss, 1985). In a data reanalysis, higher levels of hypnotizability among PTSD clients were associated with therapeutic success (Cardeña, 2000; Cardeña et al., 2000), and hypnotizability levels have been associated with avoidance symptoms (Bryant, Guthrie, Moulds, Nixon, & Felmingham, 2003). These findings have been interpreted as supportive of a diathesis/stress model in which highly hypnotizable/dissociative individuals are more likely to develop posttraumatic/dissociative conditions rather than other psychiatric conditions (Butler, Duran, Jasiukaitis, Koopman, & Spiegel, 1996). (Lynn & Cardeña, 2007, p. 170)

The research information not only provides a rationale for using hypnosis with PTSD, but also gives direction to the areas of psychotherapy where hypnosis can be applied most effectively as an adjunct. Lynn and Cardeña's (2007) evidence-based approach demonstrates how hypnosis can be combined with exposure therapy and CBT to ameliorate PTSD symptoms. This approach also provides an efficient design for evaluating the additive effect of hypnosis with a well-established therapy for PTSD. Alladin and Alibhai (2007) and Bryant *et al.* (2005) have used similar research designs to study the additive effect of hypnosis with depression and acute stress disorder respectively. The hypnotherapy component of cognitive hypnotherapy for PTSD described in this chapter integrates research from cognitive behavioural therapies, exposure therapy and imagery training. As mentioned earlier, a plethora of hypnotic techniques have been used with PTSD and some of these have been developed without regard to the latest advances in the aetiology and treatment of the disorder.

This chapter extends the work of Lynn (Lynn & Kirsch, 2006; Lynn & Cardeña, 2007) by integrating hypnosis within the framework of imagery rescripting therapy (IRT) developed by Smucker (1997; Smucker & Dancu, 1999; Smucker & Niederee, 1995; Smucker *et al.*, 1995). IRT utilises exposure and imagery training in the processing of traumatic experiences. Outcome studies (Grunert *et al.*, 2003; Smucker & Dancu, 1999) and numerous case studies offer empirical support for the efficacy of IRT in reducing PTSD symptoms, eliminating recurring flashbacks and nightmares, and modifying traumagenic schemas.

Summary

Although treatment outcome studies have demonstrated CBT and pharmacotherapy to be effective in symptom reduction, none of the treatments is effective in addressing the full range of clinical problems observed in traumatised patients. Therefore there is a need to develop multi-modal treatments for PTSD consisting of pharmacological and psychological interventions, as well as addressing interpersonal, intrapersonal and family issues and comorbid disorders. The development and administration of the multi-modal therapy should follow the guidelines recommended by the expert consensus on the treatment of PTSD (Ballenger *et al.*, 2000; Foa, Davidson & Frances, 1999). The psychoanalytical explanation of PTSD is restricted and speculative and hence therapies based on the psychodynamic principles are narrow, although helpful in resolving certain issues (e.g. guilt, symbolic meaning of the trauma). Psychodynamic psychotherapy can best serve PTSD as an adjunctive treatment.

Similarly, hypnotherapy can be most effectively utilised with PTSD as an adjunct to a multi-modal approach to therapy (Dowd, 2000; Linden, 2007; Oster, 2006). As an adjunct to the treatment of PTSD, hypnotherapy is promising because:

- Outcome studies indicate that hypnosis has an additive effect when combined with other forms of psychotherapy.
- Survivors of trauma are highly susceptible to hypnosis and hence hetero- or self-hypnosis can be utilised to modulate symptoms.

STAGES OF COGNITIVE HYPNOTHERAPY FOR POST-TRAUMATIC STRESS DISORDER

Cognitive hypnotherapy (CH) for PTSD is an evidence-based multi-modal treatment that can be applied to a wide range of traumatised patients. Although CH for PTSD represents the most comprehensive intervention, the treatment approach is a work in progress as we continue to learn more about the aetiology and treatment of PTSD. CH generally consists of 16 weekly sessions, which can be expanded or modified according to the patient's clinical needs, areas of concern, presenting symptoms and comorbid disorders. CH for PTSD involves seven stages, consisting of:

1. Clinical assessment.
2. Psychoeducation.
3. Distress reduction and affect-regulation training.
4. Cognitive interventions.
5. Emotional processing.
6. Increasing identity and relational functioning.
7. Pharmacological treatment if necessary.

These stages are based on the recommendation of a number of therapists who have proposed that treatment should follow, especially with chronic and complicated PTSD, a flexible sequence of phases: symptom stabilisation and development of the therapeutic alliance, working with traumatic memories, and integration (e.g. Cardeña *et al.*, 2000). The stages of CH are briefly described here and, wherever relevant, the strategies used for treating Roger (see case vignette) during each stage of the treatment will be illustrated. The sequence of the stages of treatment can be altered to suit the clinical needs of each patient. Before describing the stages of CH, a case vignette is presented.

Case Vignette: Roger

This is a case I treated two years ago. The details are altered to protect confidentiality and identity. Roger was referred to me by his family physician for assessment and treatment of 'trauma-related stress'. Roger consulted his family physician for anxiety, depression and sleep difficulties. He was treated with anti-depressant and hypnotic medications for six months. His sleep improved, but he still continued to experience bouts of anxiety and depression and was not ready to return to work. The family physician made the referral because he felt Roger was not coping well with his 'traumatic experience'.

Roger is a senior police officer who was assigned for six months in an Eastern European country to assist the law enforcement department in training and expanding the local police force. During this assignment Roger witnessed injustice, bloodshed, violence and mutilated victims of bombings. The most horrifying ordeal was when he was detained and interrogated for a week on allegations of spying. Roger witnessed a small village being attacked without provocation, the villagers rounded up and 'brutalised' and their property destroyed. Roger, who was staying as a guest with a trainee police officer and his family at the village, protested to the commanding officer of the operation. He was accused of being a spy and was arrested, detained and interrogated for a week. Although he was not physically tortured, he was interrogated at gunpoint for many hours at a time and he spent three days in solitary confinement without any clothes on and had to sleep on the bare floor.

Roger was 42 years old while in treatment. He has been married for 16 years and has two sons aged 12 and 10 years. Roger comes from a middle-class family; his father was a police officer and his mother was a high-school teacher. His upbringing was uneventful except for his difficult relationship with his father. His father could not tolerate weakness or any expression of emotion. Roger describes him as 'old-fashioned, authoritarian, and a heavy-handed cop'. Roger always felt uncomfortable in the presence of his father, in case he told him off about something. As a teenager Roger was very shy and did not date until he was 19. He was very conscious of his acne and for being overweight. He was average academically but excelled at sports and hence he decided to become a cop.

When Roger returned from Eastern Europe he started having flashbacks, nightmares and disturbed sleep. He felt anxious, depressed, tired and had no interest in anything. He spent most of his time in bed and maintained little communication with his family. He felt angry and hated everything, especially his job, and he did not want to go back to work.

Session 1: Clinical Assessment

The first session is devoted to history taking and clinical assessment. It is important for the therapist to take a detailed clinical history to formulate the diagnosis and identify the essential psychological, physiological and social aspects of the patient's behaviour before initiating CH. The most efficient way to obtain all this information is to use the case-formulation approach described in Chapter 2. The case-formulation approach allows the clinician to translate and tailor nomothetic (general) treatment to the individual (idiographic) patient (see Appendices B and C). It is recommended that the assessment guidelines provided by the international consensus on PTSD (Keane, Solomon & Maser, 1996) be integrated in the case formulation. The international consensus recommends obtaining the following data:

1. Information from standardised clinician-administered diagnostic interviews (e.g. SCID-PTSD module, DSM-IV-TR).
2. Ratings of trauma-related impairment and disability.
3. Aspects of the event including age, perceived life threat, injuries, harm, frequency and duration.
4. Self-report symptom instruments (e.g. Impact of Event Scale–Revised, Weiss & Marmar, 1997) with established validity and reliability.

In addition, Lynn and Cardeña (2007, p. 172) advise gathering information about personal attributes, behaviours and feelings, and thoughts that occurred before, during and after the traumatic experience, including:

1. Personal resources and limitations (e.g. capacity for insight, ability to tolerate and accept negative emotions, relevant spiritual issues, memory problems) and social support.
2. Comorbid psychological disorders and previous trauma history.
3. Changes in the person's beliefs about the self (e.g. 'I'm worthless because I didn't resist the sexual assault') and the world ('I can't trust any man') in response to the traumatic event.
4. Current triggers of post-traumatic reactions.
5. The content of flashbacks and reports of concomitant psychophysiological and emotional reactivity.
6. Successful or unsuccessful strategies used to control flashbacks.
7. Memory problems.
8. The ability to form a working alliance with the therapist.

It is also important to administer the hypnotisability scale to the patient. Alladin (2008) provides several reasons for utilizing hypnotisability measures in clinical practice, including:

1. Standardised hypnotisability tests provide an indication of the degree of hypnotic depth the patient can experience.
2. This information allows selection of appropriate treatment strategies.
3. The test allows the patient to become familiar with hypnotic-like experience prior to hypnotic induction, which helps to debunk the myths surrounding hypnosis and prepare the patient for hypnotic induction.
4. It alleviates fears and thus helps to build rapport and trust.
5. The administration of the test creates a positive psychological set and thus makes later induction of deep hypnosis easier.
6. From the test the therapist can assess the patient's response to suggestions, e.g. feeling light or heavy, which can be integrated into future sessions of hypnotherapy.

Spiegel (1993) has specifically discussed the importance of the clinical hypnotisability measure with PTSD patients.

Moreover, when assessing or treating PTSD patients, certain obstacles and special legal or ethical issues may be encountered, which need to be addressed:

1. Prior to starting the assessment, it is necessary to advise the patient of the nature and limits of confidentiality (Taylor, 2006). Confidentiality must be breached if the patient is at risk of harming self or others, the perpetrator of the trauma is at large and at risk of abusing other children, and if the patient is a minor and subjected to maltreatment. The clinician also needs to inform the patient that under some circumstances (e.g. when the patient is involved in litigation), the intake evaluation and treatment progress notes may be subpoenaed by the court.

2. In some PTSD patients, anger can be a major problem. Although many survivors of interpersonal violence harbour intense anger, the majority of them don't act out their anger. Some patients may harbour fantasies of revenge on the perpetrator and may have a plan for retribution. It is therefore important for the therapist to inquire about revenge, plan of action (e.g. buying a firearm) and history of violence (Taylor, 2006).
3. It is important to determine the physical safety of the patient. Some patients neglect their own safety, which put them at risk of revictimisation. If the patient is living in hazardous circumstances, it may be necessary to get social services or other agencies involved to provide practical assistance.
4. Unless questioned specifically, some PTSD patients are reluctant to disclose a trauma history because of shame, self-blame and the tendency to avoid disturbing topics (Kilpatrick, 1983). To overcome this obstacle, Lynn and Cardeña (2007) advise the therapist to ask straightforward and direct questions.
5. To gather all relevant information, sometimes it may be necessary to obtain collateral information from the patient's significant others to get another perspective on the patient's symptoms and functioning. Therefore it is important for the clinician to obtain the patient's permission to interview one of the patient's significant others.

The need for pharmacological intervention should also be evaluated. As noted earlier, the international consensus on the treatment of PTSD (Ballenger *et al.*, 2000; Foa, Davidson & Frances, 1999) recommended either SSRIs or psychosocial interventions as the first-line interventions; or a combination of treatment should be used when PTSD is comorbid with major depression, bipolar disorder or anxiety disorders; and if the patient fails to respond to psychosocial intervention medication can be added. It is therefore well established that some PTSD patients derive benefits from medication.

Session 2: Psychoeducation and Medication Review

As psychoeducation is considered to be a very important part of the treatment protocol, a whole session is devoted to educating the patient and answering questions. It involves teaching patients about the causes and treatment of PTSD and how the therapist and the patient can collaborate to enhance outcome. Psychoeducation is essential for obtaining informed consent; correcting misconceptions about PTSD and mental illness; dispelling misunderstandings about treatment, particularly hypnosis; discussing side-effects of both psychological and pharmacological treatments; and ensuring treatment adherence. In the absence of adequate explanation of the disorder and the treatment, it is unlikely that PTSD patients will be motivated to pursue the course of psychotherapy, especially when they might have been told that their disorder is due to a chemical imbalance. If the patient happens to be a child, the explanation should be developmentally appropriate and, in addition, the parents will have to be educated. The psychoeducation can be substantiated by advising patients to read the handout *Expert Consensus Treatment Guidelines for Posttraumatic Stress Disorder: A Guide for Patients and Families*, prepared by the Anxiety Disorders Association of America (ADAA), which can be downloaded from the internet at www.psychguides.com, or obtained by contacting ADAA on 00-1-301-231-9350. The handout describes the symptoms and treatments of PTSD and includes a self-rating questionnaire, based on DSM-IV, for identifying the symptoms of the disorder.

The majority of PTSD patients treated by psychotherapists are referred by family physicians and psychiatrists and they are likely to be on medication. Part of the psycoeducation should address the role of medication or combined (psychotherapy plus medication) treatment for PTSD, as well as the side effects. If the therapist is not well informed about medication for PTSD, the therapist should work closely with the treating physician or arrange for the physician to review or discuss the concerns regarding medication with the patient's physician.

Sessions 3–7: Distress Reduction and Affect-Regulation Training

The next four sessions are devoted to reducing the overwhelming arousal, dysphoria and emotionally laden memories experienced by PTSD patients. In order to cope with their negative emotional responses, trauma survivors resort to emotional avoidance strategies (Briere & Scott, 2006) such as suppression (of upsetting thoughts, feelings and memories); dissociation (e.g. amnesia for all or part of the stressor, depersonalisation); numbing (e.g. physiological arousal); substance abuse; or external tension-reduction activities (e.g. avoiding activities, people, places or conversations that might trigger memories of the stressor). Unfortunately these coping strategies are not only maladaptive, they also inhibit psychological recovery from the effects of the traumatic events. This section describes several hypnotic strategies for regulating destabilising affect and for dealing with overwhelming emotional and physiological distress. The hypnotic techniques described here resemble the assortment of procedures, such as grounding, relaxation training, cognitive therapy, stress inoculation and anxiety management, reported in the anxiety and trauma literature. However labelled, the goal of these strategies is to increase the patient's capacity to tolerate and down-regulate painful emotional states (Briere & Scott, 2006).

Hypnosis for Affect Regulation

As discussed in Chapter 1, CBT practitioners have tended to use relaxation training or imagery procedures rather than hypnosis. The greatest advantage of using hypnosis over relaxation training is that it provides leverage to psychological treatment (Alladin, 2006a, 2007b); that is, the hypnotic state can be easily and quickly induced in PTSD patients, who are known to be highly suggestible to hypnosis (Bryant, Guthrie & Moulds, 2001; Spiegel, Hunt & Dondershine, 1988; Stutman & Bliss, 1985). Then the hypnotic state can be utilised to produce profound mental and physical relaxation and help the patient dissociate from upsetting memories of the traumatic event to the safety and comfort of the present physical environment. Once the patient feels completely relaxed, safe and in control, the trance state can be utilised to teach the patient how to modulate emotional reactions via self-hypnosis. The four sessions of hypnosis specifically focus on inducing relaxation; demonstrating the power of the mind; ego strengthening; expanding awareness; modulating and controlling symptoms; teaching self-hypnosis; and offering post-hypnotic suggestions. Hypnosis is introduced again later in the context of emotional processing for rescripting traumatic memories. The four initial sessions of hypnosis serve as a preparatory phase for the more complex and anxiety-provoking exposure therapy that is introduced later in the treatment.

Relaxation training

One of the important goals for using hypnosis within the CH context is to induce relaxation. Trauma survivors experience high levels of anxiety and hyperaroused physiological reactions. For these reasons PTSD patients derive considerable benefit from learning relaxation techniques. Various hypnotic induction techniques can be utilised to induce relaxation. I use the *relaxation with counting method* adapted from Gibbons (1979; see Alladin, 2007b) for inducing and deepening the hypnotic trance. I have chosen this technique as it can be easily translated into a self-hypnosis technique. The hypnotherapeutic script in Appendix E (Hypnotic Induction and Ego-Strengthening: Counting with Relaxation Method) provides some examples of the types of hypnotic suggestions that can be utilised for inducing deep relaxation in PTSD patients. Roger, who had great difficulty relaxing or calming down his 'nerves', found the hypnotic relaxation procedure very useful. At the end of the first hypnotic session, he commented: 'I have never been able to relax in my entire life. The hypnosis was magic; it calmed me down so much that I switched off completely.' The majority of PTSD patients treated with CH find the relaxation experience to be empowering and confidence-boosting.

Demonstration of the power of mind

To increase the credibility of hypnosis and sense of self-empowerment, eye and body catalepsies are hypnotically induced. This procedure demonstrates the power of the mind over the body and fosters the belief that the patient can use the power of mind to control symptoms.

Ego strengthening

The principles behind ego strengthening are to decrease anxiety, increase self-esteem and self-efficacy, and gradually restore the patient's confidence in his or her ability to cope with the post-traumatic symptoms. Bandura (1977) has demonstrated that *self-efficacy*, or the expectation and confidence of being able to cope successfully, is one of the key elements in the effective treatment of anxiety disorders. Individuals with a sense of high self-efficacy tend to perceive themselves as being in control. If trauma survivors can be helped to view themselves as self-efficacious, they are less likely to avoid anxiety-provoking situations. Hartland (1971) believes that patients need to feel confident and strong enough to let go of their symptoms. The ego-strengthening suggestions are therefore specifically crafted to increase the patient's confidence, coping abilities, positive self-image and interpersonal skills (see Appendix E). However, it is important for the ego-strengthening suggestions to appear credible and logical to the patients (Alladin, 2006a, 2007b). For example, rather than stating: 'Every day you will feel better', it is advisable to suggest: 'As a result of this treatment and as a result of you practising self-hypnosis every day, you will begin to feel better.' This set of suggestions not only sounds logical, but improvement becomes contingent on continuing with the therapy and adhering to the homework.

Expansion of awareness

Hypnosis provides a powerful vehicle for expanding awareness and amplifying experience. I find Brown and Fromm's (in Hammond, 1990, pp. 322–4) technique of *enhancing affective experience and its expression* very effective in bringing underlying emotions into awareness; creating awareness of various feelings; intensifying positive affect; enhancing 'discovered' affect; inducing positive moods; and increasing motivation. The object of this procedure is to help post-traumatic patients create, amplify and express a variety of negative and positive feelings and experience. This technique instils the confidence that the post-traumatic symptoms can be modified and controlled.

To help Roger bring on his numbing experience whenever he thought about his work, under hypnosis he was suggested: 'When I count from ONE to FIVE . . . by the time you hear me say FIVE . . . you will begin to feel whatever emotion is associated with your thoughts about work.' Then Roger was helped to amplify the affect associated with work: 'When I count slowly from ONE to FIVE . . . as I count you will begin to experience the upsetting feelings more and more intensely . . . so that when I reach the count of FIVE . . . at the count of FIVE you will feel the full reaction as strongly as you can bear it . . . Now notice what you feel and you will be able to describe it to me.' Roger was then instructed to use self-hypnosis to modulate and control his reaction.

Modulating and controlling symptoms

Hypnosis is a powerful therapeutic tool for producing *syncretic cognition* (Alladin, 2006a, 2007b), which consists of a matrix of cognitive, somatic, perceptual, physiological, visceral and kinaesthetic changes. Hypnotic induction and modulation of the syncretic cognition provide dramatic proof to trau-matised patients that they can regulate and change their distressing feelings and experience. DePiano and Salzberg (1981) believe that the rapid improve-ment often observed in patients receiving hypnotherapy is partly related to the positive trance experience.

Self-hypnosis training

The goal of self-hypnosis training is to provide PTSD patients with confid-ence and skills for controlling emotional and physical symptoms outside the therapy sessions. Moreover, self-hypnosis serves as a powerful tool for countering negative thinking or negative self-hypnosis (NSH) (Alladin, 1994, 2006a, 2007b; Araoz, 1981, 1985). At the end of the first hypnotherapy ses-sion, the patient is given an audiotape or CD of self-hypnosis (consisting of the full script from Appendix D) for practising self-hypnosis at home. The homework assignment allows continuity of treatment between sessions and offers the patient the opportunity to learn self-hypnosis. The ultimate goal of psychotherapy is to help the traumatised patient establish self-reliance and independence. Self-hypnosis is a very useful tool for achieving self-reliance and personal power (Alman, 2001) and for developing self-correcting behaviours (Yapko, 2003).

The patient is also trained to induce self-hypnosis rapidly by clenching his or her preferred fist as an *anchor*. An anchor is any stimulus that evokes a consistent response pattern from a person (Lankton, 1980). The *clenched fist technique* was described by Stein (1963) and is found to be useful with anxious patients (Basker, 1979; Stanton, 1997). The fist as an anchor is easily established. When the patient is in a deep trance state, he or she is advised to become aware of the deep relaxation as well as the feeling of confidence and control. Then the patient is instructed to make a fist with the preferred hand and suggested that 'From now on, whenever you wish to feel just as you are feeling now, all you have to do it is to clench your preferred fist and anchor your mind to this experience. Moreover, from now on, whenever you get upset or anxious, you can get rid of the feeling by making a fist and anchoring your mind to this experience.' The anchoring technique is consolidated with imaginal rehearsal training and post-hypnotic suggestions. This is a 'portable' strategy: the patient can utilise it in any situation in which he or she experiences anxiety. Although any stimulus can be conditioned as an anchor, the fist acts as a powerful anchor because in most cultures making a fist evokes and symbolises self-empowerment.

Posthypnotic suggestions

Before terminating the hypnotic session, post-hypnotic suggestions are given to counter problem behaviours, negative emotions and dysfunctional cog-nitions (NSH) or negative self-affirmations. Survivors of trauma have the tendency to ruminate with negative self-suggestions (e.g. 'I will never be the same person again'; 'I can't face the world'). This can be regarded as a form of post-hypnotic suggestion (PHS), which can become part of the avoidance pattern of behaviour. To break the negative rumination it is very important to counter the NSH. Here are some examples of PHS that can be suggested to PTSD patients:

- 'Whenever you become upset in a situation, you will become more aware of how to deal with it rather than focusing on the traumatic event.'
- 'When you plan to confront an anxiety-provoking situation, you will feel less need to avoid the situation.'
- 'As you become more involved in doing things, you will feel motivated to participate in other activities.'

Clarke and Jackson (1983) consider PHS to be a form of 'higher-order conditioning', which functions as positive or negative reinforcement to increase or decrease the probability of desired or undesired behaviours, respectively. They have successfully utilised PHS to enhance the effect of in vivo exposure among agoraphobics.

Sessions 7–10: Cognitive Interventions

CBT is used to help PTSD patients alter the meaning of their traumatic events (Resick & Schnicke, 1992). CBT is particularly helpful in restructuring beliefs related to non-anxiety emotions, such as guilt, shame, embarrassment and anger (Jaycox, Zoellner & Foa, 2002; Kubany & Watson, 2002). It also helps to address unhelpful emotions such as shame and anger prior to starting exposure. For example, Jack was so enraged by the drunken driver who caused the motor vehicle accident in which he was seriously injured that he refused to focus on anxiety during exposure therapy; instead he focused on anger. Research indicates that severe anger can hinder exposure (Foa *et al.*, 1995). CBT can also facilitate processing of traumatic events and resolution of unhelpful beliefs in patients who are unable or unwilling to complete exposure. Cognitive restructuring teaches patients to systematically replace unhelpful thoughts with more helpful and realistic thoughts. It helps PTSD patients to recognise and modify their negative beliefs and perceptions about self, others and the environment that emanated from the trauma. Trauma survivors, especially victims of interpersonal violence, have the tendency to self-blame, thus causing guilt, shame and embarrassment. For example, a rape victim may believe 'It was my fault' or 'I asked for it'. They also overestimate the risks and dangers. Roger believes 'The world is not a safe place', 'You can't walk down the street without being mugged'. The overestimation of danger causes phobic reactions and avoidance behaviour.

As discussed in Chapter 4, CBT uses some very well-known and tested reason-based models such as Socratic logic-based dialogues and Aristotle's method of collecting and categorising information about the world (Leahy, 2003). CBT therapists engage their patients in scientific and rational thinking by guiding them to examine the presupposition, validity and meaning of their beliefs that lead to their anxiety, depression and avoidance behaviour. As CBT techniques are fully described in several excellent books (e.g. Beck, 1995) and a detailed description of the sequential progression of CBT within the CH framework is provided elsewhere (Alladin, 2007b) and in Chapter 4, they are not described in detail here. Figure 5.1 provides an example of how to utilise the Cognitive Restructuring (ABCDE) form (Appendix B) to restructure the dysfunctional beliefs ('I can't handle this', 'I will not be able to cope', 'The world is unsafe' and 'I will get shot at') held by Roger.

The following transcript illustrates how Roger was guided by the therapist to re-evaluate and change his maladaptive belief about the world ('The world is unsafe') that was produced from his traumatic experience.

Th = Therapist, R = Roger
Th: Roger, what do you mean by 'The world is unsafe'?
R: You can't go out there, you may get killed.
Th: What do you mean by 'out there'?
R: Well, you can't go out in the street without getting killed or mugged.
Th: So, let me get it right what you are saying. You believe that if you go out in the street, you will either get killed or mugged.
R: Precisely.
Th: How much do you believe in the belief that you will get shot or mugged when you go out in the street?
R: Totally, one hundred per cent.
Th: What kind of a thinking error is this?
R: All-or-nothing thinking, magnification and I'm overgeneralising.

(This transcript is from Roger's third session of CBT. From his three sessions of CBT and homework assignments, Roger is well versed in the types of cognitive distortions that anxious people ruminate with, as described by Burns, 1999. See Alladin, 2007b for the sequential progression of CBT within the context of CH.)

Th: So you are aware that your thinking is inaccurate.
R: Yes, but I can't help it. I know I live in a fairly safe neighbourhood, but my mind keeps going back to Eastern Europe. I get confused. My mind keeps going back as if I'm still there. It's so crazy.
Th: Do you see the connection between your thinking and your negative reactions?
R: Yes, it's so dumb. Whenever I think of going out, I think of the dangerous situations we faced in Eastern Europe, people getting shot, arrested and blown up. But this is so dumb, I am not going to get attacked or shot going to the store.
Th: So your thinking gets confused. When you think of going out to the store, you think you are in Eastern Europe.
R: Yes, but I can't help it.
Th: Having the thinking that you are in Eastern Europe and exposed to dangers is not deliberate on your part. You don't think this way on purpose. As a result of your

DATE	A ACTIVATING EVENT	B IRRATIONAL BELIEFS	C CONSEQUENCES	D DISPUTATION	E EFFECT OF DISPUTATION
	Describe actual event, stream of thoughts, daydream etc. leading to unpleasant feelings	Write automatic thoughts and images that came in your mind. Rate beliefs or images 0–100%	1. **Emotion:** Specify sad, anxious or angry. Rate feelings 1–100% 2. **Physiological:** Palpitations, pain, dizzy, sweat etc. 3. **Behavioural:** Avoidance, in bed 4. **Conclusion:** Reaching conclusions, self-affirmation	Challenge the automatic thoughts and images. Rate belief in rational response/image 0–100%	1. **Emotion:** Rerate your emotion 1–100% 2. **Physiological:** Changes in bodily reactions (i.e. less shaking, less tense etc.) 3. **Behavioural:** Action taken after disputation 4. **Conclusion:** Reappraise your conclusion and initial decision. Future beliefs in similar situation

| Nov 09/05 | A worked example: Planning going to the local grocery store | 1. I can't handle this (100)
2. I will not be able to cope (100)
3. The world is unsafe (100)
4. I will get shot at (90) | 1. Anxious (100), scared (100), depressed (90), angry (90)
2. Agitated, trembling, heart pounding, sweating
3. Don't want to go to the store
4. I will never get out of this | 1. How do I know I won't be able to handle this, I am not there yet? It is true that when I went to the store last week I felt nervous and shaky, but I managed to survive. There's no reason why I can't do it again (70).
2. Again, I am not there yet, how do I know I can't cope? I may feel anxious or uncomfortable, but this does not mean I will lose control. I have never lost control (80).
3. The world is a big place, some part of the world is dangerous, but there are also places where it is relatively safe (90). My neighbourhood is relatively safe (100).
4. This is not true. The neighbourhood is safe. It's possible to get shot at, but it is unlikely to happen in this place (100). I am exaggerating my fear (100). | 1. Less scared (10), less anxious (20), less depressed (20), no longer feeling angry (0)
2. Feeling relaxed
3. Decided to go to the store
4. It is possible to get shot, but it's unlikely that anyone will shoot me in this neighbourhood |

Figure 5.1 Cognitive Restructuring (ABCDE) form completed by Roger

traumatic experiences, your mind has developed many associations with the fearful and dangerous situations you were in. Also you learned to think automatically about danger, even in situations where there is no danger. Does this make sense to you?

R: Yes, but how do I get out of this?

Th: As we talked before, we use disputation or reasoning. When you are thinking of going to the store and the thought crosses your mind that you will be mugged or shot, how would you reason with this statement?

R: I can remind myself that I'm not in Eastern Europe, my assignment is over. I am at home now, and this is a safe environment.

Th: That's excellent. You have to separate 'then' from 'now'. You have to reason that you are in a safe environment now, even if your thinking keeps going back to Eastern Europe.

R: I guess I always knew my thinking was wrong, but the feelings are so real that you begin to go along with your feeling, rather than thinking with your head. Funny, this is what cops are taught to do.

Th: What kind of a thinking error is this, when you are thinking with your feeling?

R: Emotional reasoning. You are right, I need to use my head more than my feeling.

Th: That's right, you have to continue to assess the link between your thinking and your feeling. Try to identity the cognitive distortion and then reason with it.

As a result of this session Roger was able to modify his maladaptive beliefs as shown in Figure 5.1. Some therapists often wonder whether to use hypnotherapy or CBT first when treating PTSD. Although the choice of the initial mode of therapy is determined by the clinical needs of the patient, it is recommended that CBT be introduced first if the PTSD patient is overly preoccupied with dysfunctional cognitions and non-anxiety symptoms, and to resort to hypnotherapy if the patient is overly overwhelmed with anxiety, flashbacks and hyperarousal.

Sessions 11–14: Emotional Processing

Imaginal exposure is incorporated in CH to help PTSD patients process their traumatic memories. Although imaginal exposure may sound simple and straightforward, the success of the procedure with PTSD depends on two critical factors (Zayfert & Becker, 2007). First, the clinician should have a solid understanding of the process of imaginal exposure and should have the experience to be able to titrate the process to match the patient's emotional level of comfort. Second, the clinician should have complete confidence in the procedure so that patients can be encouraged to stay on course despite their struggle and lack of habituation. On the other hand, the clinician should be sensitive not to emotionally overtax the patient or give in to the patient's avoidance behaviour – a middle-of-the-road approach is required, which comes with experience.

Lynn and Cardeña (2007) give three main reasons why exposure therapy is effective with post-traumatic patients:

1. Exposure provides a direct route to accessing and modifying *fear structures* and minimising avoidance. Traumatic experiences can lead to the development of fear structures or networks in memory that are activated by certain stimuli or reminders of the trauma, leading to escape and avoidance, which interferes with the processing and integration of the traumatic content (Foa & Rothbaum, 1998; Foa, Steketee & Rothbaum, 1989). Repeated exposure to what is feared in a safe environment leads to habituation and adaptive reorganisation of the fear structure.
2. Exposure reduces anxiety and restructures maladaptive thinking. As exposure is conducted in a safe and supportive environment, with the waxing and waning of fears, positive self-suggestions and expectancies (e.g. 'I can handle this') are engendered. This positive attitude or perceived self-efficacy (Bandura, 1977) decreases anxiety and alters the maladaptive beliefs that maintain the avoidance behaviour.
3. Exposure provides a safe environment for patients to re-evaluate the traumatic event and their reactions to it. The re-evaluations lead to changes in cognitive distortions. For example, during exposure Roger realised that it was not his fault that he did not stop the raiding of his friend's village. In fact, he recognised that it was his intervention (confrontation with the commander of the raid) that led to his own arrest. Roger had the dysfunctional belief that 'I am a coward. I did nothing to stop the destruction'. Lynn and Cardeña (2007) believe that exposure has the potential to change the patient's narrative: as 'Meichenbaum (Meichenbaum, 1994; Meichenbaum & Fong, 1993) has observed, the entire narrative in which the traumatic event is embedded can change with retelling or reexperiencing in the direction of greater self-acceptance and a more realistic assessment of the dangerousness of the environment and the likelihood of retraumatization' (Lynn & Cardeña, 2007, p. 173).

Hypnotic Reprocessing Therapy

Hypnosis is applied to exposure therapy in the context of imagery rescripting therapy (IRT). The goal of IRT is to alleviate PTSD and related clinical symptoms by eliminating intrusive traumatic flashbacks, altering traumagenic beliefs and schemas (e.g. powerlessness, hopelessness, vulnerability) and enhancing the victim's ability to self-calm and self-nurture (Grunert *et al.*, 2003). IRT is an imagery-based, cognitive treatment that employs exposure, *not* for habituation but for activating the images, emotions and beliefs associated with the traumatic memories. Grunert *et al.* (2003) regard exposure in IRT to be a means to an end; that is, for activating the trauma memory as a means of enhancing cognitive restructuring rather than an end in itself. Therefore the focus of IRT is on both activation and modification of the traumatic images and associated maladaptive attributions, beliefs and schemas (e.g. guilt, anger, shame, self-blame, powerlessness). The trauma-related 'corrective information' in IRT is processed both visually and verbally during high states of emotional arousal within the context of a Socratic intrapersonal dialogue between the patient's 'traumatised self' and 'survivor self'.

IRT consists of four sequential components: imaginal exposure; imaginal rescripting; self-calming and self-nurturing; and emotional-linguistic processing. Each of these IRT components can be easily integrated with some of the well-known hypnotic techniques (e.g. split-screen technique, 'Comforting the Child' technique) utilised in the management of PTSD.

There are three fundamental reasons for integrating hypnosis with IRT in the management of post-traumatic symptoms. First, as discussed before, a plethora of hypnotic strategies have been imported to CBT, exposure therapy and psychodynamic therapy of PTSD. With the exception of using hypnosis with exposure therapy (Lynn & Cardeña, 2007; Lynn & Kirsch, 2006), the rationale for integrating hypnosis with CBT or psychodynamic therapy is not clear. Moreover, it is not clear how the hypnosis effect changes when it is combined with other forms of psychotherapy for PTSD. IRT provides an empirical therapeutic context wherein hypnotic techniques can be easily integrated with relaxation training and imaginal exposure. It is also known how the components of IRT produce change in post-traumatic symptoms. As discussed earlier, hypnosis is a more powerful technique for producing syncretic cognition and facilitating regression than relaxation training. Moreover, there is a mutual relationship between hypnosis and PTSD:

> There is some evidence that patients with PTSD are higher than average in hypnotisability (Cardeña, 2000). This may mean that high hynotisability predisposes a person to develop PTSD, or that PTSD renders people more hypnotisable. Spiegel and Cardena (1990) draw a parallel between PTSD and hypnosis. For them, the three major components of hypnosis are absorption, dissociation and suggestibility. They compare these components to (respectively) the intrusive reliving of traumatic events, 'psychic numbing', and hypervigilence and heightened sensitivity to environmental events, all of them symptoms that are observed in PTSD. (Heap & Aravind, 2002, pp. 423–4)

From the above, it would appear theoretically and conceptually logical to utilise hypnosis in the management of post-traumatic symptoms, particularly flashbacks, numbing and hyperarousal. As noted before, Brom, Kleber and Defare (1989) demonstrated that hypnosis can be effective in reducing post-traumatic symptoms, especially flashbacks, in the context of behaviour therapy, systematic desensitisation and psychodynamic psychotherapy.

Secondly, IRT has been found to be effective with a variety of post-traumatic conditions. Therefore it will be easy to compare the relative effectiveness of IRT with hypnosis and without hypnosis. Thus, the combination of IRT with hypnosis provides an opportunity to study the additive effect of hypnosis with PTSD.

Thirdly, hypnosis facilitates non-conscious and non-linguistic information processing. For these reasons, Smucker, Weis and Grunert (2002, p. 85) use imagery training, rather than traditional exposure protocol, in their treatment of PTSD:

> The use of imagery as a therapeutic strategy in treating trauma victims has been advocated by clinicians from a variety of theoretical orientations. Van der Kolk and van der Hart (1991) have noted that traumatic memories and their associated meanings are encoded as vivid images and sensations and are not accessible through linguistic retrieval alone, regardless of the victim's age at the time of the trauma. This finding corroborates the claims of many trauma victims who report difficulty with linguistically accessing and processing their traumatic experiences. It further has implications for the use of imagery as a primary therapeutic agent in the treatment of PTSD. Since much of the cognitive-affective disturbance associated with traumatic memories (e.g., intrusive recollections, recurring flashbacks) is embedded in the traumatic images themselves, directly challenging and modifying the traumatic imagery becomes a powerful, if not preferred, means of processing the traumatic material (Smucker, 1997).

Since hypnosis, imagery and affect are all predominantly mediated by the same right cerebral hemisphere (Ley & Freeman, 1984), imagination is easily intensified by hypnosis (Boutin, 1978). Hypnosis thus provides a powerful modality for imagery training, conditioning emotional responses and restructuring experience. Hypnotic imagery has been used for systematic desensitisation; restructuring of cognitive processes at various levels of awareness or consciousness; exploration of the remote past (regression work); and directing attention on positive experiences. In addition to facilitating diverse emotional experiences, hypnosis also provides a vehicle for exploring and expanding experience in the present, the past and the future. Such strategies can enhance divergent thinking and facilitate the deconstruction of dysfunctional 'realities' (Alladin, 2008). Hypnosis allows direct entry into accessing and organising emotional and experiential information, largely served by the right cerebral hemisphere (in right-handers). By engaging the right hemisphere, the hypnotic experience is intensified, providing strong validation of reality (Alladin, 2008).

As humans, we do not validate reality by the way we think, but by the way we feel. When an anxious patient is feeling panicky, although this may be due to irrational beliefs (e.g. 'I'm going to lose control'), because the feeling is real to the person experiencing it, the anxious reality ('I can't cope') is validated or consolidated as part of conceptual reality. The induction of an intense positive experience via hypnosis provides the validation of an alternative or positive reality. The best way to change an experience is to produce another experience. Hypnosis provides rapid induction of an alternative or competing reality. Hypnosis also allows access to psychological processes below the threshold of awareness, thus providing a means of exploring and restructuring non-conscious cognitions and experience related to the symptoms. In addition, hypnosis provides a vehicle whereby cortical and subcortical functioning can be accessed and integrated. Since the subcortex is the seat of emotions, access to it provides an entry into the organisation, processing and modification of primitive emotions.

Imaginal exposure

This phase involves recalling and re-experiencing of the entire traumatic event, as experienced by the patient in the form of recurring flashbacks, nightmares or other intrusive recollections. Before starting the procedure, the rationale for using hypnotic exposure is thoroughly discussed with the patient and this rationale is often repeated during the exposure process. It is important for the therapist to communicate his or her confidence in the procedure and inform the patient that exposure can be anxiety provoking during the early stages of treatment. It is emphasised that the patient's sense of control during the exposure is an essential element in the success of the procedure. The patient is reassured that, armed with the skills of affect regulation and mind-over-body control acquired from the initial sessions of hypnotherapy, he or she will be able handle the imaginal exposure. The patient is further reassured that the therapist will be present throughout the sessions to provide support and address any concerns from the patient.

I use the following script, based on Meadows and Foa (1998), to describe the rationale for using imaginal exposure with post-traumatic conditions. To provide clarity, the script that was tailored for Roger is described here:

Now that you have learned to regulate your affect and reason with your maladaptive beliefs, we are ready to do imaginal exposure. This technique encourages you to relive the traumatic experience in your memory. I know that you think about your experience in Eastern Europe quite a lot. In our session today, we are going to confront the memories in a different way. Currently, when you think about your experience you feel upset and therefore you try to push it away. It is understandable that you want to avoid thinking about it, since it was such a distressing experience for you. Unfortunately, as you have already noticed, trying not to think about it does not work very well, it keeps coming back. Some of your symptoms, like the nightmares, the intrusive thoughts and flashbacks, are signs that you have not dealt with the memories of the experience yet. This is why they are so upsetting to you and they keep coming back.

In imaginal exposure, I will encourage you to deliberately confront your thoughts and images related to your traumatic experience without pushing them away. Reliving the traumatic experience in your memory lets you process the experience, so that you can file it away in your mind like any other bad memory. The exposure will also demonstrate to you that you can let yourself think about it, without losing control or going crazy. This will give you control over the memories, rather than the memories controlling you. You will also discover that

> the anxiety you experience when you think about your experience in Eastern Europe decreases, just like it does when you watch a frightening movie several times.

After discussing the rationale, the patient is encouraged to close his or her eyes and induce deep relaxation via self-hypnosis. The patient is instructed to use an ideomotor signal (the same signal as used in previous hypnosis sessions) to indicate when the patient is deeply relaxed. The therapist then deepens the hypnotic trance by using a counting method and suggests: 'However deep is your trance level, you will still hear everything I say, you will be aware of everything around you, and you will be able to speak when requested to do so.' Then the therapist asks the patient to re-enact the trauma by visualising and verbalising aloud the entire traumatic memory in the present tense, as if it were occurring at that moment. If multiple traumatic memories recur, the patient is advised to focus on the most distressing one. The patient is instructed to monitor and report his or her SUD level (subjective units of distress rated on a 0–100 scale; 0 = no anxiety or distress, 100 = worst level of anxiety or distress), as well as numbing or sense of dissociation, about every 10 minutes. This information allows the therapist to be aware of the current emotional state of the patient.

I offer the following suggestions at the beginning of the imaginal exposure, based on a script from Smucker, Weis and Grunert (2002, pp. 87–8):

> You have now become so deeply relaxed and you are in such a deep hypnotic trance that your mind has become so powerful and so sensitive to what I say, that you will be able to imagine, feel and experience everything I ask you to imagine, feel and experience. I will ask you to recall the painful and distressing memories as vividly as possible. It's important for you to describe the traumatic event in the present tense as if it were happening now, right here. If you start to feel uncomfortable and want to shut off the image, I will help you stay with it. About every 10 minutes I will ask you about your SUD level. Please answer quickly as it's important for you not to leave the image. Do you have any questions before we start?
>
> Now I want you to go back in time and place and remember the event that was most distressing to you (*since Roger was exposed to several traumatic events, it was important to focus on one event at a time*). Visualise the beginning of the traumatic scene and describe what you experience, tell me about the feelings you are having and the kinds of thoughts that go through your mind.

While conducting hypnotic exposure, it is important to help the patient vividly recall the memories and the experiences of the traumatic event, but not to regress fully (avoid revivification) back to the event. The patient should be grounded in the present while processing the emotional memories. The therapist should continually titrate the trance level to prevent complete dissociation from the present (here and now). One way of doing this is to continually suggest to the patient: 'However absorbed and involved you become in your imagination, part of you knows that you are in my office and you are simply thinking about the event.' At the end of the exposure, the patient is debriefed and any questions that the patient may have are addressed in a reassuring and succinct manner.

The primary task of the therapist during the exposure procedure is to titrate the hypnotic level and provide a safe and supportive environment to allow the patient to visualise the traumatic event while re-experiencing the distressing feelings associated with it. The therapist helps the patient to 'stay with' the painful imagery as the patient decides on the details he or she wants to describe. Smucker, Weis and Grunert (2002) emphasise that the therapist's role should be facilitative rather than directive during the imaginal procedure. Except for being verbally reflective, or restating what the patient said, the therapist should not intervene or ask for more details about the traumatic scene. At the end of the re-enactment of the traumatic memory, after the debriefing, the patient is encouraged to induce self-hypnosis. Then the therapist deepens the trance and offers post-hypnotic suggestions, such as: 'As a result of this exposure therapy, every day your fear will become less and less.' Here is a hypnotic exposure script from Lynn & Kirsch (2006, pp. 166–7) that can be easily adapted to the needs of your individual patient:

Now that you have a better understanding of what you will gain by learning to contend with flashbacks, and learning to accept your past, it is time to practise exposure to learn how to coexist with and ultimately master the disturbing memories and images that have their roots in your past. Go deeper now into your hypnosis, knowing at the deepest levels of your being that you will be safe in this room, even though your mind tricks you into relating to the past as if it were present. On this deep level, you will know that that was then, and this is now. And it is safe 'in the now'. Each time you practise exposure, it will get easier for you to experience what you fear. Like when you watch a tape of a scary movie the first time, at the scariest part you may feel like jumping out of your skin. But if you were to watch it over and over, your fear would diminish with each viewing. When it's time, you will turn the imaginary tape on by imagining you are watching the scene on a video on your mental TV. You can imagine dials that can be used to control the degree of emotion you feel during the scene, and you can zoom in to observe details you wish to focus on. If the emotion gets to be too much for you, simply dial it down, take a deep breath, and be sure to remind yourself you are safe in the present. But keep the emotional intensity turned up as high as you can tolerate it. Soon I will ask you to let the mental tape unroll and play the scene from beginning to end. I'd like to hear all about your experience, in the first person and in present tense, all the details you wish to share at this point . . . what the scariest moment is . . . what you are thinking and feeling. If you go a bit too fast, I will tell you to roll the tape in slow motion. You can control the speed with a remote control . . . fast . . . slow . . . but let's keep it as slow as you can go, so you experience everything to the fullest extent you are capable of at this point in time. Create it, feel it, live it, but deep within yourself, all the while you know that it is you who is letting the tape roll . . . you who is doing it, and you who will control it. And you will know that the event is not actually occurring in the present, but in your mind and nowhere else. At the end of the tape, you will go deeper and deeper into your hypnosis, letting yourself relax completely, relax completely, calm and at ease, taking away from the scene what you can, what you will, learning what you can . . . growing as a person in subtle or perhaps not so subtle ways. Learning and growing. Learning to feel comfortable with your experience of life, what is pleasant and what is not so pleasant. Now let's let the scene roll. If I tell you to stop the scene, you will be able to stop it immediately. Quickly and easily. Negative emotions associated with the scene will break up, dissipate, like clouds in the wind, as you let them go.

Lynn and Cardeña (2007) recommend repeating this script for three to nine sessions, until the scene can be experienced with a SUD rating of no more than 20 (on a 0–100 scale). In the process of the exposure therapy, other traumatic scenes such as childhood sexual abuse can emerge. In such a case the trauma can be targeted in subsequent sessions.

Imaginal rescripting

The second phase of HRT involves the creation of a 'mastery image'. This is done immediately after the completion of the imaginal phase. The mastery imagery phase is an extension of the exposure imagery. The procedure starts with the visualisation and verbalisation of the traumatic memory. Once the traumatic imagery is at its emotional peak, the patient is asked to visualise his or her 'survivor' self today entering the traumatic scene to assist the 'traumatised', 'victimised', 'injured' self (Smucker, Weis & Grunert, 2002). The primary goal of the mastery imagery phase is to replace victimisation imagery with mastery or coping imagery. In some instances, the survivor today may need to 'confront' a perpetrator (if a perpetrator is involved in the traumatic scene) to 'rescue' the 'traumatised' self from the traumatic scene. It is crucial that patients select their own coping strategies during the mastery phase. If a patient is unable to visualise himself or herself as a survivor, the patient is advised to imagine deploying help from others (e.g. friend, spouse, police officer) to rescue the 'victim'. Again, the therapist refrains from dictating to the patient what to do; instead a client-centered approach is used. Smucker (1997) found patient-generated coping imagery to promote greater patient empowerment than coping or mastery imagery coming from the therapist.

The *split screen technique* is often used in hypnotherapy to make the traumatic event more bearable (Cardeña *et al.*, 2000; Spiegel, 1981). The split screen technique involves projecting (Lynn & Cardeña, 2007, p. 181):

> images of memories of the trauma on the left side and on the right side something they did to protect themselves or someone else (e.g., fight back, scream, protest, lying still). If patients blame themselves for a sexual assault, for example, or feel they did not resist enough, they can be told that not resisting is an automatic and common survival strategy in the face of mortal danger, and is entirely understandable in such instances. As Cardeña et al. (2000) state, 'The image on the right may help patients realize that while they were indeed victimized, they were also attempting to master the situation and displayed courage during a time of overwhelming threat' (p. 257).

Self-calming/Self-nurturing

After the completion of the mastery imagery, the self-nurturing imagery is introduced. The induction of self-nurturing imagery facilitates the survivor today to interact directly with the 'traumatised' self. Smucker, Weis and Grunert (2002, p. 89) use a series of questions to facilitate the 'survivor-traumatised self' interactive imagery:

- What would you, the survivor today, like to do or say to your 'traumatised' self?
- Can you see yourself doing (or saying) that?
- How does your 'traumatised' self respond?
- How do you, the survivor today, respond to your 'traumatised' self?

Once the survivor today has offered sufficient nurturance to the 'traumatised' self, the imagery is ended: 'Now you can let the imagery fade away and you can open your eyes.'

If the trauma occurred during childhood, hypnosis can be used to glean meaning from a childhood traumatic event by viewing it from an adult perspective. For this purpose the *'Comforting the Child'* technique can be used, as scripted by Lynn and Cardeña (2007, pp. 181–2).

Now you can see yourself watching a movie . . . a movie of something from your past . . . something that we have talked about before, but you want to know more about . . . to learn more about . . . to reclaim your past . . . to learn from it . . . you can watch this scene . . . an old traumatic scene . . . the scene of [insert situation] . . . something you remember but want to learn more about . . . you can watch it from beginning to end . . . and learn from it . . . learn how it affected you . . . learn what decisions you made as a result of it . . . and learn how you can move beyond . . . perhaps to love and wholeness . . . perhaps to understanding . . . and forgiving [as appropriate to the patient] . . . learn more about you . . . and what you can be now, in the present . . . What is really interesting about this movie is that you can float right into the picture . . . or walk right

into it . . . you can comfort the child . . . you can reassure the child . . . you can communicate with the child on many levels . . . you can touch the child . . . or hold the
child . . . embrace the child . . . or just look lovingly at the child . . . with the eyes of
wisdom and knowing . . . and forgiveness . . . and protection and care . . . whatever
you want to say or do is entirely up to you . . . but you have a feeling . . . a sense that
you know what is right to do . . . what is the next best thing to do. (Lynn & Kirsch,
2006, p. 171)

If the child made some decisions at the time of the event . . . talk to the child
about them . . . you are more experienced than the child . . . you have more understanding . . . you have more empathy . . . you have more insight . . . the child is wise
too . . . and can understand . . . yet the child needs your nurturing and your guidance,
your adult perspective . . . talk to it . . . let it know how you feel . . . what you think.

Soon you will be ready to let go of this scene . . . yet to hold onto the child and feel
it hold onto you . . . just right . . . so tight . . . you need to care for this child . . . it needs
to let you know how it feels . . . what it thinks . . . you can do this . . . take some time
to do this now . . . [60 seconds]. Now you can step out of the scene, take with it what
you want . . . the drama of life will continue with you richer for the learning . . . for
the witnessing . . . wondering in what small ways you will be enriched . . . so much
still to learn . . . so much time . . . so much time (Lynn & Kirsch, 2006).

Given the risk of suggested memories and confabulation, Lynn and Cardeña
(2007) recommend working with a target event that is well remembered and
discussed prior to using the 'Comforting the Child' technique.

Emotional-linguistic processing

The fourth phase of HRT is facilitated after a brief pause, during which the
patient is allowed to readjust and any arising questions addressed. Again
the process can be facilitated by asking such questions as (Smucker, Weis &
Grunert, 2002, p. 89):

- What was that like for you?
- What was it like to see yourself today coping in the traumatic situation?
- What was it like for you, the survivor today, to interact with your 'traumatised'
  self?
- What have you learned from the imagery session today?

During this phase of exposure, the therapist reviews the patient's ability to
self-calm and self-nurture when anxious or distressed. The therapist also col-
laborates with the patient to explore various self-calming strategies that the
patient can use or experiment with between sessions. Homework assignments

related to imaginal exposure form a very important component of exposure therapy. Each imagery session is taped and the patient is advised to listen to the audiotape at home between sessions and to try new acquired skills of self-calming and self-nurturing in new upsetting situations. The between-session homework involves five components:

- Listening daily to the self-hypnosis audiotape.
- Continuing to complete the Cognitive Restructuring (ABCDE) forms.
- Listening daily to the audiotape/CD of the most recent imagery session.
- Recording the SUD level every 10 minutes while listening to the imagery training audiotape.
- Documenting efforts to self-calm and self-nurture whenever feeling upset.
- Record the number of traumatic flashbacks, nightmares and intrusive recollections experienced between sessions.

Smucker, Weis and Grunert (2002, p. 90) consider the imagery training to be accomplished when patients are able to:

- Replace their traumatic/victimisation imagery with self-generating mastery/coping imagery, whereby they can visualise themselves successfully coping with the traumatic situation or the perpetrator.
- Rescue their 'traumatised' or 'victimised' self from the traumatic situation.
- Create self-calming and self-nurturing imagery.
- Utilise mastery imagery skills with other potentially difficult or upsetting situations outside the session.

If these goals are not achieved, it would mean the patient may still be experiencing recurrent recollections, flashbacks or nightmares, thus requiring further imagery rescripting sessions.

Session 15–16: Increasing Identity and Relational Functioning

Above and beyond post-traumatic stress, cognitive distortions and affect dysregulation, trauma can produce chronic problems in identity and interpersonal problems (Briere & Scott, 2006). Identity and relational difficulties in chronic PTSD patients are often viewed by clinicians as borderline personality disorder. While there is a significant link between trauma and some enduring psychological disturbances, not all of the problems are related to dysfunctional personality. Many of the identity and interpersonal problems may represent reactions, accommodations or coping strategies for dealing with chronic childhood maltreatment. CH for PTSD, therefore, devotes some sessions to addressing identity and relational problems, especially if these difficulties are identified in the case formulation (see Cognitive Hypnotherapy Case Formulation and Treatment Plan, Appendices C and D).

Identity Problems

Briere and Scott (2006) have identified several problems associated with an inability to access and gain from an internal sense of self among survivors of early severe childhood trauma:

- Inability to determine one's own needs or entitlements.
- Unable to maintain a consistent sense of self or identity in the context of strong emotions or the presence of dominant others.
- Lacking an internal reference point at times of stress.
- Unable to predict one's own reactions or behaviour in various situations.
- Having no direct access to a positive or nurturing sense of self.

The intervention involves providing safety, supporting self-validity and encouraging self-exploration.

Providing safety

To be able to explore internal thoughts, feelings and experiences, the traumatised patient requires an environment where he or she can feel safe physically and psychologically. Such a safe environment is created by the presence and client-focused stance of the therapist. Hypnosis can further enhance the patient's sense of safety. When in trance, the patient can be helped to create a sense of safety by offering the following suggestions:

You have now become so relaxed, you are in such a deep hypnotic trance, that your mind and your body feel calm, peaceful and very relaxed. Just continue to feel this beautiful sensation of peace and tranquility . . . relaxation and calm flowing through your mind and your body . . . giving you such a pleasant feeling, such a beautiful sensation, that you feel you are drifting into a deeper and deeper hypnotic trance . . . as if, for now, all your worries and cares have disappeared. Since you are relaxing, since this is your time out, put everything on hold, for now . . . meaning, although you are aware of everything, you are not concerned or preoccupied with anything. Although you are aware of everything, you can let go, you can let your mind and body relax completely. So just continue to feel free from all the worries and cares you had before . . . just continue to feel free from all the anxiety and tension you felt before . . . just continue to feel free from all the upsetting and depressive feelings you felt before . . . just continue to feel free from all the stress you experienced before . . . just continue to feel free from the frustration, irritation and anger you felt before. Just continue to enjoy this beautiful sensation of peace and tranquility, relaxation and calm flowing through your mind and body . . . that you feel so calm, so peaceful, sense of well-being, feeling safe, feeling secure. Just continue to enjoy these feelings . . . feeling safe and secure.

Once this 'pleasant state of mind' is created, the patient is encouraged to speak of any concerns he or she may have. Prior ending the session the patient is provided post-hypnotic suggestions to solidify the pleasant state of mind and to encourage taking calculated risks; that is, the patient is encouraged to face some of the situations he or she was avoiding. If the patient has developed phobias from the traumatic experience, exposure in vivo may be necessary.

Supporting self-validity

Apart from taking a client-focused therapeutic approach, it is important for the therapist to convey to the traumatised patients that their needs and perceptions are intrinsically valid. This may appear to contradict the CBT tenet of challenging a patient's negative self-perceptions and other cognitive distortions. Briere and Scott (2006, pp. 151–2) provide directions on how to challenge a patient's perception and beliefs without invalidating them:

> the approach advocated . . . is not to argue with the client regarding his or her 'thinking errors' about self, but rather to work with the client in such a way that he or she is able to perceive incorrect assumptions and reconsider them in light of his or her current (therapy-based) relational experience. Although the therapist typically will not validate the client's self-rejection (for example, the belief that one does not have entitlement to self-rejection and caring treatment by others), he or she will provide a therapeutic experience that contradicts such thoughts.

For instance:

> although the client may view himself or herself as not having rights to self-determination, these self-perceptions will be contrary to the experience of acceptance and positive regard experienced in the therapeutic session.

During chronic abuse, especially during childhood, because attention is usually focused on the abuser's needs (e.g. he or she will be angry or violent), the victim learns the abuser's view of reality. In such a context the survivor's needs of reality become irrelevant, or dangerous when asserted. Again Briere and Scott (2006, p. 152) provide therapeutic strategies of how to help the patient develop a coherent and positive view of the self:

> In a client-focused environment, however, reality becomes more what the client needs or perceives than what the therapist demands or expects. In such an environment, the client is more able to identify internal states, perceptions, and needs, and discover how to 'hang on to' these aspects of self even when in the presence of meaningful others (that is, the therapist). By stressing to the client that his or her experience is the ultimate focus, and by helping the client to identify and label his or her internal feelings and needs, the therapist helps the client to build a coherent and positive model of self – much in the way parents would have, had the client's childhood been more safe, attuned, and supportive.

Encouraging self-exploration

Most of the self-exploration work is usually done during hypnotic reprocessing therapy (HRT). In the context of resolving identity problems, the therapist allows the patient to gain a greater sense of self-reference or internal topography by repeatedly asking the patient about his or her ongoing internal experience throughout the course of the session. The therapist gently inquires about the patient's experiences, feelings and reactions during and after the victimisation, as well as the thoughts and conclusions emanating from the treatment process. It is also important for the patient to discover what he or she thinks and feels about the trauma and the current situations, and how he or she thinks and feels about himself or herself as distinct from how others think or feel.

Relational Difficulties

One of the earliest impacts of abuse and neglect is manifested in the child's internal representations of self and others. A child who has been maltreated may conclude that he or she is intrinsically unacceptable, malignant and deserving of punishment or disregard, views others as inherently dangerous, rejecting or unavailable, and reaches the conclusion that he or she is helpless, inadequate or weak (Allen, 2001). These early inferences about self and others are thought to produce a generalised set of expectations and assumptions referred as an *internal working model* (Bowlby, 1982) or *relational schemas* (Baldwin et al., 1993). These core schemas, often referred to as *attachment styles* (Bowlby, 1988), affect the individual's later capacity to form and maintain meaningful connections and attachments with other people.

The relational difficulties, to some extent, are dealt with during affect-regulation training, cognitive interventions and HRT. When the relational issues are specifically addressed in the later sessions, the therapeutic approach is more client centred. The fostering of a safe, soothing and supportive environment facilitates the disclosure and reframing of dysfunctional relational cognitions. However, it should be noted that some core relational schemas based on early trauma 'are often relatively nonresponsive to verbal information or the expressed views of others later in life, since they are encoded in the first years of life, and thus are preverbal in nature' (Briere & Scott, 2006, p. 154). For example, the patients who believe, based on early learning, that they are unlikable or unattractive to others, or that others are not to be trusted, will not easily change such views based on other people's declarations that they are valued by them or they can be relied on (Briere & Scott, 2006). Regression and reframing work assisted by hypnotherapy is of assistance here.

Pharmacological Intervention

There is no specific session devoted to pharmacotherapy. Issues related to medication are continually reviewed during the sessions. As mentioned before, PTSD is associated with enduring neurochemical and psychophysiological changes that lead to substantial impairment and distress. When the symptoms are severe, First and Tasman (2004, p. 934) recommend the use of medication rather than focusing on 'trauma-focused psychotherapy'. Although the first-line medications are the selective serotonin reuptake inhibitors (SSRIs), First and Tasman (2004) suggest a sequencing approach to using medication with PTSD as outlined in Table 5.1 earlier in the chapter. SSRIs, including fluoxetine, sertraline (e.g. Davidson *et al.*, 2001) and paroxetine (e.g. Marshall *et al.*, 1998) have broad-spectrum properties across the full symptom range of PTSD and they have been applicable with survivors of all the major classes of trauma, such as combat, sexual violence, non-sexual violence and accident. Moreover, they have been helpful to patients with or without comorbid depression (e.g. Davidson *et al.*, 2001). However, these drugs do not address avoidance behaviour and interpersonal issues. Therefore medication should be combined with CBT or exposure therapy as proposed by the expert consensus in the management of PTSD. As medication may be necessary, non-medical therapists should work closely with the treating physician or arrange for the physician to review the medication with the patient.

SUMMARY

The chapter reviewed the current theories and treatments of PTSD. As yet there is no single unifying theory of PTSD and there is no single effective treatment for all the post-traumatic symptoms. The international panel of experts on PTSD provides very useful guidelines for the management of PTSD, especially in the context of comorbid disorders.

CH provides a multi-faceted approach to treating PTSD. The hypnotherapy component of CH is integrated with IRT to establish a valid and empirical foundation for using hypnosis with PTSD. Although there is some evidence that hypnosis serves as a useful adjunct to CBT and exposure therapy of PTSD, more research is required to understand how hypnosis effects change. The integration of hypnosis with exposure therapy and IRT, since these two techniques for PTSD are empirically validated, provide a very useful design for studying the additive effect of hypnotherapy with PTSD.

CHAPTER 6

COGNITIVE HYPNOTHERAPY WITH PSYCHOCUTANEOUS DISORDERS

INTRODUCTION

The literature on the psychological aspects of skin disorders is sparse. This is surprising considering that a large number of patients with various skin disorders present wide-ranging psychological consequences and many skin conditions lie between the fields of psychiatry and dermatology. It is estimated that at least one third of dermatology patients have psychological or psychosocial issues associated with their chief complaint (Koo *et al.*, 2003). The interface between psychiatry and dermatology is manifested (Koo & Lee, 2003):

- When an underlying psychopathology in the absence of real skin disorders plays an aetiological role in the development of such conditions as delusional parasitosis and neurotic excoriations.
- When psychological factors such as emotional stress exacerbate bona fide skin conditions (e.g. acne or eczema).
- When patients with skin disorders develop secondary psychological or psychosocial problems (e.g. resulting from the disfigurement caused by the skin problems).

The DSM-IV-TR (American Psychiatric Association, 2000) has come a long way in recognising and classifying the subspeciality of Psychocutaneous Disorders. However, the primary clinical features of skin disorders are still considered to be organic and the treatment of choice is largely medical or physical. This chapter will review the psychocutaneous disorders classified in the DSM-IV-TR (APA, 2000) and outline some general principles, involving multi-modal and multi-disciplinary approaches, for working with dermatological patients. Then the rest of the chapter will describe in detail a sample treatment package, cognitive hypnotherapy (CH) for acne vulgaris, consisting of alternative and adjunctive methods of treatment. The CH described can be easily tailored for the treatment of other skin disorders.

DESCRIPTION AND CLASSIFICATION OF PSYCHOCUTANEOUS DISORDERS

Arnold (2005) describes psychocutaneous disorders as dermatological diseases that are affected by psychological factors and psychiatric illnesses in which the skin is the target of disordered thinking, behaviour or perception. The DSM-IV-TR (APA, 2000) classifies psychocutaneous disorders into five categories, consisting of:

1. Psychological factors affecting medical condition.
2. Somatoform disorders.
3. Delusional disorder, somatic type.
4. Impulse-control disorders.
5. Factitious disorders.

Each of these categories of disorder is briefly reviewed, highlighting the role of psychological factors in the genesis, exacerbation and maintenance of the disorder. The treatment for each disorder is also reviewed very briefly.

Psychological Factors Affecting Medical Condition

Psychological factors affecting medical condition or psychophysiological disorders are subdivided into atopic dermatitis, psoriasis, alopecia areata, uticaria and angioedema, and acne vulgaris.

Atopic dermatitis

Atopic dermatitis is a chronic skin disorder characterised by inflammation (eczema), dry skin and severe itching (pruritus). Due to excessive scratching, lichenification, excroriations and infection frequently occur. Atopic dermatitis is a common disorder and it usually starts in early infancy, childhood or adolescence, and is frequently associated with a personal or family history of atomic dermatitis, allergic rhinitis or asthma (Ginsburg et al., 1993). Approximately 1–3% of all adults and 5–20% of all children are affected by the disease (Gieler et al., 2003) and it is estimated that the prevalence has increased by 10% over the past decade (Rothe & Grant-Kels, 1996).

Although there is a genetic predisposition to atopic dermatitis, environmental factors such as food allergy, contact irritants, stress and so on frequently trigger or exacerbate the disease (Ehlers, Stangier & Gieler, 1995). Patients with atopic dermatitis appear to have a lower response threshold to pruritic stimuli than control subjects, and hence a vicious cycle of itching, scratching and lesion aggravation frequently develops and contributes to the chronicity of the disease (Gupta & Gupta, 1996). Psychological factors seem to be an important factor in the modulation of the disease. For example, stressful life events are known to precede the onset or exacerbation of the condition and stress may have an effect on the condition through an interaction between the central nervous system (CNS) and the immune system (Buske-Kirshbaum, Geiben & Hellhammer, 2001). Kodama *et al.* (1999) investigated the relationship between atopic dermatitis and stress in a large population of adult patients (N = 1457) who suffered the consequences of the 1995 Hanshin earthquake. They found that 38% of the patients from the severely hit region and 34% from the moderately hit region were affected with atopic dermatitis, compared to 7% from a control group without stress. A similar relationship between stress level and the severity of atopic dermatitis has been found in children (Absolon *et al.*, 1997; Daud *et al.*, 1993).

There is also a relationship between atopic dermatitis and psychopathology. Several controlled studies have shown patients with atopic dermatitis to be more anxious and depressed compared to clinical and disease-free control groups (e.g. Hashiro & Okumura, 1997). There is evidence that anxiety and depression exacerbate atopic dermatitis by amplifying itch perception (Gupta *et al.*, 1994) and eliciting scratching behaviour (Hashiro & Okumura, 1997). Psychological stress appears to affect the epidermal permeability barrier homeostasis, resulting in inflammation and pruritus (Garg *et al.*, 2001).

Because increased distress, anxiety and depression are associated with atopic dermatitis, Arnold (2005) recommends psychiatric intervention as part of the overall management of patients with atopic dermatitis. The main goal of psychiatric treatment with atopic dermatitis is to reduce itching, scratching, anxiety, depression and social avoidance. Psychiatric interventions include psychological therapies and psychotropic medications. Psychological interventions such as relaxation training, habit reversal training and cognitive behaviour therapy, when used as adjuncts to standard medical care, produce significant reduction in anxiety and depression (Ehlers, Stangier & Gieler, 1995). Anti-depressants with histamine antagonism, such as topical 5% doxepin cream and trimipramine 50 mg/day, have been found to reduce itching and scratching.

Hypnotherapy, in one form or other, has been used since ancient times to assist in the healing of skin disorders. Stewart and Thomas (1995), in a clinical trial, treated 18 adults with extensive atopic dermatitis who had been resistant to conventional medical treatment with hypnotherapy. The results showed significant reduction in itch, scratching, tension and sleep disturbance, and 40%, 50% and 60% decreases in the use of topical corticosteroid at 4, 8 and 16 weeks respectively. Sokel *et al.* (1993), in a controlled trial with children with atopic dermatitis, also found favourable results for hypnotherapy.

Psoriasis

Psoriasis is a common, chronic disease of the skin, characterised by circum-scribed silvery and glossy lesions mainly on the elbows, knees and scalp. Approximately 2% of the adult general population, equally common in men and women, is affected by the disease (Christophers & Mrowietz, 1999). The pathogenesis of psoriasis involves the skin-repair system, the inflammatory defence mechanisms and the immune system. Both genetic and environmental factors such as cold weather, physical trauma, acute bacterial and viral infec-tions, corticosteroid withdrawal, beta-adrenergic blockers and lithium seem to contribute to the manifestation of the disease (Arnold, 2005; Christophers & Mrowietz, 1999). Moreover, stressful life events and various psychosocial factors can trigger the onset or exacerbation of the psoriasis. Several studies have shown the appearance of new lesions (Farber & Nall, 1974) and exacer-bation of psoriasis at a time of worry and stressful events (Fava *et al.*, 1980). The study by Fava *et al.* found a correlation between stressful events and the appearance or exacerbation of lesions in 80% of psoriatic patients. However, most patients report disease-related stress, rather than major life events or gen-eral levels of distress, to trigger their episodes of psoriasis. The disease-related stress results from the cosmetic disfigurement and social stigma of psoriasis. Moreover, the psoriasis-related stress seems to result from the psychosocial difficulties inherent in the interpersonal relationships of patients with psori-asis rather than the severity and chronicity of the psoriasis activity (Fortune *et al.*, 1977).

Although it is not clear how stress influences the inflammatory and prolif-erative processes of psoriasis, the nervous, endocrine and immune systems may be involved. Farber (1995) has proposed that the descending autonomic information from the central nervous system might be transmitted to sensory nerves in the skin, resulting in the release of neuropeptides such as substance P, which could initiate and maintain the inflammatory response in psoriatic lesions.

Psoriatic patients have high levels of anxiety and depression and significant comorbidity with several personality disorders such as schizoid, avoid-ant, passive-aggressive and compulsive personality disorders (see Arnold, 2005). The association between psoriasis and psychopathology has led to the development of a comprehensive approach to treatment consisting of both pharmacological and psychosocial interventions. Controlled trials have shown cognitive behavioural therapy, hypnosis, imagery training, meditation and relaxation training to be effective in reducing psoriatic activities (Fortune *et al.*, 2002; Gaston *et al.*, 1991; Shenefelt, 2000; Zachariae *et al.*, 1996). Shenefelt (2000), from his review of the effectiveness of hypnotherapy with dermatology, concluded that hypnosis as a complementary therapy has a positive effect on psoriasis, and it is particularly useful for resistant psoriasis associated with emotional factors.

Alopecia areata

Alopecia areata (AA) accounts for 2% of new dermatological outpatient visits in the United States (Price, 1991). AA is characterised by non-scarring hair loss in patches from the scalp. Although the scalp is usually involved, hair loss can also occur from the eyebrows, eyelashes, beard and different part of the body. The pathogenesis of AA involves immunological and genetic factors (Olsen, 1999), but it can be exacerbated by stress and comorbid anxiety and depression (see Gupta & Gupta, 2003). Gupta, Gupta and Watteel (1997) found a strong correlation between high stress reactivity and depression in AA patients (p < .001). However, few controlled trials of psychopharmacology and psychotherapy have been conducted with AA. Although the initial results are encouraging, more controlled trials are needed (see Arnold, 2005).

Hypnosis has been used to teach AA patients how to control high stress reactivity (Shenefelt, 2000). Although anecdotal reports have indicated favourable results of hypnotherapy with AA, the small clinical trial (N = 5) by Harrison and Stepanek (1991) showed significant growth of hair in only one patient; three had slight increase in hair growth; and one had no change. However, all the five patients improved in terms of the psychological variable. From this study, Shenefelt (2000) concludes that hypnotherapy may be more appropriate as a complementary therapy than a primary alternative treatment for AA.

Urticaria and angioedema

Urticaria, or hives, involves the superficial dermis and is characterised by edematous plaques that are accompanied by intense itching. Angioedema occurs when the edema spreads into the deep dermis, subcutaneous or submucosa layers. Urticaria occurs in approximately 15–20% of the general population and most patients with acute urticaria respond to treatment of the underlying cause, usually infection or intolerance to specific drugs or food. The manifestations of urticaria result from the release of vasoactive mediators in the skin, primarily histamine from mast cells or basophils (Soter, 1999). The cause for chronic idiopathic urticaria is unknown, it responds poorly to usual dermatological treatments, and its adverse effects on the quality of life are comparable to that of patients with chronic heart disease (O'Donnell *et al.*, 1997).

Psychiatric factors are known to be involved in the development of adrenergic urticaria and the 'halo-hives' that result from acute emotional stress, caused by increased levels of plasma noradrenaline and adrenaline, are easily resolved by propranolol (Haustein, 1990). The relationship between chronic idiopathic urticaria and psychiatric factors is less clear. However, controlled trials have shown anti-depressant medications to be effective in the management of chronic idiopathic urticaria (e.g. Gupta & Gupta, 1995). Hypnosis has been the main psychological intervention for chronic idiopathic urticaria.

In a controlled study of hypnosis with relaxation therapy with 15 patients with chronic urticaria of 7.8 years' average duration, within 14 months six patients had resolved and another eight improved, with decreased medication requirements reported by 80% of patients. These findings led Shenefelt (2000) to conclude that in selected individuals, hypnosis may be useful as a complementary or even alternative therapy for chronic urticaria.

Acne vulgaris

This common sebaceous gland disease is described under hypnotherapy for psychocutaneous disorders later in the chapter.

Somatoform Disorders

The somatoform disorders category of the DSM-IV-TR (APA, 2000) classification of psychocutaneous disorders includes:

1. Chronic idiopathic pruritis.
2. Idiopathic pruritus ani, vulvae and scroti.
3. Body dysmorphic disorders.

Chronic idiopathic pruritus

Pruritus, or the sensation of itch, is a common symptom of skin disorders and other internal disorders such as chronic renal disease, diabetes or biliary disease. Chronic idiopathic pruritus and pruritus ani, vulvae and scroti result from central nervous mechanisms (Arnold, 2005). Recent stressful life events and degree of depression seem to be correlated with an increased ability to detect itch, and tricyclic anti-depressants can relieve chronic idiopathic pruritus (Gupta *et al.*, 1994). Cognitive behavioural therapy (Welkowitz, Held & Held, 1989), habit reversal training (Rosenbaum & Ayllon, 1981) and hypnosis (Ament & Milgram, 1967; Scott, 1960) have been found effective in interrupting the itch–scratch cycle, thus preventing the complications of long-term scratching. For example, Ament and Milgram (1967) reported on a man with chronic myelogenous leukemia whose intractable pruritus improved significantly with hypnotic suggestions. Therefore hypnosis can be used as a complementary therapy for intractable pruritus (Shenefelt, 2000).

Body dysmorphic disorders

Body dysmorphic disorder (BDD), also known as dysmorphophobia, is a relatively common psychiatric disorder encountered by dermatologists. BDD patients are preoccupied with the belief that some aspects of their appearance are unattractive, deformed or 'not right' in some way (Phillips, 1996). The most common areas of concern are the skin and hair, and approximately 12%

of patients seeking treatment for concerns about the skin or hair meet criteria for BDD (Phillips *et al.*, 2000). Although the areas of concern appear normal or minimal, the patients perceive them to be significantly flawed, very unattractive and very distressing, thus causing excessive worries and anxiety. Most patients with BDD have poor insight or are delusional, not recognising that the flaw they perceive is actually minimal or non-existent (Phillips & Dufresne, 2003). Normally, these patients do not benefit from reassurance from their physicians or therapists and the majority of them have ideas or delusions of reference; that is, they think that other people take special notice of their supposed defect and level criticism against them. Many patients with BDD pick their skin in an attempt to improve their appearance.

Most BDD patients have other comorbid psychiatric disorders, including major depression, obsessive-compulsive disorder, social phobia, substance abuse and personality disorder (see Phillips & Dufresne, 2003). Because of the underlying psychiatric aetiology, BDD patients do not respond to standard dermatological treatment. Serotonin-reuptake inhibitors have been found to be effective with BDD (e.g. Phillips, Albertini & Rasmussen, 2002), even with patients with delusional BDD. Behaviour therapy and CBT have been found to be effective with the majority of the patients with BDD (see review by Phillips & Dufresne, 2003).

Delusional Disorder, Somatic Type

The most common types of delusional disorder of the somatic type seen by dermatologists are delusional parasitosis, delusional dysmorphosis and delusional bromosis.

Delusional parasitosis

Delusional parasitosis is characterised by a fixed, false conviction that one is infested with living organisms and it typically occurs as a single somatic delusion with no other impairment of thought process. Patients with delusional parasitosis consult dermatologists because their delusions often involve a cutaneous invasion (Arnold, 2005). The differential diagnosis of delusional parasitosis includes various medical disorders (e.g. diabetes mellitus), neurological conditions (e.g. multiple sclerosis), other psychiatric disorders (e.g. schizophrenia) and long-term substance abuse (e.g. amphetamines). Patients with delusional parasitosis are reluctant to accept psychiatric referral for fear of being told that the infestation is not real.

The most common psychiatric treatment for delusional parasitosis involves the use of the potent neuroleptic pimozide (Hamann & Avnstorp, 1982) and 50% of the patients on pimozide have been reported to show full remission of their delusions (Trabert, 1995). Psychotherapy has not been found to be effective with delusional parasitosis (Freinhar, 1984).

Delusional dysmorphosis

The patient with delusions of dysmorphosis is convinced that his or her body is ugly, misshapen or disproportionate in a certain part. Patients with delusional dysmorphosis seek treatment from dermatologists and plastic surgeons to rectify the abnormality.

Delusional bromosis

Patients with delusions of bromosis believe that they emit a foul odour from the skin or bowel. The treatment data for delusions of dysmorphosis and bromosis are limited. However, the most common approach to treatment is pharmacological, involving selective serotonin-reuptake inhibitors (SSRIs) and pimozide (see Arnold, 2005).

Impulse-Control Disorders

Although the spectrum of self-induced dermatological conditions is very wide, DSM-IV-TR (APA, 2000) subdivides impuse-control disorders related to dermatology into psychogenic excoriation, trichotillomania and onychonphagia.

Psychogenic excoriation

Psychogenic excoriation or neurotic excoriation is a disorder characterised by self-induced skin lesions from excoriating the skin in response to skin sensations or an urge to remove an irregularity on the skin (Arnold, 2005; Van Moffaert, 2003). Approximately 2% of dermatology outpatients present with psychogenic excoriation (Gupta, Gupta & Haberman, 1987) and the lesions are usually found in areas that the patient can reach easily, such as the face, upper back, and upper and lower extremities. Patients with psychogenic excoriation suffer from an irresistible urge to excoriate the skin to remove imaginary foreign substances (Cotterill, 1981). Once the process of self-picking has begun, the damaged tissue from scratching, or a focal itch or other sensation in uninvolved skin, may initiate scratching, and gradually the itch–scratch cycle takes a life of its own (Van Moffaert, 2003). The underlying psychopathology may vary with patients, but the most common findings are obsessive-compulsive disorder, anxiety and depression (see Arnold, 2005). Psychogenic excoriation is usually treated with anti-depressant medications or anti-psychotic agents (Gupta & Gupta, 1998).

Psychological treatment of psychogenic excoriation appears to be promising, but is limited to case reports (Deckersbach *et al.*, 2002). Two case studies (Hollander, 1959; Shenefelt, 2000) report on the successful use of hypnosis with acne excoriée. Hollander (1959) used post-hypnotic suggestions to achieve control of acne excoriée in two cases. Shenefelt (2000) used hypnotic suggestions to alleviate the picking of acne in a 32-year-old woman who has been picking at the acne lesions on her face for 15 years.

Trichotillomania

Trichotillomania is a disorder of chronic pulling out of one's hair and it causes substantial distress and impairment in functioning, leading to alopecia, most commonly involving the scalp hair but also eyelashes, eyebrows, pubic hair and other body hair (Arnold, 2005). Patients may pull hair in response to negative affective cues (e.g. anxiety) or during sedentary contemplatory activities (e.g. reading) and it may occur automatically (with less awareness) or in a focused way (to decrease tension; Stein *et al.*, 2003). Patients with trichotillomania commonly have comorbid anxiety, mood, substance abuse or dependence, eating, and cluster B and C personality disorders (Arnold, 2005; Stein *et al.*, 2003). SSRIs are considered the first line of choice for medication in the treatment of trichotillomania (Vythilingum & Stein, 2001), although controlled trials of SSRIs have not proven persuasive (O'Sullivan, Christensen & Stein, 1999). CBT and hypnosis have been found to produce a favourable outcome with trichotillomania. From his review of hypnotherapy with skin disorders, Shenefelt (2000) concludes that hypnotherapy may serve as a useful complementary therapy for trichotillomania.

Onychonphagia

Onychophagia, or repetitive nail biting, if severe, can lead to significant medical and dental problems, such as hand infection and paronychia. Clomipramine and behaviour therapy have been found effective with onychophagia (see Arnold, 2005). Several hypnotherapeutic approaches (see Hammond, 1990, pp. 429–31) have been described for dealing with nail-biting, but empirical studies are lacking. Wagstaff and Royce (1994) investigated a single session of hypnotherapy with nail-biting, emphasising the benefits of stopping the habits and the use of self-suggestion. Seven of eleven subjects, compared to one subject from the control group, stopped biting their nails at five-week follow-up. The results of this preliminary trial indicate that hypnotherapy can be used as an alternative treatment for onychophagia, although more empirical studies are needed.

Factitious Disorders

Factitious dermatological disorders include dermatitis artefacta or factitious dermatitis and psychogenic purpura.

Dermatitis artefacta

Dermatitis artefacta or factitious dermatitis is a disorder in which patients intentionally produce skin lesions in order to assume the sick role (Arnold, 2005). The lesions range from minimal aggravations of a previous genuine dermatosis to intentional cutaneous self-injury, which may be life-threatening because of gangrene or generalised infection (Van Moffaert, 2003). Dermatitis artefacta occurs in about 0.3% of dermatology patients (Gupta, Gupta & Haberman, 1987) and the onset is usually triggered by severe psychosocial stress involving loss, threatened loss or isolation (Stein & Hollander, 1992). Dermatitis artefacta occurs in several psychiatric disorders, including schizo-affective psychosis, monosymptomatic hypochondriacal psychosis, substance abuse, severe anxiety and borderline personality disorder (see Van Moffaert, 2003).

As no controlled trials of the treatment of dermatitis artefacta have been published, the choice of treatment is based on anecdotal experience (Arnold, 2005). Patients with dermatitis artefacta are generally reluctant to be referred to a psychiatrist or psychologist as they deny the self-inflicting nature of their lesions. However, within the context of a good therapeutic alliance, the patient may be open to be referred to a mental health specialist.

Psychogenic purpura

Psychogenic purpura is a rare skin condition characterised by spontaneous appearance of recurrent bruising (purpura). Although psychogenic purpura can be caused by autoerythrocyte sensitisation and conversion reaction, the most likely causation seems to be factitious disorder (Arnold, 2005).

PRINCIPLES OF PSYCHOCUTANEOUS MANAGEMENT

An international group of dermatologists and psychiatrists has developed a consensus statement on the care and management of psychodermatological disorders (Koo et al., 2003). Psychodermatology is defined as a discipline that strives to encourage a comprehensive and humanistic approach to the management of dermatology patients with psychological overlays to their chief complaints (Koo et al., 2003). The main goals of the consensus statement are to promote delivery of quality care, and to help other health professionals understand the complexities of dermatological disorders, particularly the interface between psychiatry and dermatology.

The International Consensus on Care of Psychodermatological Patients advocates six steps to patients' care:

1. Establishing a clear definition of psychodermatological conditions.
2. Forming a good patient–doctor relationship.
3. Having a clear rationale for integrating psychological treatment.
4. The importance of determining an accurate diagnosis.
5. Sensitivity around referral to a psychiatrist.
6. Provision of comprehensive treatment consisting of psychopharmacology, behavioural therapy, psychotherapy, supportive group treatment and stress reduction.

As the cognitive hypnotherapy approach to treatment described in this chapter integrates these six components, each of the components is briefly described below.

Defining Psychodermatological Disorders

Psychodermatological disorders refer to the various conditions that interface between dermatology and psychiatry (Koo *et al.*, 2003). These conditions range from real skin disorders that are exacerbated by emotional stress (e.g. acne vulgaris) to severe self-inflicted skin lesions precipitated by serious underlying psychopathology (e.g. dermatitis artefacta). The field of psychoneuroendocrinimmunodermatology (see Zane, 2003) has evolved to explain the mechanisms underlying the complex interactions between stress and the body in terms of the effects on the endocrine, immune and nervous systems. The psychodermatological conceptualisation also provides a biopsychosocial model of care, emphasising the role of both psychopharmacological and psychological approaches to treatment.

Importance of a Good Patient-Care Provider Relationship

Without establishing good rapport and a therapeutic alliance, it will be almost impossible to formulate an accurate diagnosis and effective treatment regimen. The International Consensus of Care recommends three approaches that the care provider can exercise to build a positive alliance with the patient with a psychocutaneous condition:

- Ensure that the patient does not feel rejected, judged, trivialised or abandoned and deliver the optimal care respectfully.
- Be empathic and convey the message that the message that the practitioner knows what the patient is going through.
- Provide hope and demonstrate a willingness to help.

Determination of Accurate Diagnosis

It is important to make an accurate diagnosis. Without correct diagnosis the treatment ordered is likely to be ineffective and this may demoralise the patient, who may already be frustrated and disappointed. The following guidelines may enhance the accuracy of the diagnosis.

- Rule out primary dermatological or other organic disorders that may be masquerading as a psychocutaneous disorder.
- Do not base a psychiatric diagnosis on skin findings only. Use positive psychiatric findings to make a psychiatric diagnosis.

- Ascertain the nature of the underlying psychopathology, such as anxiety, depression, obsessive-compulsive disorder, personality disorder, psychosis and so on, as the choice of psychopharmacological or psychological intervention will be determined by the underlying psychiatric condition.
- Identify and differentiate between the categories of psychocutaneous disorders: (1) psychophysiological disorders (bona fide skin disorders exacerbated by psychological stress, e.g. acne, eczema or psoriasis); (2) primary psychiatric disorders (e.g. neurotic excoriation or trichotillomania); (3) secondary psychiatric disorders (e.g. anxiety or depression); and (4) cutaneous sensory disorders (e.g. dysesthesia).
- Assess for substance abuse.
- In some cases, skin biopsies or stool analysis for ova and parasites may be necessary.

Sensitivity Around Referral to a Mental Health Practitioner

Although, as a routine, psychocutaneous cases should be referred to a psychiatrist, psychologist or other mental health practitioner, sensitivity should be exercised when making such a referral:

- A psychiatric referral should be discussed and should be made with care and empathy.
- The dermatologist should establish a working relationship with a mental health practitioner so that the patient's care is coordinated.
- When a patient refuses to see a psychiatrist regularly, the dermatologist can continue to provide psychological care in consultation with the psychiatrist, especially when the psychological issues are less serious.
- In cases where the underlying psychopathology is serious and the patient refuses to see a psychiatrist, the dermatologist should exercise extra urging.

Comprehensive Management

A multi-disciplinary treatment approach is recommended. In the absence of a multi-disciplinary team, the treatment should be multi-modal, consisting of psychopharmacology, cognitive behaviour therapy and hypnotherapy.

COGNITIVE HYPNOTHERAPY WITH ACNE VULGARIS

Cognitive hypnotherapy (CH) adopts a multi-modal approach to the treatment of psychocutaneous disorders and integrates the six steps to patients' care advocated by the International Consensus on Care of Psychodermatological Patients (Koo *et al.*, 2003). The CH strategies for treating acne vulgaris are described in detail to illustrate how CH can be systematically utilised with specific psychocutaneous disorders.

Acne vulgaris (referred to as acne in the rest of the chapter) is the most common of all skin disorders. It is a sebaceous gland disorder characterised by a variety of skin lesions, including comedones (non-inflamed bumps), papules, pustules and modules (Arnold, 2005). The lesions occur largely over the face, neck, upper chest and shoulders, and the main complications of the lesions are either pitted or hypertrophic scars. Most cases of acne occur at puberty, although the onset may be delayed into the third and fourth decade. It is estimated that over 90% of adolescent males and 80% of adolescent females are affected by the condition (Rademaker, Garioch & Simpson, 1989).

Although the cause of acne is not known, it is believed to be caused by changes in the hair follicle and the sebaceous glands of the skin that produce sebum. The oily substance plugs the pores, resulting in whiteheads or blackheads (acne comedonica) and pimples (acne papulopustulosa). The changes in the hair follicles and sebaceous glands can be produced by multiple factors, including hormonal changes, sebum production, bacterial colonisation (Brown & Shalita, 1998) and psychological stress (Chiu, Chou & Kimball, 2003; Gupta & Gupta, 2003). Two recent surveys (Green & Sinclair, 2001; Yosipovitch et al., 2007) have reported the close chronological association between the exacerbation of acne and episodes of emotional stress. Green and Sinclair (2001) surveyed 215 sixth-year medical students and found 67% of the students to associate the cause of their acne with stress. The study by Yosipovitch et al. (2007) involved 94 secondary-school students surveyed during high stress (prior to mid-year exams) and low stress (during summer holidays) conditions. The results demonstrated that 23% of the teenagers who were under high levels of stress increased the severity of their acne. These studies suggest there is a significant association between stress and severity of acne.

While it is generally accepted that psychological stress is involved in the pathogenesis of acne, there has been little research to understand the mechanisms behind this relationship. Several writers (e.g. Koo & Smith, 1991; Strauss & Thiboutot, 1999) have proposed the release of adrenal steroids, which affect the sebaceous glands, as responsible for stress-induced aggravation of the acne. The study by Yosipovitch et al. (2007) examined whether the levels of sebum, the oily substance that coats the skin and protects the hair, increase during times of stress and whether they are related to acne severity. The results showed that sebum production did not differ significantly between the high-stress and low-stress conditions. However, the researchers found that students who were reporting high stress were 23% more likely to have increased severity of acne papulopustulosa (pimples). Therefore, the levels of stress were not linked to severity of acne comedonica (white- or blackheads) but to increased severity of pimples (acne papulopustulosa). From these findings, the researchers concluded that acne severity associated with stress may not be related to sebum quantity, but to other factors such as inflammation. Extension of this important study conducted by Yosipovitch et al. (2007) is likely to further elucidate the mechanisms involved in the link between stress and exacerbation of acne.

Nevertheless, it is generally accepted that acne is a psychophysiological disorder. A psychophysiological disorder (previously known as a psychosomatic disorder, and referred to as psychological factors affecting medical condition in the DSM-IV-TR) is characterised by a genuine physical pathology such as asthma, hypertension, migraine headache and peptic ulcer that is caused or worsened by emotional factors (Davison *et al.*, 2005). Acne falls within the psychophysiological category, since patients frequently complain of acne flare-ups when they experience frustration, stress or anxiety (Lee & Koo, 2003). Moreover, severe acne is associated with increased anxiety and poor self-image (Koo & Smith, 1991). Acne can also seriously affect social and occupational functioning and cause significant psychological distress and body image concerns (Gupta *et al.*, 1990). The scarring and disfiguring caused by acne can lead to depression and suicidal ideation (Gupta & Gupta, 1998), which in turn can exacerbate the acne. Most frequently patients with acne predominantly focus on their experience and the psychosocial consequences of having acne than on the physical pathology. As a result, acne patients suffer more from self-consciousness, embarrassment, low self-esteem and suicidal ideation than from the physical symptoms of pain and bleeding (Koo *et al.*, 2003).

Although acne is considered to be a psychophysiological disorder, pharmacological intervention is the main approach to treatment. A topical dermatological therapeutic agent such as isotretinoin (Accutane) is normally used if the symptoms are not promptly controlled by antibiotics. Although isotretinoin is shown to be effective with acne, some anecdotal reports have shown exacerbation of depression, suicidal ideation, suicide attempts and suicide (Jick, Kremers & Vasilakis-Scaramozza, 2000). In some cases, depressed patients have shown improvement in their acne after treatment of depression with paroxetine (Moussavian, 2001).

Given the contribution of emotion and stress to acne, treatments aimed at reducing stress, anger, anxiety and depression have been found to be beneficial. Biofeedback-assisted relaxation and cognitive imagery training have been found to reduce acne severity significantly compared with medical control groups (Hughes *et al.*, 1983). Similarly, hypnosis has been found to be beneficial in reducing potential complications of acne (Shenefelt, 2000). Using post-hypnotic suggestions, Hollander (1959) helped two patients control acne excoriée, a condition in which patients habitually pick their lesions. Whenever either patient felt like picking her face, she was instructed to remember the word 'scar' and to refrain from picking by saying 'scar' instead. The excoriations reduced significantly, although the underlying acne did not resolve. This report indicates hypnosis to be a useful treatment for reducing excoriation.

To summarise, the interplay between acne and psychiatry can be manifested at three levels:

1. Emotional stress can exacerbate the acne.
2. As a consequence of their acne, some patients can develop psychiatric conditions such as depression, social phobia and low self-esteem.
3. Some patients with such primary psychiatric conditions as obsessive-compulsive disorder and psychosis may become preoccupied with their acne (e.g. acne excoriée).

Stages of Cognitive Hypnotherapy (CH) for Acne

CH for acne consists of 11 stages:

1. Assessment and case formulation.
2. Hypnotic induction and deepening.
3. Restoring autonomic balance.
4. Mind over body training.
5. Ego strengthening.
6. Symptom management.
7. Imagery training for healing.
8. Post-hypnotic suggestions.
9. Cognitive behaviour therapy.
10. Problem-solving skills.
11. Self-hypnosis training.

Assessment and Case Formulation

As described in previous chapters, the assessment is carried out in the context of a case-formulation approach (Appendices B and C; see Chapter 2). However, the patient should be asked to describe the areas of the skin that are affected by the acne. This provides the basis for further detailed assessment of the symptoms at each location and enables the therapist and the patient to have a common, shared understanding of which body parts are affected by the acne (White, 2001). The therapist should also inquire about remissions and flare-ups and how the patient reacts to these behaviourally (e.g. scratching, rubbing), cognitively and emotionally. It is also important to gather information about the patient's beliefs about the skin, the acne and its treatment, and other people's reaction to it. The therapist should also briefly screen for obvious psychopathology that may significantly interfere with the management of the acne.

Hypnotic Induction and Deepening

The hypnotic procedure is targeted at the three main components of acne:

1. Physiological changes (inflammation).
2. The subjective experience of having acne (anxiety, depression, shame, embarrassment).

3. The behaviour motivated by the acne (e.g. scratching, rubbing, social withdrawal).

Any formal or informal method of hypnotic induction and deepening can be used. I have adopted the *relaxation with counting method* from Gibbons (1979), which is easily adapted for self-hypnosis training (see Appendix E for a complete script for induction and deepening). The session is audiotaped or made into a CD to facilitate home practice.

Restoring Autonomic Balance

One of the main objectives of using hypnosis is to induce a deep sense of relaxation and restore autonomic balance. By learning to relax, acne sufferers are able to reduce sympathetic arousal and enhance feelings of self-efficacy and control (Bernstein, Borkovec & Hazlett-Stevens, 2000). Moreover, by inducing relaxation, hypnosis reduces anxiety and creates a feeling of well-being. These experiences create a sense of control, promote positive expectancy and strengthen the therapeutic alliance. The hypnotic script presented below provides suggestions for ameliorating the acne, based on a credible or scientific rationale (physical relaxation and emotional calmness). These suggestions are provided when the patient is in a fairly deep trance.

Hypnotic Script for Ameliorating Skin Condition via Relaxation

You have now become so deeply relaxed ... and you are in such a deep, deep hypnotic state ... that your mind has become so sensitive and so receptive to my suggestions ... that everything that I tell you ... will go straight into your unconscious mind. And they will become fully embedded there ... so that they will continue to help you, even when you are not listening to your tape ... so that your skin will continue to heal ... until it is healed up completely.

As you listen to your tape daily ... you will become more relaxed ... and less tense each day. Relaxing your nervous system is the first step towards healing your skin. As the skin and the nervous system are derived from the same material, there is a close connection between the skin and the nervous system. Therefore anything that affects your nervous system, affects your skin. So as you listen to your tape daily ... your skin and your nervous system will become less tense ... and more relaxed every day.

Your skin also acts as a medium through which strong emotions are expressed. We become flushed when we are angry ... we blush when we are embarrassed or confused ... and itch when our desires are frustrated. In fact, the skin reacts very quickly to feelings . . . and because the skin is so readily available to us . . . we often tend to take our aggression or frustration out on our skin.

As you listen to your tape every day . . . you will learn to let go . . . therefore, you will stay calm even when you are upset and frustrated . . . So, your skin will stay calm and relaxed.

Moreover, when you have a skin problem . . . the problem causes upset to your nervous system, which in turn affects the blood flow to your skin . . . and causes irritation to your skin condition. This vicious cycle causes dysregulation of your sweat glands. The dryness, irritation and inflammation of your skin condition are caused by this dysregulation of your sweat glands . . . which may encourage bacteria and fungi to grow in your skin. All these factors interfere with the healing process.

By listening to your self-hypnosis tape every day . . . you will be able to produce a deep sense of relaxation . . . thus restoring proper balance to the functioning of your skin . . . so that the proper blood circulation in your skin will be restored . . . and the proper activity of the sweat glands will be established.

Mind over Body Training (Trance Ratification)

Hypnosis provides a commanding tool for demonstrating the credibility of psychological therapy for acne. The more credible and the more powerful the treatment is perceived to be by the patient, the better the treatment outcome (DePiano & Salzberg,1981). When the patient is in a fairly deep hypnotic trance, eye and body catalepsies (associated with the challenge to open the eyes and get out of the chair or couch) are induced to demonstrate the power of the mind over the body. These demonstrations ratify the power of the hypnotic intervention and provide confidence to the acne patient that the skin condition can be ameliorated.

Ego Strengthening

When experiencing hypnosis, ego-strengthening suggestions are offered to acne patients to increase self-confidence, self-esteem and optimise treatment effect. The enhancement of feelings of self-confidence and self-esteem produces positive expectancy and perceived self-efficacy (Bandura, 1977). If acne sufferers can be helped to view themselves as having the ability to control their symptoms, they will perceive the future as hopeful. The most popular method for increasing self-efficacy within the hypnotherapeutic context is to provide ego-strengthening suggestions. According to Hartland (1971), ego-strengthening suggestions 'remove tension, anxiety and apprehension, and . . . gradually restore the patient's confidence in himself and his ability to cope with his problems'. Appendix E provides a list of ego-strengthening suggestions that can be adapted for use with acne sufferers. However, to ensure credibility and acceptance of the ego-strengthening suggestions, it is important for the ego-strengthening suggestions to be crafted in such a way that they appear credible and logical to the acne patient.

For example, rather than stating 'your acne will disappear', it is advisable to suggest:

> As a result of this treatment and as a result of you listening to your self-hypnosis tape every day, you will begin to relax and learn to let go. And every day as you listen to your tape, you will begin to feel more and more deeply relaxed, less tense, less anxious and less upset, so that every day your mind, your body and your nerves will become more and more relaxed. As a result of this deep relaxation, every day, your mind, your body and your nerves will become stronger and healthier. As a result of this, your acne will become less severe, until it will disappear completely.

Not only does this set of ego-strengthening suggestions sound logical, but improvement becomes contingent on continuing with the therapy and listening to the self-hypnosis tape daily

Symptom Management

Hypnotherapy provides a powerful tool for producing *syncretic cognition* (Alladin, 1994, 2007b), which consists of a variety of cognitive, somatic, perceptual, physiological, visceral and kinaesthetic changes under controlled conditions. Hypnotic production and modulation of these changes provide acne patients with dramatic proof that they can change their feelings and experience, thus providing hope that they can alter their skin conditions. After two or three sessions of hypnosis and ego strengthening, the Shower Technique is introduced to manage the symptoms. The nearby box is an example of the kind of relaxation suggestions that can be given to the patient to gradually reduce the acne.

The Warm Shower Technique

You have now become so deeply relaxed ... you are in such a deep hypnotic trance ... that your mind has become so powerful and so sensitive to what I say ... that you will be able to feel, experience and imagine everything I ask you to feel, experience and imagine.

Now I want you to imagine you are having a warm shower. Imagine the warm water is flowing over your face ... over your back ... flowing over the affected areas of your face ... flowing over the affected areas of your back. Feel the warm water gently moving and spreading over all the affected areas of your face . . . flowing and spreading all over the affected areas on your back.

Imagine you are gently massaging the affected areas while the warm water is flowing . . . and you feel the warm water producing a sense of comfort . . . easing away the irritation . . . easing away the tenderness . . . easing away the rash bumps . . . allowing the skin to heal up. As the comfort spreads over all the affected areas . . . imagine the underlying texture of the skin is changing . . . is softening . . . and becoming more and more normal. You feel your skin changing and becoming more relaxed . . . feeling more comfortable . . . feeling normal. Continue to imagine gently rubbing the warm water to the affected areas in your face and your back until you feel a sense of complete comfort and relief. As the skin feels very relaxed and very comfortable . . . imagine the skin is healing up.

As you imagine the warm water flowing and spreading over your skin, you feel the irritation . . . the discomfort . . . the tenderness . . . and the rash bumps dissipate. As the tenderness and discomfort leave, the skin energy is left to continue the healing. Imagine the injured and irritated skin cells are healing up . . . and new cells are forming on the surface.

The above suggestions can be repeated, modulated and expanded to produce the desired effects. As a result of this hypnotic procedure, many acne sufferers have reported dramatic improvement of their skin. DePiano and Salzberg (1981) maintain that the rapid positive changes experienced by patients undergoing hypnotic procedures are partly due to the profound behavioural, emotional, cognitive and physiological changes brought on by the trance experience.

Imagery Training for Healing

Imagery training is used within the context of the Warm Shower Technique to promote healing of the skin. Once the acne patient is able to induce the warm feeling by visualising having the warm shower, the therapist capitalises on this experience to promote healing of the skin. The suggestions are worded to associate warmth of the skin with increased circulation of blood, which appears logical to the patient.

Script for Healing the Skin

As you continue to imagine the warm water flowing over your skin, become aware of the areas where your skin is affected. Soon you will be able to feel a warm sensation in the areas where your skin is affected. This warm sensation is

(Continued)

due to the fact that the blood circulation has increased in the areas where you feel warm. This extra blood flow is going to bring more oxygen and more nutrition to the areas where your skin is affected. Below the surface of the skin . . . imagine the blood flow is increasing . . . the increased blood flow is bringing more oxygen, more nutrition . . . nourishing the healthy tissue growing on the skin.

For the next few minutes just become aware of the sense of comfort in your skin . . . imagining the skin becoming healthy . . . and new skin replacing the damaged skin. As you listen to the tape every day . . . the soothing and the healing of the skin will continue . . . even when you are not listening to the tape. And each time you listen to the tape . . . the healing and regrowth of your skin will become more activated . . . until the healing is complete . . . the affected skin replaced by healthy new skin.

Post-hypnotic Suggestions

Post-hypnotic suggestions are regarded as a very necessary part of the therapeutic process, as they encourage the patient to carry new possibilities into their future experience (Yapko, 2003). In the treatment of acne, post-hypnotic suggestions serve to ratify the hypnotic experience, promote self-hypnosis, counter problem behaviours (e.g. scratching, rubbing, social avoidance), prevent negative emotions, and forestall dysfunctional cognitions that may trigger, exacerbate or maintain the skin condition. The following post-hypnotic suggestions can be used with acne sufferers. These post-hypnotic suggestions are worded in such a way that they sound logical to patients and they convey a contingent relationship between their behaviour (e.g. listening to the self-hypnosis tape) and the outcome.

Post-hypnotic Suggestions for Acne

As a result of this treatment . . . as a result of listening to your tape every day . . . you are going to feel stronger and fitter in every way. Your circulation will improve . . . particularly the circulation through the little blood vessels that supply the skin. Your heart will beat more strongly . . . so that more blood will flow through the little blood vessels in the skin . . . carrying more oxygen . . . and more nourishment to the skin. Because of this . . . your skin will become much better nourished . . . it will become healthier . . . more normal in texture . . . and the rash will gradually diminish . . . until it fades away completely . . . leaving the underlying new skin perfectly healthy and normal in every way. And . . . as you become more relaxed every day . . . your nervous system will become stronger and steadier . . . so that you will become much less sensitive . . . much less easily irritated . . . therefore your skin will become less upset, less irritated.

Cognitive Behaviour Therapy

Acne is considered a psychophysiological disorder as its physical pathology is worsened by emotional reaction (Lee & Koo, 2003). Given that there is a strong relationship between emotion and acne, the treatment should be aimed at reducing anger, frustration, anxiety and depression. Similarly, there is a strong relationship between stress and acne.

Cognitive behaviour therapy (CBT) is used with acne patients in order to help them deal more effectively with stress and negative emotional reactions. CBT directs acne sufferers to examine the role their thoughts play in generating stress and negative affect. Three to five sessions may be spent on CBT and this treatment is particularly helpful to acne patients with comorbid anxiety or depression. The CBT approach used with acne patients is similar to the sequential format of CBT described with depression in Chapter 3. More specifically, acne patients use the Cognitive Restructuring (ABCDE) form (Appendix B) to identify the circumstances (events) in which their acne flares up. Once the acne-related situations are identified, the patient is coached to identify and restructure the dysfunctional cognitions (see Chapter 3) related to the situations. Cognitive targets may be stress-generating *thoughts* (e.g. 'I can't deal with this situation') or an underlying *belief* or *assumption* (e.g. 'I'm ugly and scarred, no one wants to go out with me') that distils the meaning or theme from many stress-generating thoughts. As discussed in the context of migaine headaches (Chapter 4), the goal of CBT is to train patients to 'catch' their stress-generating thoughts, 'thereby controlling stress and other negative effects, and to render the patient less vulnerable to stress-related negative effect' (Holroyd, 2006, p. 262).

CBT can also be utilised to deal with scratching the affected areas of the skin. In an attempt to help patients with skin disorders refrain from the urge to scratch the skin, White (2001) engages his patients in self-dialogue examining the short-term and long-term consequences of scratching as in the nearby box.

CBT for Controlling Itching

Although my automatic reaction is to scratch, I have discovered the following disadvantages:

- It only helps for a few minutes.
- When I delay it, the itch and urge subside.
- I am starting to get scars from where I have been bleeding.

(Continued)

I can try to:

- Do something, anything else with my hands.
- Place my hands on itchy areas if I need to at first.
- Phone someone – do something to take my mind off it.
- Apply cream.

Problem-Solving Skills

As mentioned above, psychosocial stressors can make acne flare up. Moreover, these stressors can maintain the symptoms. Lasek and Chren (1998) have examined the quality of life of adults with acne. They found acne patients to have decreased dating; decreased eating out; decreased participation in sports; increased unemployment; and impaired academic performance. In order to improve their quality of life, the therapist may have to teach acne patients various problem-solving skills to deal effectively with these situations. Hypnosis can be used for increasing self-esteem and self-efficacy.

Self-Hypnosis Training

The main goal of teaching patients self-hypnosis is to help them develop self-correcting behaviour (Yapko, 2003) and achieve self-reliance and personal power (Alman, 2001). Therefore it is important to teach self-hypnosis to patients with chronic skin conditions. At the end of the first hypnotherapy session, the patient is provided with an audiocassette or CD of self-hypnosis that the patient can use to practise self-hypnosis at home, as homework. This homework assignment provides continuity of treatment between sessions and allows the patient the opportunity to learn self-hypnosis. The self-hypnosis component of hypnotherapy for acne is devised to induce relaxation, promote autonomic balance, increase self-esteem and produce symptom amelioration.

Complex cases

Insight-oriented or exploratory hypnotic techniques can be used when the patient does not respond to the usual treatment protocol. This approach allows the therapist and the patient to explore intrapersonal dynamics and the unconscious origin or purposes of the skin condition. Chapter 4 describes in detail how to conduct insight-oriented hypnotherapy.

SUMMARY

This chapter described the interface between psychiatry and dermatology, and outlined the general principles involved in multi-disciplinary approaches to working with dermatological patients. Psychocutaneous disorders were briefly described to give the reader background information on the major skin disorders classified in the DSM-IV-TR (APA, 2000). The rest of the chapter focused on acne vulgaris to illustrate how cognitive hypnotherapy can be utilised in the treatment of psychocutaneous disorders. The multi-modal treatment described in the chapter can be simply tailored to the treatment of other skin disorders. The cognitive hypnotherapy protocol used for treating acne vulgaris can be subjected to empirical validation very easily.

CHAPTER 7

COGNITIVE HYPNOTHERAPY IN THE MANAGEMENT OF SOMATISATION DISORDER

INTRODUCTION

Somatoform disorders are characterised by complaints of bodily symptoms that suggest physical defects or dysfunctions, but no physiological bases for these symptoms are found. The symptoms are not under voluntary control and they are believed to be caused by psychological factors. The DSM-IV-TR (American Psychiatric Association [APA], 2000) lists seven types of somatoform disorders, namely pain disorder, body dysmorphic disorder, hypochondriasis, conversion disorder, somatisation disorder, undifferenti-ated somatoform disorder and somatoform disorder not otherwise specified. The goal of this chapter is to review the aetiology and existing empirical treat-ments for somatisation disorder and then to describe *cognitive hypnotherapy* for somatisation disorder, a multi-modal treatment approach that combines cognitive behaviour therapy with hypnosis. But before focusing on somatisa-tion disorder, the other types of somatoform conditions are briefly reviewed to provide readers some background information on the whole spectrum of somatoform syndromes. The treatment cognitive hypnotherapy approach described here for somatisation disorder can be easily adapted to the treatment of other forms of somatoform conditions.

PAIN DISORDER

In pain disorder, the chief complaint is pain, and psychological factors are known to play an important role in the onset, maintenance and severity of the pain. Pain disorder causes significant distress and impairment, and the patient may be unable to work and may become dependent on paink-illers or tranquillisers (Davison *et al.*, 2005). The lifetime prevalence for pain disorder in the general population is 12% and twice as many women as men suffer from the condition (Thomassen *et al.*, 2003). The pain experienced by pain disorder patients may have a temporal relationship with some stress or conflict, or it may provide secondary gain in the form of avoidance behaviour or gaining sympathy. As the pain worsens and remains unresolved, the associated morbidity, such as functional disability, increased health services utilisation, inappropriate treatment with medications, excessive evaluations and higher rates of psychiatric disorders, increases (see Clark & Chodynicki, 2005). Moreover, patients with medically unexplained chronic pain are at risk of iatrogenic consequences, excessive diagnostic tests, inappropriate medication and unnecessary surgery.

As pain is always influenced by psychological factors, it is often difficult to differentiate between somatoform pain and medically accountable pain. It is also not easy to decide when a pain transcends into a somatoform pain. However, from the way the patients describe their pain, an experienced clinician can deduce an accurate diagnosis. For example, patients with physically based pain seem to be more specific about the locality of the pain, give a more detailed sensory account of the pain and link their pain more clearly to situations (e.g. physical activities) that increase or decrease the pain (Adler *et al.*, 1997). Patients with pain disorder, on the other hand, are less specific about the location of their pain, they provide vague or less detailed descriptions of the pain experience, the pain is often triggered by emotional or conflict situations and, at times, the pain can dramatically occur or disappear. By definition, pain disorder is associated with psychological factors, and both classical and operant learning may be involved in the aetiology of the condition (Cloninger, 1993). In terms of classical conditioning, neutral settings such as the workplace or the bedroom, where the pain was initially experienced, come to evoke pain-related behaviour. In terms of operant conditioning, pain-related complaints may be reinforced by increased attention and sympathy, relief from unpleasant activities, monetary compensations and the pleasurable effects of analgesics. The gate control theory of pain developed by Melzack and Wall (1983) provides a useful model for understanding how psychological processes are involved in the perception of pain (King, 1994).

The major goals in the treatment of pain disorder are to reduce 'pain-related behaviour' and encourage activity. King (1994) warns clinicians not to use sedative-anxiety drugs and opioids with pain disorder. He proposes judicious use of analgesics on a fixed interval schedule so as not to reinforce pain-related behaviours and recommends psychological interventions such as biofeedback, relaxation training, operant conditioning, cognitive behaviour therapy and hypnotherapy. Hypnosis is particularly effective as it induces deep muscle relaxation and helps the patients 'dissociate' from the pain (First & Tasman, 2004). A well-known hypnotic method for dissociating from the pain is to suggest to the patient that the pain and the affected part are being separated, or to suggest that the pain is 'somewhere else', for example in another part of the room (Heap & Aravind, 2002, p. 358). Another popular hypnotic technique for dissociating from pain is to become detached from the whole body, as described in detail by Barabasz and Watkins (2005, pp. 236–7).

BODY DYSMORPHIC DISORDER

The essential feature of body dysmorphic disorder (BDD) is the preoccupation with an imagined defect in appearance or a markedly excessive concern with a minor physical anomaly that is accompanied by significant distress or impairment in social or occupational functioning (APA, 2000). Some patients with BDD spend hours each day checking on their defect or looking at themselves in mirrors. Other patients take steps to avoid being reminded of the defect by eliminating mirrors from their homes or camouflaging the defect (Davison *et al.*, 2005). These concerns can be so distressing that some patients seek plastic surgery. Approximately 5% of patients seeking cosmetic surgery have BDD. The onset of the condition is usually in late adolescence, occurring mostly in women, and it is frequently comorbid with depression, obsessive compulsive disorder, social phobia, substance abuse and personality disorders (Corove & Gleaves, 2001; Veale, De Haro & Lambrou, 2003). Although a number of sociological, psychological and neurobiological theories of BDD have been proposed (First & Tasman, 2004), the aetiology of BDD is poorly understood. Some theorists view it as a variant of an eating disorder or a form of obsessive compulsive disorder; others argue that it can be regarded as delusional disorder, or a symptom of other psychiatric disorders (see Davison *et al.*, 2005).

Treatment strategies for BDD have included cosmetic surgery, pharmacotherapy, psychotherapy and a combination of medication and psychotherapy. Corove and Gleaves (2001), from their review of the treatment outcome literature with BDD, found cognitive behavioural strategies to be effective with both the symptoms of BDD and the associated features. Although the effectiveness of hypnosis-based interventions for BDD has not been empirically tested, hypnosis appears to be an effective form of adjunctive treatment for body image related to eating disorders (Barabasz & Watkins, 2005; Hammond, 1998). Perhaps similar kinds of procedures may be utilised with BDD. Finally, some studies suggest that selective serotonin reuptake inhibitors (SSRIs) can be effective in some cases in reducing obsessional thoughts and compulsive behaviours (Phillips & Najjar, 2003).

HYPOCHONDRIASIS

Hypochondriasis is characterised by persistent fears of having a serious disease based on the misinterpretation of one or more bodily symptoms despite medical reassurance (APA, 2000). Although the disorder can begin at any age, the onset is most commonly in early childhood and about 5% of the general population is affected by the condition (Asmundson *et al.*, 2001). Hypochondriasis patients have a high rate of psychiatric comorbidity, including generalised anxiety disorder, dysthymia, major depressive disorder, somatisation disorder and panic disorder (Barsky, Wyshak & Klerman, 1992). These patients tend to be frequent consumers of medical services and the potential exists for them to sustain iatrogenic damage from repeated investigations.

The aetiology of hypochondriasis is not fully understood. However, the cognitive theory is often cited as the most acceptable explanation of hypochondriasis. This theory holds that individuals with hypochondriasis over-react to ordinary physical sensations and minor abnormalities, such as irregular heartbeat, sweating, occasional coughing, a sore spot or stomach ache, seeing these as evidence for their belief that there is something seriously wrong with them (Davison *et al.*, 2005). Currently, the trend in hypochondriasis research is to focus on health anxiety rather than on hypochondriasis per se. Asmundson *et al.* (2001, p. 4) define health anxiety as 'health related fears and beliefs, based on interpretations, or perhaps more often, misinterpretations, of bodily signs and symptoms as being indicative of serious illness'. Health anxiety is not limited to hypochondriasis but can also be linked with anxiety and mood disorders, and it represents both hypochondriasis and illness phobia.

Psychological treatment, namely cognitive behaviour therapy, is considered the first-choice intervention with hypochondriasis (Looper & Kirmayer, 2002). Some hypochondriacal patients have shown positive effects from antidepressant medication such as clomipramine, fluvoxamine, imipramine and paroxetine (First & Tasman, 2004). Heap and Aravind (2002) have suggested the use of hypnotherapy with hypochondriasis in terms of direct symptom control, correcting attentional biases and correcting interpretative biases.

CONVERSION DISORDER

Conversion disorders are characterised by symptoms or deficits affecting voluntary, motor or sensory function that are suggestive of, yet are not fully explained by, a neurological or other general medical condition or the direct effects of a substance (First & Tasman, 2004). Psychological factors are known to be associated with symptom onset, exacerbation or maintenance. The psychological nature of the symptoms is clearly demonstrated by the fact that they appear suddenly in stressful situations, allowing the individual to avoid some activity or responsibility or to receive badly wanted attention (Davison *et al.*, 2005). However, the symptoms are not intentionally produced or feigned; that is, the individual does not consciously contrive a symptom for external rewards, as in malingering, or for the intra-psychic rewards of assuming the sick role, as in factitious disorder (First & Tasman, 2004). The term *conversion* was originally used by Freud, who hypothesised that the psychic energy of a repressed instinct was diverted into sensory-motor channels and blocked functioning. Freud thus viewed anxiety and psychological conflict as converted into physical symptoms.

Prevalence rates of conversion disorder are estimated to be approximately 0.3% in the general population, 1–3% in medical outpatients and 1–4.5% in hospitalised neurological and medical patients respectively (Toone, 1990). The onset is typically in adolescence and more women than men are given the diagnosis (Davison *et al.*, 2005).

Conversion disorder is difficult to treat because the patients do not believe that there is anything wrong with them psychologically. Many forms of therapy, including behavioural, cognitive behavioural, suggestion-based, psychodynamic, physical and biofeedback, have been used with conversion disorder. Although case-based anecdotal evidence has been advanced to support effectiveness, there is no agreement about the most effective therapy for conversion symptoms (Moene *et al.*, 2003). To examine the effectiveness of hypnotherapy with conversion disorder, Moene *et al.* (2003) randomly assigned 44 outpatients with conversion disorder, motor type, to either hypnosis or a waiting-list condition. They found hypnosis to be effective in reducing motor disability and behavioural symptoms associated with the motor conversion. Chaves (1996) provides a detailed description of utilising hypnotic strategies with somatoform disorders, which can be easily adapted to conversion disorder.

SOMATISATION DISORDER

Clinical Characteristics and Epidemiology of Somatisation Disorder

Somatisation disorder, historically referred to as hysteria or Briquet's syndrome, represents DSM-IV-TR's distillation of the long and convoluted struggle to define the complex, multi-faceted syndrome first described by Paul Briquet in 1859. In DSM-IV-TR, somatisation disorder is characterised by multiple somatic complaints, with no apparent physical cause, for which medical attention is sought (Davison *et al.*, 2005). To meet DSM-IV-TR criteria, the patient must have

1. A history of at least four pain symptoms in different sites or functions (e.g. head, abdomen, back, joints, extremities, chest, rectum, during menstruation, during sexual intercourse or during urination).
2. Two gastrointestinal symptoms other than pain (e.g. nausea, bloating, vomiting other than during pregnancy, diarrhoea or intolerance of several different foods).
3. One sexual or reproductive symptom other than pain (e.g. sexual indifference, erectile or ejaculatory dysfunction, irregular menses, excessive menstrual bleeding, vomiting throughout pregnancy).
4. One pseudoneurological symptom or deficit (e.g. those of conversion disorder).
5. Symptoms started before the age of 30 years and persisted over a period of several years.

These symptoms are more pervasive and impairing than the complaints of hypochondriasis and the specific symptoms vary across cultures. For example, the disorder has been found to be more prevalent in cultures where overt emotions are discouraged (Ford, 1995). The lifetime prevalence of somatisation disorder ranges from 0.2% to 2.0% among women and less than 0.2% in men from the general population (APA, 2000). The prevalence rate is much higher (1–5%) in the medical setting, as patients with somatisation disorder actively seek medical help (Simon & Gureje, 1999). The condition typically starts in early childhood and seems to run in families; it is found in about 20% of the first-degree relatives of index cases (Guze, 1993).

Somatisation disorder is characterised by excessive medical and psychiatric complaints. As many as 75% have comorbid Axis I diagnoses, including major depressive disorder, dysthymia, panic disorder, simple phobia and substance abuse (Katon et al., 1991). Up to 50% of patients with somatisation disorder are estimated to meet criteria for a lifetime diagnosis of major depressive disorder (Simon & Von Korff, 1991). Personality disorders – Cluster B (antisocial, borderline, histrionic and narcissistic) diagnoses in psychiatric settings and Cluster C (avoidant, dependent and obsessive compulsive) in primary care settings – are also common in patients with somatisation disorder (Rost et al., 1992). Many patients with somatisation disorder may also have medically explained symptoms. For example, cancer patients may have comorbid somatisation symptoms. Moreover, patients with somatisation disorder often have multiple social problems and chaotic lifestyles characterised by poor interpersonal relationships, disruptive or difficult behaviour, substance abuse and significant occupational and social impairment (see Abbey, 2006). Somatisation disorder is a chronic but fluctuating disorder, seldom remitting completely, and many patients experience iatrogenic disease or injury secondary to unnecessary diagnostic investigations, polypharmacy and polysurgery (Abbey, 2006). One study found patients with somatisation disorder to utilise nine times the US per capita health cost (Smith, Monson & Ray, 1986). Pilowsky (1969) uses the phrase 'abnormal illness behaviour' to describe the dysfunctional behaviours (disproportionate use and misuse of healthcare services) in which patients with hypochondriasis and somatisation engage. According to Pilowsky, inppropriate healthcare-seeking behaviour is motivated by fear of disease and/or the potential rewards of the 'sick role' (Woolfolk & Allen, 2007).

The abnormal illness behaviour of patients with somatisation disorder is also seen in the home and occupational settings. Because of their discomfort, fatigue and/or fears of exacerbating their symptoms, somatisers withdraw from both productive and pleasurable activities. Allen et al. (2006) found 36–83% of these patients to be unemployed and 18–60% to be receiving disability payments from either their employers or the government. In fact, the functional impairments are so substantial that patients with somatisation disorder spend between two and seven days in bed per month (Katon et al., 1991).

Integrated Model of Somatisation Disorder

Many theories have been proposed to explain the cause of somatisation disorder, but none has provided a complete scientific theory based on empirical research. To date, Brown (2004) has attempted to provide the most unified and comprehensive conceptual model of somatisation disorder, based on theories and research from mainstream cognitive psychology. In particular, his model is derived from research on the role of different attentional mechanisms in shaping contents of consciousness and controlling thought and action. This model informs and guides the cognitive hypnotherapy approach to treating somatising symptoms described in this chapter. Brown's model is not a new model of somatisation disorder, but an extension of the existing models. His model is integrative in the sense that it accommodates the basic elements of dissociation, conversion and somatisation concepts within a common explanatory framework. However, the model is not restricted to somatisation disorder, it attempts to explain the functional somatisation involved in several DSM-IV somatoform and dissociative disorders, including pain disorder, conversion disorder, somatisation disorder, dissociative amnesia and dissociative fugue. Brown's model provides a general account that can be accommodated to each specific somatoform syndrome. Moreover, although there are common mechanisms underlying different medically unexplained symptoms, each case is likely to be moderated by a variety of factors and hence the same processes may not be involved in the creation and maintenance of similar cases. The model is briefly reviewed here, with the emphasis on somatisation disorder.

Brown's integrative model of medically unexplained symptoms has two principal aims: it provides a precise and mechanistic account of how it is possible to experience compelling symptoms in the absence of underlying pathology; and it clarifies how the development and maintenance of unexplained symptoms are moderated by different risk factors (Brown, 2004). The model can be conveniently discussed under five headings:

- attention, consciousness, and control
- alterations in perception and control
- origins of rogue representations
- development of symptom chronicity
- body-focused attention

Attention, consciousness and control

Information processing involves a complex chain of sensory, perceptual, semantic and memorial analyses. At any given time, the *cognitive system* is inundated with information and it is the function of the *attentional system* to direct action and select relevant information for further processing. This selection process draws from the most active information available in sensory, perceptual and memorial systems triggered by the receipt of sense data to produce control of routine behaviour and further processing at higher levels of the system. The parallel spread of activation in perceptual and memorial systems generates a number of perceptual hypotheses, each representing a possible interpretation of the stimulus world based on previous experience (Marcel, 1983). The most active perceptual hypothesis is then selected by the primary attentional system (PAS) to provide a working account of the environment for the control of action. However, the PAS is influenced by several factors, including the nature of the available sense data; the activation of competing and complementary representations in memory; the selection threshold of perceptual hypotheses in question; and top-down input from high-level attention (Brown, 2004). In this model, routine behaviours are controlled automatically or without conscious effort by the underlying *schemata* (hierarchical systems of cognitive representations) or by the secondary attentional system or volitional (conscious) moderating cognitions that indirectly affects the schemata.

Alterations in perception and control

The cognitive processing research has a number of implications for understanding somatisation disorder. First, it suggests that behaviours are governed by non-volitional control systems and therefore functional dissociation between experience and action can occur easily. Second, it demonstrates that subjective awareness is a construction or interpretation of the world rather than a reflection of objective reality. This indicates that at times there may be no direct mapping between sensory data and the contents of subjective experience, as illustrated by such phenomena as hallucinations, misperceptions, hypnosis, placebo effects, certain illusions and defence mechanisms (Hilgard, 1977; Wall, 1993). These phenomena underscore the fact that perceptual experience can be over-determined by prior information (e.g. memories) stored in the schemata and they represent a compelling model for somatisation disorder. In this model, unexplained symptoms arise when the PAS chronically selects inappropriate information during attentional selection and automatic control processing. In other words, although the sensory data is misrepresented, the subjective experience is considered valid (i.e. 'real' symptoms) because the individual does not have introspective access to the inferences made during the creation of experience and control of action. The nature of the resulting symptom is determined by the kind of information involved in the process.

The model proposed by Brown (2004) is consistent with contemporary dissociation theory, which asserts that unexplained symptoms are generated preconsciously by an attentional gating mechanism (e.g. Ludwig, 1972; Sierra & Berrios, 1999). It also captures Janet's (1889) original idea that unexplained symptoms reflect a distortion in awareness resulting from information that has become 'stuck' in the cognitive system. More importantly, the model assumes that there is horizontal dissociation between different levels of processing in the cognitive system. This assumption explains the paradox inherent in all somatoform symptoms that the patients are not able to control their perception, cognition or action despite repeated and honest attempts to exert control.

Origins of rogue representations

Brown (2004) uses the concept of 'rogue representation' to explain the psychogenic nature of unexplained symptoms. Somatoform complaints are not caused by disturbances in the neural hardware; they constitute alterations in body image generated by misrepresentation of information in the cognitive system. In the model, the term rogue representation is used as a generic label for the inappropriate information selected by the PAS. It is asserted that 'any kind of information within the cognitive system concerning the nature of physical symptoms can provide a template for the development of an unexplained complaint' (Brown, 2004, p. 802). Rogue representations are acquired from different sources, including direct exposure to physical states in the self (somatisation patients often have a history of physical illness); indirect exposure to physical states in others (many somatisers have been exposed to abnormal levels of illness in the family environment); sociocultural transmission of information about health and illness ('genuine' symptoms are often shaped by sociocultural conceptions of illness); and direct verbal suggestion (autosuggestions or heterosuggestions can produce hypnotic phenomena akin to somatoform symptoms).

Development of symptom chronicity

Given that we all possess rogue representations for a potential somatoform complaint, the model identifies self-focused attention to account for differential effect and the chronicity of the condition. According to the model, any factors that serve to increase symptom-focused attention will contribute to the development and maintenance of medically unexplained symptoms. These factors include misattribution of symptoms to physical illness (patients' experience of symptoms and their behavioural responses to them strongly influence the interpretation of symptomatology), negative affect (increasing symptom-focused attention), illness worry and rumination (leading to 'cognitive-attentional syndrome' characterised by chronic rumination, worry and symptom focus; maladaptive coping; and reduction of central processing resources), illness behaviour (engagement in 'checking', medical consulting, information seeking, reassurance seeking, avoidance and doctor shopping, directing more attention towards the body) and certain personality traits (e.g. negative affectivity, high hypnotic susceptibility).

Body-focused attention

Somatisation patients report a significantly higher incidence of chronic emotional and physical abuse relative to comparison subjects (e.g. Brown, Schrag & Trimble, 2005). The model considers body-focused attention to be a means of avoiding the affect and cognitive activity associated with such traumatic events as physical, sexual or emotional abuse. The development of somatic symptoms also provides a way of expressing negative affect without acknowledging its psychosocial source. Moreover, the symptoms may be maintained by additional advantages conferred to the individual, such as secondary gains, positive reinforcement (e.g. greater emotional support) and negative reinforcement (e.g. prevention of revictimisation).

Treatment Outcome Research

The treatment approaches, either pharmacological or psychosocial, for somatisation disorder have been targeted more at the management of the symptoms than at curing the illness (First & Tasman, 2004).

Pharmacological treatment

Despite the frequent use of medication and the sizeable body of research on the pharmacological treatment of somatisation disorder, the evidence for long-term efficacy of medication with somatisation disorder is lacking (Woolfolk & Allen, 2007). However, data from controlled clinical trials provide (moderately effective) support for using amitriptyline, duloxetine (reuptake inhibitors of both serotonin and norepinephrine), alosetron and tegaserod (serotonergic medications) and St John's wort for reducing somatisation and associated symptoms (Woolfolk & Allen, 2007; for detailed reviews see Arnold, Keck & Welge, 2000; Jailwala, Imperiale & Kroenke, 2000; Klein, 1988; Whiting *et al.*, 2001).

Psychosocial treatment

Psychosocial interventions for treating somatisation disorder that have been subjected to controlled studies include short-term dynamic therapy, relaxation training, exercise regimens, behaviour therapy, cognitive therapy and cognitive behavioural therapy. The data indicate that, in general, psychosocial interventions are moderately effective in reducing the physical symptoms associated with somtisation spectrum disorders and the improvements persist as much as a year after the treatment (Woolfolk & Allen, 2007). However, none of the psychosocial interventions appears to be superior to any of the others. Woolfolk and Allen (2007) believe that the lack of difference in efficacy between the psychosocial treatments may be due to a great deal of overlap of techniques among the interventions (e.g. relaxation, changing of maladaptive behaviour, problem-solving strategies, physical exercise and so on).

Allen *et al.* (2006) have examined the efficacy of cognitive behaviour therapy (CBT) with full somatisation disorder. They conducted a randomised, controlled treatment trial in which 84 patients diagnosed with full somatisation disorder received either augmented standard medical care (ASMC) or 10 sessions of CBT. The ASMC consisted of standard medical care supplemented by psychiatric consultations, which is considered to be evidence-based practice (Mayou *et al.*, 2005). The CBT comprised relaxation training, behaviour modification, emotional awareness, cognitive restructuring and interpersonal skills training. The results showed that CBT produced significant improvements in somatisation symptoms and functioning over and above those obtained from augmented standard medical care. The improvements were observed immediately after the 10-session treatment phase and persisted for a year. To date, this is the only psychological treatment that has been shown to be effective with somatisation disorder in a methodically adequate randomised controlled trial.

Based on the findings of their study, Woolfolk and Allen (2007) have developed a multi-faceted psychosocial treatment approach, called *affective cognitive behavioural therapy* (ACBT), for treating somatoform disorder. ACBT includes cognitive, experiential, interpersonal and behavioural interventions. This treatment approach is consonant with the biopsychosocial conceptualisation of somatisation disorder that emphasises the interaction of physiology, cognition, emotion, acceptance, behaviour and environment in the causation and maintenance of the symptoms. Cognitive hypnotherapy (CH), described in the rest of the chapter, integrates the components of ACBT with hypnotherapy in the management of somatisation disorder.

COGNITIVE HYPNOTHERAPY FOR SOMATISATION DISORDER

As the model of somatisation disorder described in this chapter includes elements of dissociation, conversion and somatisation, it would appear intuitive to utilise hypnotherapy in the management of the medically unexplained symptoms. Although there is no randomised clinical trial of hypnosis-based treatment for somatisation disorder reported in the literature, there are several reasons for combining hypnosis with CBT.

First, many early psychiatric luminaries such as Charcot, Janet, Breuer and Freud successfully treated somatoform disordered patients with hypnosis and noted the similarity between hypnotic response and somatisation (Moene *et al.*, 2003). Recent brain-imaging studies have supported the proposition that there are common neurological processes shared by hypnotic responding and somatoform symptoms (Halligan *et al.*, 2000; Marshall *et al.*, 1997). These findings have led many contemporary theorists to propose that hypnotic interventions may be useful in the treatment of somatoform disorders.

Second, because there are similarities in the neurological mechanisms involved in hypnosis and somatoform disorders, somatisation patients might be particularly responsive to hypnotic suggestions. It is well established that patients with somatoform disorders have high hypnotic capacity. For example, Bliss (1984) found conversion patients to score an average of 9.7 on the Hypnotic Induction Profile (HIP) 12-point scale. This finding was corroborated by Maldonado (1996a, 1996b), which led him to hypothesise that patients with conversion disorder may be using their own capacity to dissociate to displace uncomfortable emotional feeling onto a chosen body part, which then becomes dysfunctional. Therefore Maldonado and Spiegel (2003) propose that since the hypnotic phenomena may be involved in the aetiology of some somatoform symptoms, hypnosis can be used to control the symptoms. Maldonado and Spiegel suggest that hypnosis can be used with somatoform disorders both as a diagnostic tool and as an adjunct to treatment.

Third, somatoform symptoms can be elicited during hypnosis (Thornton, 1976), thus creating positive expectancy and credibility of the hypnotic procedures.

Fourth, as discussed earlier in this chapter, hypnotic susceptibility, dissociation and conversion play an important role in the aetiology of somatisation disorder. Within this conceptualisation of somatisation, it makes logical sense to use hypnosis to manage the symptoms.

Fifth, hypnotherapy has been reported by many authors to be effective in the management of somatoform disorders (e.g. Frankel, 1994; Maldonado & Spiegel, 2003). Although, to date, no randomised controlled clinical trial of hypnotherapy for somatisation disorder has been reported in the literature, the hypnosis-based treatment utilised by Moene *et al.* (2003) for conversion disorder can be easily adapted to the treatment of somatisation. In their randomised controlled clinical trial of hypnosis-based treatment for conversion disorder, motor type, Moene *et al.* (2003) found hypnosis to be effective in reducing motor disability and behavioural symptoms associated with motor conversion.

There are also several empirical reasons for combining hypnosis with CBT in the management of somatisation disorder. A literature review (Schoenberger, 2000), meta-analysis (Kirsch, Montgomery & Sapirstein, 1995) and empirical studies (Alladin & Alibhai, 2007; Bryant *et al.*, 2005) have demonstrated that when hypnotherapy is combined with CBT in the management of emotional disorders, the effect size increases. Moreover, well-controlled studies of hypnotherapy in the management of a variety of medical conditions have demonstrated the clinical efficacy of hypnosis (Lynn *et al.*, 2000; Pinnell & Covino,

2000). The effectiveness of hypnosis in the management of pain has been even more remarkable. For example, a meta-analysis of controlled trials of hypnotic analgesia demonstrates that hypnotherapy can provide relief for 75% of the patients studied (Montgomery, DuHammel & Redd, 2000). The treatment effect was largest for the patients who were highly suggestible to hypnosis. The National Institute of Health Technology Assessment Panel on Integration of Behavioural and Relaxation Approaches into the Treatment of Chronic Pain and Insomnia (1996) reviewed outcome studies on hypnosis with pain and concluded that there is strong research evidence that hypnosis is effective with chronic pain. Similarly, a meta-analysis review of contemporary research on hypnosis and pain management (Montgomery, DuHamel & Redd, 2000) documented that hypnosis meets the American Psychological Association criteria (Chambless & Hollon, 1998) for being an efficacious and specific treatment for pain, showing superiority over medication, psychological placebos and other treatments.

More recently, Elkins, Jensen and Patterson (2007) reviewed 13 controlled prospective trials of hypnosis for the treatment of chronic pain, which compared outcomes from hypnosis for the treatment of chronic pain to either baseline data or a control condition. The data from the review indicates that hypnosis interventions consistently produce significant decreases in pain associated with a variety of chronic pain problems (cancer, low back problems, arthritis, sickle cell disease, temporomandibular conditions, fibromyalgia, physical disability and mixed aetiologies, e.g. 15 lumbar pain, 7 rheumatological pain, 3 cervical pain, 1 peripheral neuropathy, 1 gynaecological-related pain). Also, hypnosis was generally found to be more effective than non-hypnotic interventions such as attention, physical therapy and education. Similarly, Hammond (2007), from his review of the literature on the effectiveness of hypnosis in the treatment of headache and migraine (see Chapter 4), concluded that hypnotherapy meets the clinical psychology research criteria for being a well-established and efficacious treatment for tension and migraine headaches. Hammond pointed out that hypnotherapy 'is virtually free of the side effects, risks of adverse reactions, and ongoing expense associated with accompany medication treatments'.

CH for somatisation disorder combines CBT and hypnotic strategies and the treatment is extended over 16 weekly sessions of one hour each. CH for somatisation disorder is specifically designed in a structured way to test for the clinical usefulness of adding a hypnotherapy component to the CBT protocol evaluated by Allen *et al.* (2006). An additive design involves a strategy in which the treatment to be tested is added to another treatment to determine whether the treatment added produces an incremental improvement over the first treatment (Allen *et al.*, 2006). The 16 weeks of CH, which draw heavily from Woolfolk and Allen (2007), comprise hypnotherapy, self-hypnosis, behaviour modification, cognitive restructuring, emotional awareness, positive mood induction and interpersonal skills training.

SESSION 1

The first session is devoted to clinical assessment and goal setting. Before initiating CH it is important for the therapist to take a detailed clinical history to formulate the diagnosis and identify the essential psychological, physiological, social and environmental aspects of the patient's behaviours within a biopsychosocial framework. As many somatisation patients have complex symptom histories, assessment should be seen as a process that occurs throughout the treatment (Woolfolk & Allen, 2007).

Clinical Assessment

The most efficient way to obtain all this information is to take a case-formulation approach as described in Chapter 2. The main function of the case formulation is to devise an effective treatment plan. Moreover, the case-formulation approach allows the clinician to translate and tailor a nomothetic (general) treatment protocol to the individual (idiographic) patient. Alladin (2007b) has described in great detail how to conduct cognitive hypnotherapy case formulation in order to select the most effective and efficient treatment strategies. This approach emphasises the role of cognitive distortions, negative self-instructions, irrational automatic thoughts and beliefs, schemas and negative ruminations or negative self-hypnosis. By conceptualising a case, the clinician develops a working hypothesis on how the patient's problems can be understood in terms of the integrated model of somatisation disorder described by Brown (2004). This model provides a compass or a guide to understanding the treatment process. The evidence suggests that matching of treatment to particular patient characteristics increases outcome (Beutler, Clarkin & Bongar, 2000).

In order to identify the mechanisms that underlie the somatising patient's problems, the eight-step case formulation derived from the work of Alladin (2007b), Ledley, Marx and Heimberg (2005) and Persons, Davidson and Tompkins (2001) can be used. The eight components summarised in Table 7.1 are described in detail below. Appendix C provides a generic template for a CH case-formulation and treatment plan and Appendix D provides a completed example of a CH case-formulation and treatment plan for Jackie (a depressed patient).

Goal Setting

As most somatisation patients have a long history of unexplained medical symptoms, repeated medical examinations and investigations, and various medical and psychosocial interventions without significant outcome, they feel confused, frustrated, helpless and suspicious about ever getting better,

Table 7.1 Eight-step cognitive hypnotherapy case formulation for somatisation disorder

---

1. List the major symptoms and problems in functioning.
   - Lifetime medical and psychiatric histories and social, physical and occupational information are thoroughly reviewed. It is important to examine the symptoms as part of the larger biopsychosocial context and liaise closely with the treating physician or psychiatrist in order to avoid unnecessary piecemeal medical testing. Self-rating measures such as the Somatic Symptom Questionnaire (SSQ; Woolfolk *et al.*, 1998) and the Severity of Somatic Symptoms Scale (SSS; Allen *et al.*, 2001) can be used to screen and assess the severity of the symptoms. As somatisation patients have high rates of emotional distress, it is advisable to assess for concomitant psychopathology, particularly anxiety and depression.
2. Formulate a formal diagnosis.
   - To make an accurate diagnosis, a structured interview such as the Structured Clinical Interview for DSM-IV Axis I Disorders (SCID; First *et al.*, 1997) or the Composite International Diagnostic Interview (CIDI; World Health Organization, 1994) is recommended.
3. Formulate a working hypothesis.
   - Hypothesise the underlying mechanism producing the listed problems.
4. Identify the precipitants and activating situations.
   - List triggers for current problems and establish connections between the underlying mechanism and triggers of current problems.
5. Explore the origin of negative self-schemas.
   - Establish the origin of core beliefs from childhood experience, early adverse negative life events, or the manifestation of initial somatic symptoms. History of treatment (treatment failures and uncertainty of unexplained symptoms) and genetic predisposition (diathesis) may also provide various cognitive distortions related to the illness.
6. Summarise the working hypothesis.
   - Indicate how triggers lead to onset or exacerbation of symptoms, how the patient reacts emotionally and behaviourally, and how others react.
7. Outline the treatment plan.
   - Outline treatment goals and indicate the measures that will be used to monitor progress. List intervention modalities that will be utilised and indicate the frequency of treatment sessions. Also outline the adjunctive therapies that will be prescribed.
8. Identify strengths and assets and predict obstacles to treatment.
   - List the strengths and assets that may enhance the treatment effect. It is also important to identify and predict obstacles that may interfere with outcome.

---

believing that the doctors have given up on them. The clinicians need to be sensitive to these feelings and sentiments and the patient's suspicion can be alleviated by setting realistic goals. I find discussion of the following treatment goals reassuring to patients and it conveys a sense of realistic hope.

- The treatment may not cure the condition, but it will help to ameliorate the symptoms.
- The treatment approach is skills based; that is, the focus is on teaching the patients how to manage their symptoms.
- The treatment requires full collaboration between the patient and the therapist.
- The therapist serves as a guide or instructor and the patient is encouraged to become fully engaged not just in learning the skills but in trying them out.
- To a large extent, treatment gains are contingent on homework. The homework is an essential part of the intervention. The homework allows continuity between sessions and it helps build confidence and disrupt patterns of behaviour that might not have been useful in the past. Moreover, the homework consolidates skills learnt and the physiological changes produced by hypnosis.

SESSION 2

Session 2 focuses on:

1. Review of the week.
2. Discussing the rationale for treatment.
3. Providing an overview of the treatment.
4. Establishing rapport.
5. Reviewing the patient's physical symptoms.
6. Introducing the symptom-monitoring forms.
7. Assessing for hypnotic suggestibility.

Reviewing the Week

Although each treatment session is agenda driven and fairly structured, the therapist should create opportunities to allow the patient to express concerns or opinions. One of the ways to address this issue is to review the week at the beginning of each session, before setting the agenda for the session. The review should cover impressions of the last session (what was useful or not useful), the intensity of symptoms or level of distress during the week, level of activities, social interaction and other concerns.

The main focus of the review in the second session centers on the impression of the last session and goals of the treatment. Reviewing the impression of the first session allows patients the opportunity to express their attitudes (negative or positive), reservations or optimism about the treatment and the therapeutic goals.

Rationale of Treatment

Having a clear understanding of the rationale for utilising a specific treatment generates therapeutic alliance, positive expectation and compliance in patients. The rationale for using CH with somatisation disorder is discussed around several topics in a simple language.

- The physiological and psychological consequences of acute and chronic stress are discussed.
- How stress and emotional upsets trigger, exacerbate and maintain physical symptoms are described. It is pointed out that although their symptoms are physical, even though medically unexplained, they can be affected by stress and emotional factors.
- How physical symptoms, pain and distress can become stressors in themselves is also described.
- The definition and clinical usefulness of hypnosis are discussed. In the treatment of somatisation disorder, hypnosis is used for inducing relaxation and a sense of well-being; stress management; amelioration of symptoms; promoting healing; and teaching self-hypnosis techniques for self-management of symptoms.
- The role of cognitions in emotional disturbance is discussed and the importance of cognitive therapy is highlighted.
- The importance of interpersonal skills and the involvement of significant other in therapy is mentioned.
- Finally, the role of homework and behavioural activation is discussed.

Overview of Treatment

- The frequency and duration of the treatment are outlined. The treatment consists of 16 weekly one-hour sessions.
- The collaborative and skills-based approach to the treatment is emphasised.
- The importance of learning and practising self-hypnosis techniques for symptom management is stressed. Part of the practice involves listening to the self-hypnosis CD on a daily basis.
- CBT will also involve homework consisting of selective reading, recording of thinking, practising cognitive restructuring and increasing behavioural activities.
- It is also explained that some sessions will be joint sessions with a significant other person and some of the homework may involve practising social and interpersonal skills.

Establishing Rapport

When treating somatisation patients, it is of paramount importance to build a therapeutic alliance. This can be achieved by

- Adopting an empathic and non-confrontational stance.
- Listening empathically to the patient's distress and description of the symptoms.
- Validating the patient's suffering and efforts to cope with the symptoms.
- Acknowledging the patient's frustration and disappointments with lack of success in various interventions.

- Stressing the patient's physical discomfort within a biopsychosocial model rather than pointing out that the symptoms are due to psychgological factors.
- Describing the rationale for using CH without contradicting the patient's understanding of his or her symptoms (Woolfolk & Allen, 2007).

If the patient does not buy into CH, the therapist can inquire and address the patient's concerns and reservations; review the effectiveness of CBT and hypnotherapy with somatisation disorder, particularly pointing out the cortical changes produced both by CBT and hypnosis; and encourage the patient to watch videos or CDs on hypnosis that illustrate the power of the mind over the body, especially in regard to controlling acute (e.g. surgery under hypnosis) and chronic pain. If the patient attributes his or her symptoms to an unknown biological mechanism or to toxic aspects of the physical environment, Woolfolk and Allen (2007, p. 87) suggest stressing to the patient that even if the symptoms are caused by some organic pathology or environmental agents, stress is likely to exacerbate them. Such an explanation helps create variations in the patient's explanation of the symptoms.

Reviewing Symptoms

- Review the major physical and psychological symptoms listed during the case formulation under Problems List (see Appendices C and D).
- Assess the discomfort and impairment caused by each symptom.
- Identify the antecedents (onset or trigger) and consequences of each symptom.
- Explore the patient's hypotheses about the causes of the symptoms.
- Identify the patient's thoughts and feelings about the symptoms, noting dysfunctional beliefs.
- Inquire about the outcome and treatment the patient had received for each symptom.

Introducing Symptom-Monitoring Forms

The rationale for and frequency of completing the symptom-monitoring forms are discussed. The patient is introduced to the Somatic Symptom Questionnaire (SSQ; Woolfolk *et al.*, 1998), the Severity of Somatic Symptoms Scale (SSS; Allen *et al.*, 2001), the Beck Anxiety Inventory (Beck & Steer, 1993c), Beck Hopelessness Scale (Beck & Steer, 1993b) and the Beck Depression Inventory – Revised (Beck, Steer & Brown, 1996). One of the forms, preferably either the SSQ or the SSS, is completed in the session to give the patient an idea of how to complete it. For homework, the patient is encouraged to fill in the forms.

Assessing Hypnotic Suggestibility

A standard hypnotic suggestibility test is administered to assess the patient's level of hypnotic suggestibility. I routinely use the Barber Suggestibility Scale

(BSS; Barber & Wilson, 1978/79) with somatisation patients. Within the CH case-conceptualisation model, somatizers are considered to be highly suggestible to hypnosis (Bliss, 1984), which may present as a risk factor in the aetiology of some somatoform symptoms (see Maldonado & Spiegel, 2003). Although the concept of hypnotic suggestibility is controversial, it is my belief that somatisation patients with low capacity to experience hypnosis may not derive maximum benefit from hypnotherapy. For such patients relaxation or imagery training can be substituted for hypnosis. The standard tests not only indicate which patient is highly suggestible, but the assessment also serves as an experiment to discover what kinds of suggestions the patient responds to. Such information guides the therapist in crafting and delivering congruent induction, and hypnotic and post-hypnotic suggestions. For example, if a patient obtained his or her highest score on 'arm heaviness' and lowest score on 'arm levitation' on the Barber Suggestibility Scale, then it would be more appropriate to use suggestions of heaviness for hypnotic induction, deepening and post-hypnotic suggestions regarding self-hypnosis (Alladin, 2007b, p. 103).

SESSIONS 3–4

In the third session the week is reviewed; homework is examined; hypnosis is introduced; and homework is assigned (self-hypnosis CD, monitoring symptoms and increasing physical activities).

Reviewing the Week

The impressions of the last session, particularly opinions regarding hypnosis and the biopsychosocial nature of the symptoms, are reviewed.

Examining Homework

The intensity of symptoms or level of distress during the week, what was useful or not useful, level of activities, social interaction and other concerns are considered.

Introducing Hypnotherapy

CH for somatisation disorder deviates from the treatment manual developed by Woolfolk and Allen (2007) by utilising hypnotherapy instead of relaxation training. As with other disorders described in this book, the hypnotherapy component is used to provide leverage to the psychological treatment (Alladin, 2006a, 2007b) and prevent relapses (Alladin, 2006b; Alladin &

Alibhai, 2007). Hypnotherapy is specifically utilised with somatisation disorder to induce relaxation; produce somatosensory changes; demonstrate the power of the mind; expand awareness; for ego strengthening; to teach self-hypnosis; provide post-hypnotic suggestions; and access non-conscious psychological processes. The main focus of Sessions 3–5 is to demonstrate to the patient that hypnosis can be easily utilised to induce relaxation and gain a sense of control. Sessions 6–7 concentrate on symptom amelioration and Sessions 8–9 are sdevoted to cognitive restructuring under hypnosis and unconscious exploration.

Relaxation training

One of the main goals for using hypnosis with somatisation disorder is to induce relaxation. Somatisation patients experience high levels of anxiety, as there is an overlap between somatisation disorder and anxiety disorders. First and Tasman (2004, pp. 980–1) noted that patients with somatisation disorder

> frequently complain of many of the same somatic symptoms as individuals with anxiety disorders, such as increased muscle tension, features of autonomic hyperactivity, and even discrete panic attacks. Likewise individuals with anxiety disorder may report irrational disease concerns and such somatic complaints as those involving gastrointestinal function that are commonly seen in somatization disorder.

Moreover, patients with chronic pain have elevated muscle tension (which causes a muscle-pain cycle; Linton, 1994) and generalised physiological arousal or reactivity (Rief, Shaw & Fichter, 1998). For these reasons somatisation patients derive significant benefits from learning relaxation techniques. Relaxation has been found to interrupt the muscle-pain cycle (Linton, 1994) and reduce generalised physiological arousal or reactivity (Rief, Shaw & Fichter, 1998) in chronic pain patients.

By learning to relax, somatisation patients can decrease sympathetic arousal or over-activity, manage the physiological responses associated with symptoms, reduce stress and enhance feelings of self-efficacy and control (Bernstein, Borkovec & Hazlett-Stevens, 2000). Moreover, by inducing relaxation, hypnosis reduces anxiety and creates a feeling of well-being, thus providing somatisers with the evidence that they can relax, calm down, modify their symptoms and feel different. These experiences create a sense of control and promote positive expectancy and a strong therapeutic alliance.

A variety of hypnotic methods are available for inducting relaxation (e.g. see Allen, 2004). I use the *relaxation with counting method* adapted from Gibbons (1979; see Appendix E) for inducing and deepening the hypnotic trance.

I have chosen this technique as it is easily adapted for self-hypnosis training (Alladin, 2007b). The majority of somatisation patients find hypnotic induction very relaxing and empowering and are very surprised to discover that it is so easy to relax and let go. Furthermore, this experience gives them the confidence that they can interrupt the anxious sequences/cycles in their lives. The hypnotherapeutic script in Appendix D provides some examples of the types of hypnotic suggestions that can be utilised for inducing deep relaxation.

Producing somatosensory changes

Hypnosis serves as a powerful psychotherapeutic tool for producing a holistic experience or *syncretic cognition* (Alladin, 2006a), which consists of a variety of cognitive, somatic, perceptual, physiological, visceral and kinaesthetic changes. Hypnotic induction and modulation of the syncretic cognition provide dramatic evidence to the somatisation patients that feelings and affect can be regulated, thus providing hope that the symptoms too can be altered and modulated. DePiano and Salzberg (1981) believe that this positive experience is largely responsible for producing rapid and profound changes in behavioural, emotional, cognitive and physiological changes in some patients following the induction of the hypnotic experience.

Demonstration of the power of mind

Various hypnotic procedures such as catalepsy, hallucination and amnesia can be induced to demonstrate inner control in patients. I normally induce eye and body catalepsies to exhibit the power of the mind over the body. Such demonstrations reduce scepticism over hypnosis, foster positive expectancy and instil confidence in patients that they can produce significant physical and behavioural changes (see Chapter 3). Reducing scepticism and inculcating hope are particularly important when treating patients with somatisation disorders. These patients have a long history of treatment failures and are accustomed to dismissal by various healthcare providers. Demonstration of the catalepsies establishes the credibility of psychological therapy for somatisation disorder and ratifies the importance of hypnotherapy. The more credible and the more powerful the treatment is perceived to be by the patient, the better the treatment outcome is likely to be (DePiano & Salzberg, 1981).

To avoid failure, induction of eye and body catalepsies is recommended when the patient is in a deep trance state. Here is an example of the script that can be used to induce eye and body catalepsies while the patient is in a fairly deep trance.

You have now become so deeply relaxed and you are in such a deep hypnotic trance, that your mind has become so powerful and so sensitive to what I say, that you will be able to feel, experience and imagine everything I ask you to feel experience and imagine.

Now, I would like you to focus on your eyes. Imagine your eyes are tightly glued together and your eyelids are heavy, heavy as lead. Your eyelids feel heavy, heavy and glued together, as if they are welded together. Your eyelids are so heavy, glued together, welded together, so that when I count ONE to THREE, you will not be able to open your eyes, however hard you try. But you will find this experience quite amusing rather than alarming, and not being able to open your eyes indicates how powerful your mind is.

ONE . . . your eyes feel glued together.

TWO . . . your eyelids are glued together, they are welded together.

THREE . . . your eyes are so tightly glued together that you feel you can't open your eyes. The more you try, the more they become glued together, making it impossible for you to open your eyes. Try . . . notice you can't open your eyes. Try harder . . . noticing that you can't open your eyes . . . *(when you see the patient is struggling to open his/her eyes say)* this shows how powerful your mind is.

And now I would like you to focus on your body. Imagine you have been lying in this chair for years. You have been lying in the chair for so long that you feel you are part of the chair. Your body feels heavy, solid, rigid, and you weigh a ton. You are so heavy, that you feel you are stuck in the chair . . . so that when I count ONE to THREE, at the count of THREE you will not be able to get out of the chair.

ONE . . . Your whole body feels heavy, solid and rigid . . . and you feel like you weigh a ton . . . feeling stuck in the chair.

TWO . . . Your legs and feet feel heavy and stuck in the chair. Your back feels heavy and stuck in the chair. Your shoulders, your neck and your head feel heavy and stuck in the chair.

THREE . . . Your whole body feels stuck in the chair and you feel you have become part of the chair . . . and you feel gravity is pulling you down so that you feel you can't get out of the chair. Try . . . notice that you can't . . . try harder, notice that you can't . . . *(if the patient is struggling say)* this shows that your mind is so powerful.

(The cataleptic responses are fed to the patient to reinforce the power of mind over body and sense of inner control.)

Let me explain to you what have achieved here. You produced eye and body catalepsies. By eye catalepsy, I mean that you paralysed your eyelids . . . that you can't open them. By body catalepsy, I mean that you paralysed your body . . . that you can't get out of the chair. If you can achieve this through the power of your mind, then you will be able to use this power to overcome or manage your difficulties. In the next few sessions we will be showing you how to use the power of your mind to work with your symptoms.

Expansion of awareness

Because of the focus on their symptoms, somatisation patients tend to focus on a narrow range of experience. Hypnosis can be utilised to expand their awareness and amplify their experience. Although *enhancing affective experience and its expression* (Brown & Fromm, 1986, in Hammond, 1998, pp. 322–4), described in Chapter 4, is generally used with depression, it can be adapted to somatisation disorder. The technique is very effective in bringing into awareness underlying emotions, creating awareness of various feelings and intensifying positive affect. The discovery of the ability to experience a variety of affect provides somatisers with the confidence that they can feel different and modify their symptoms. Alladin (2007b) has argued that hypnosis, by creating positive affect, can produce anti-depressive pathways.

Goldapple *et al.* (2004) provided functional neuroimaging evidence to show that CBT produces specific cortical regional changes in treatment responders. Similarly, Kosslyn *et al.* (2000) have demonstrated that hypnosis can modulate colour perception. Their investigations showed that hypnotised subjects were able to produce changes in brain function (measured by PET scanning) similar to those that occur during visual perception. These findings support the claim that hypnotic suggestions can produce distinct neural changes correlated with real perception. Moreover, Schwartz (1976) has provided electromyographic evidence that depressive pathways can be developed through conscious negative focusing. His investigation led him to believe that if it is possible to produce depressive pathways through negative cognitive focusing, then it would be possible to develop anti-depressive or happy pathways by focusing on positive imagery (Schwartz, 1984). From the foregoing evidence it would not be unreasonable to infer that the positive affect and images, coupled with ego-strengthening suggestions, produced by the hypnosis and positive mood induction technique might have exerted some cortical changes in the brains of depressives subjected to repetitive positive hypnotic experience.

Ego strengthening

The main purposes of providing ego-strengthening suggestions to somatisation patients are to increase confidence, coping abilities, positive self-image, interpersonal skills, self-esteem and self-efficacy (Alladin, 2007b; Hartland, 1971). As ego strengthening involves repeating positive suggestions to oneself, these suggestions can become embedded in the unconscious mind, exerting an automatic influence on feelings, thoughts and behaviour (Heap & Aravind, 2002). Ego strengthening is incorporated in hypnotherapy to enhance the patient's self-confidence and self-worth (Heap & Aravind, 2002). Bandura

(1977) has provided experimental evidence that *self-efficacy*, the expectation and confidence of being able to cope successfully with various situations, enhances treatment outcome. Individuals with a sense of high self-efficacy tend to perceive themselves as being in control. If somatisers can be helped to view themselves as self-efficacious, they are likely to feel hopeful about the future and this will motivate them to actively pursue the treatment.

The hypnosis script in Appendix E provides a list of generalised ego-strengthening suggestions that can be routinely used in hypnotherapy with a variety of medical and psychological conditions. However, when working with patients with somatisation disorder, it is important to word the ego-strengthening suggestions in such a way that they appear credible and logical. For example, rather than stating 'every day you will feel better', it is advisable to suggest 'as a result of this treatment and as a result of you listening to your self-hypnosis tape/CD every day, you will begin to feel better'. This set of suggestions not only sounds logical, but improvement becomes contingent on continuing with the therapy and listening to the self-hypnosis CD daily (Alladin, 2006a, 2006b, 2007b). For example:

> You are now so deeply relaxed . . . you are in such a deep hypnotic trance . . . that you are going to feel physically stronger and fitter in every way. At the end of the session . . . and every time you listen to your CD . . . you will feel more alert . . . more wide awake . . . more energetic . . . Every day as you learn to relax . . . you will become much less easily tired . . . much less easily fatigued . . . much less easily discouraged . . . much less easily upset . . . much less easily depressed. As you relax your mind and body every day by listening to your CD . . . your mind, your body and your nerves will become stronger and healthier . . . and as a result of this your symptoms will become less severe, less frequent, until they disappear completely.

Post-hypnotic suggestions

Post-hypnotic suggestions (PHS) are given to counter problem behaviours, negative emotions and dysfunctional cognitions that can be regarded as a form of negative self-hypnosis (NSH; Alladin, 2007b; Araoz, 1981). Patients with somatisation disorder tend to ruminate with negative self-suggestions, particularly when experiencing symptoms (e.g. 'The pain is terrible, I can't stand it') or when feeling anxious (e.g. 'I will not be able to cope') or depressed (e.g. 'I will never get better'). These self-statements can be regarded as a form of PHS, which can become part of the pain, anxiety and depressive cycle. Nolen-Hoeksema and her colleagues (see Nolen-Hoeksema, 2002) have provided empirical evidence that individuals who ruminate a great deal about their symptoms have more negative and distorted memories of the past, the present and the future. To break this ruminative cycle it is vital to counter the NSH.

Here are some examples of PHS that can be offered to somatisation patients to counter NSH:

- When you are in pain, you will become more aware of how to deal with it rather than focusing on the consequences of the pain.
- When you decide to take action to improve your future, you will feel motivated to increase your level of activities.
- As you become involved in your activities, you will begin to enjoy doing more things.

Many clinicians (e.g. Alladin, 2007b; Yapko, 2003) consider PHS to be a very necessary part of the therapeutic process as it motivates patients to explore new experiences and try out new behaviours in the future. Hence, many clinicians use PHS to shape their patients' behaviour. For example, Clarke and Jackson (1983) regard post-hypnotic suggestion as a form of 'higher-order-conditioning', which functions as positive or negative reinforcement to increase or decrease the probability of desired or undesired behaviours, respectively. They have successfully utilised post-hypnotic suggestions to enhance the effect of in vivo exposure among agoraphobics.

Self-hypnosis training

CH provides training in self-hypnosis, practice in self-help skills and continuity of self-care between the treatment sessions. At the end of the first hypnotherapy session, the patient is provided with a CD of self-hypnosis training (consisting of the full script from Appendix E) designed to induce deep relaxation and a sense of well-being; bestow ego-strengthening suggestions; and impart post-hypnotic suggestions. Learning self-help skills trains somatisation patients in establishing self-reliance and independence. According to Alman (2001), training in self-hypnosis provides a powerful means of achieving self-reliance and personal power.

Increasing Activities

Because of their physical pain and emotional discomfort, many somatisation patients withdraw from potentially pleasurable and fulfilling activities, such as work, social activities, hobbies and exercise (Woolfolk & Allen, 2007). Therefore an essential component of CH is to encourage patients to gradually increase their vocational, recreational, social and self-care activities. Increasing activities is particularly important with unemployed or single patients (those living on their own). These patients can be encouraged to engage in meaningful activities such as volunteering their time, taking a class or doing favours for friends or family, and to reconnect with others by telephoning or e-mailing, returning to church or temple or joining a club (Woolfolk & Allen, 2007). The increase in activities can be enhanced by giving post-hypnotic suggestions.

Homework

- Complete the symptom-monitoring form each day.
- Listen to the self-hypnosis CD every day.
- Increase physical activities.

SESSIONS 5–7

These three sessions concentrate on reviewing the week; reviewing homework; introducing hypnotic strategies for symptom amelioration; and assigning homework. The main focus of these two hypnotherapy sessions is to teach patients how to utilise different hypnotic strategies to produce amelioration in symptoms.

Reviewing the Week

- The patient's impression of hypnosis, particularly the power of mind–body demonstration, is discussed.
- The reaction and response to self-hypnosis training are reviewed.
- The impact of self-hypnosis training is examined, especially in relation to the profile obtained from daily completion of the symptom-monitoring form.
- Increase in level of activities is monitored.

Reviewing Homework (Symptoms, Self-Hypnosis, Increase in Activities)

- Review the patient's reaction to completing the symptom-monitoring form on a daily basis. If the patient is having difficulties completing the form on a daily basis, validate and normalise the concern, and discuss the rationale for completing the form.
- Examine the impact that daily completion of the symptom-rating form has on the patient.
- Review progress with the self-hypnosis training and sensitively deal with the obstacles and concerns the patient may have about listening to the self-hypnosis CD daily.
- Discuss the impact of self-hypnosis on symptoms, paying attention to both somatic and psychological symptoms (e.g. anxiety and depression).

Introducing Hypnotic Strategies for Symptom Amelioration

The mind–body demonstrations (eye and body catalepsies) and self-hypnosis training during the past two weeks have prepared the patient for the next stage of hypnotherapy. The two hypnotherapy sessions focus specifically on modifying symptoms and the sessions include several hypnotic strategies, including deep relaxation; symptom transformation; dissociation of body parts; and complete dissociation. Although many other hypnotherapeutic techniques can be utilised, I have selected these four techniques because somatisation patients find these fairly easy for self-practice, and they can be easily replicated by other therapists. The strategies are illustrated by describing the techniques used with Rick. Rick is a 39-year-old man with multiple unexplained medical symptoms who meets the DSM-IV-TR criteria for somatisation disorder. His symptoms include tension headaches, pain and ringing inside his ears, temporomandibular joint pain (TMJ), low back pain, pain in his knees, abdominal pain, nausea, constipation, numbness in his face and legs, and feeling weak and dizzy at times. He also has sleep-onset insomnia and symptoms of anxiety and depression.

Deep relaxation

As mentioned earlier, relaxation interrupts the muscle-pain cycle (Linton, 1994) and reduces generalised physiological arousal and reactivity (Rief, Shaw & Fichter, 1998). At this point in therapy, the relaxation response is used to modify or ameliorate the symptoms. When Rick is in a fairly deep trance (he is very susceptible to hypnosis), the following suggestions are used to decrease or eliminate his symptoms:

> You have now become so relaxed, you are in such a deep hypnotic trance, that your mind and your body are completely relaxed. Just continue to feel the beautiful sensation of peace and tranquillity, relaxation and calm flowing through every part of your mind and body.
>
> Feel this beautiful sensation of peace and tranquillity, relaxation and calm flowing through every muscle in your body, relaxing every muscle in your body, easing every muscle in your body.
>
> Feel this beautiful sensation of peace and tranquillity, relaxation and calm flowing through every nerve in your body, relaxing every nerve in your body, easing every nerve in your body.
>
> Feel this beautiful sensation of peace and tranquillity, relaxation and calm flowing through every part of your mind, relaxing every corner of your mind.
>
> Now you feel this beautiful sensation of peace and tranquillity, relaxation and calm flowing through every part of your mind and body, relaxing every part of your mind and body . . . giving you such a pleasant feeling all over your mind and your body . . . such a soothing feeling all over your mind and your body . . . that you feel all the pain and all the discomfort easing away.

Whenever the focus of the treatment is on ameliorating or decreasing the symptoms, it is advisable for the therapist to monitor the intensity of pain or discomfort regularly. This involves three steps:

1. Establish the level of pain or discomfort at the beginning of the session. I routinely use a subjective rating scale: 'On a scale of 0 to 10, 0 being no pain and 10 representing the worst pain, where is your pain now?'

2. Set up an ideomotor signal: 'As you are relaxing, occasionally I will be asking you some questions so that I know how you are feeling. But you don't have to speak to me. We can communicate with signals so that we don't disturb your relaxation. Whenever I ask you a question, if the answer is YES, just nod your chin up and down, and if the answer is NO, just shake your head side to side. So if I ask you a question and the answer is YES, you will automatically, without any effort, nod your chin up and down, and if the answer is NO, you will automatically, without any effort, shake your head side to side... and we will be able to communicate without disturbing your relaxation.'

3. During the treatment procedure, assess the level of pain or discomfort regularly or when necessary: 'Where is your pain now? I will say some numbers and nod your head when your pain coincides with the number.'
   Just continue to enjoy this beautiful sensation of peace and tranquillity, relaxation and calm, flowing through every part of your mind and body. Do you feel completely relaxed, both mentally and physically? *(Rick nods his head. If the patient indicates NO, the suggestions are repeated until the YES signal is received.)* Where is your pain now? Eight, Seven, Six, Five, Four *(Rick nods his head. At the beginning of the session, his pain was at SEVEN. The relaxation suggestions are repeated until the pain or discomfort is at ZERO. If the pain or discomfort is not eliminated completely by the end of the session, the patient is reassured and given feedback about the progress.)*

The relaxation technique described above focuses on the whole body. At times, it is necessary to focus on one part of the body at a time. This approach is required when the patient has pain or discomfort in one or two areas of the body, or when the pain is so severe that the patient is not able to lessen the discomfort via general relaxation. On a few occasions Rick came to the sessions with either severe headache or severe low back pain. The technique for working with head pain is described in detail in Chapter 4. Here are the suggestions used for working with low back pain.

> You have become so deeply relaxed and you are in such a deep trance that your mind and body feel completely relaxed. And now we are going to focus on your back. Where is the pain now? *(Rick nodded it is at 7.)* That's good, it reduced from 9 to 7. Now we are going to help you reduce the pain further.
>
> Now focus on the upper part of your back. Just become aware of the feeling and sensation in your upper back, neck and shoulders. Let your upper back, neck and shoulders go limp, loose and slack. You feel all the muscles in your neck, your shoulders and your upper back becoming limp, loose and slack. You feel all the nerves in your neck, your shoulders and your upper back are becoming limp, loose and slack. You feel all the bones and joints in your neck, your shoulders and your upper back are becoming limp, loose and slack.
>
> As all the muscles, all the nerves, all the bones and joints loosen up, you feel all the tension, all the pressure from your muscles in your neck, shoulders and upper back loosening up, giving you such a soothing feeling, that your neck, your shoulders and your upper back feel very relaxed and comfortable. Do

your neck, shoulders and upper back feel relaxed and comfortable? *(Rick nods YES.)*

And now we are going to focus on your lower back. Where is the pain now? *(Rick nods to 5. Although the pain is located in his lower back, the initial focus was on his upper back as it is easier to relax a part of the body that is free of pain. The induction of the relaxation on his upper back reinforces the belief that he can equally relax his lower back, though he is in pain.)* Just become aware of the feeling and the sensation in your lower back. Let your lower back go limp, loose and slack. You feel all the muscles in your lower back becoming limp, loose and slack. You feel all the nerves in your lower back becoming limp, loose and slack. You feel all the bones and joints in your lower back becoming limp, loose and slack.

As all the muscles, all the nerves, all the bones and joints loosen up, you feel all the tension, all the pressure from your muscles in your lower back loosening up, giving you such a soothing sensation, that your lower back feels very relaxed and comfortable. And as you feel the tension and the pressure easing away from your lower back, you feel the pain easing away. And soon your lower back will feel so comfortable that you feel all the pain eased away. Where is the pain now? *(Rick nods at 4. The suggestions are repeated until the pain is cleared completely or almost completely.)*

While in trance, Rick was offered post-hypnotic suggestions to reinforce the benefits of the relaxation procedure and to gain self-mastery of the technique:

As a result of this treatment and as a result of you listening to your CD every day, every day your mind, your body and your nerves will become more relaxed and less tense. As a result of this your symptoms will become less and less frequent, less and less severe, until they will disappear completely. And when you have pain or discomfort, you will be able to ease these very easily either by relaxing or listening to your CD.

Symptom transformation

Several hypno-behavioural strategies, including distraction, pain displacement, symptom substitution, causal reinterpretation, hypno-analgesia, pattern interruption, symptom reinterpretation and reframing, time distortion, non-judgemental focus of awareness and deliberate increase of pain, can be used to transform or alter the perception of the symptoms (see Eimer & Freeman, 1998, pp. 298–302 for more detail). All of these strategies may not be applicable to every somatisation patient. It is advisable to try each of these techniques with a patient and stick to the strategy that is most appealing and natural to that patient. To enhance the treatment effect, post-hypnotic suggestions are given:

With practice, you will be able to transform your symptom *(state symptom, e.g. pain)* into . . . *(state the imagery used, e.g. an itch)* and as a result of this your symptom will become less uncomfortable and less bothersome to you . . . so that you will become less focused on your symptom and more interested in what you are doing.

Dissociation of body parts

On occasions, relaxation and symptom transformation may not be suffi-cient to reduce certain symptoms, especially if the symptoms are severe. Under these circumstances dissociation of body parts can be utilised. For example, Rick can easily decrease most of his symptoms via relaxation, but the pain in his knees and the numbness in his legs show little improve-ment. However, he finds the detachment of his legs, knees and feet very effective. I find an adapted version of the script from Barabasz and Watkins (2005, p. 237) very effective in temporarily dissociating certain parts of the body:

> You have now become so deeply relaxed, and you are in such a deep trance, that your mind has become so powerful and so sensitive to what I say, that you will be able to imagine, feel and experience everything I ask you to imagine, feel and experience.
>
> Now I want you to imagine that your legs and your feet are detaching from your body. Soon they will become completely detached from your body, and your legs and your feet will no longer be part of you. The legs and the feet have no feeling or movement. You cannot move your legs or your feet, because they are no longer connected to you. You feel that there is a space between the ends of your feet and the beginnings of your legs. Therefore, there is no connection between your legs and yourself. Because they are no longer within your own being, they no longer have the power to send you painful or uncomfortable impulses. They are dead and attached like a board to your lower body. You experience no sensations coming from them. Do you experience any sensation coming from them? *(Rick indicated NO by shaking his head side to side.)*

Rick was also given post-hypnotic suggestions that with practice he will be able to detach his legs and feet from his being, and as a result of this he will be able to have more and more control over the pain in legs and feet and the numbness in his knees.

Complete dissociation

As somatisation patients have multiple symptoms, dissociation of the whole body may be desirable at times. The script for the whole body dissociation is similar to the suggestions used for dissociating certain body parts.

> Now I want you to imagine your whole body is detaching. Soon your whole body will become completely detached from you. Your body will no longer be part of you. Your body has no feeling or movement. You cannot move your body because it is no longer connected to you. You feel that there is no connection between you and your body, your body is detached, totally detached. Because your body is totally detached and is no longer part of your own being, it no longer has the power to send you painful or uncomfortable impulses. Your body is detached and you experience no sensations coming from your body. Do you experience any sensation coming from your body? *(Rick indicated NO by shaking his head side to side.)*

Homework

- Complete the symptom-monitoring form each day.
- Listen to the self-hypnosis CD every day.
- Practise using deep relaxation to ameliorate symptoms.
- Practise transforming symptoms.
- Practise dissociating each part of the body that is of concern.
- Practise dissociating the whole body.
- Increase physical activities.

SESSION 8

The main goal of the eighth session is to teach self-hypnotic techniques for symptom amelioration and promoting healing. In addition, as usual, the week is reviewed and further homework is assigned.

As described with migraine headache (Chapter 5) and acne vulgaris (Chapter 6), imagery training is used to promote healing of the areas where the pathophysiology supposedly exists. When focusing on his IBS symptoms, Rick is advised to imagine dipping his hand into a bucket full of warm water and once he experiences that his hand is warmed up, he is instructed to gently place his hand over his abdomen and imagine the sensation of warmth transferring to his gut (for more details of gut-directed hypnotherapy for IBS, see Gonsalkorale, 2006):

> Imagine that the warmth from your hand is transferring to your gut and soon you will feel a warm sensation inside your gut. Let me know when you feel this warm sensation inside your gut. *(After a short pause, Rick nodded his head.)* You feel that this warm feeling is spreading inside your gut. As this warm sensation spreads inside your gut, you feel your gut becoming more and more relaxed, more and more comfortable. The warm feeling inside your gut is due to the fact that the blood circulation inside your gut has increased. Imagine that the

blood flow is increasing inside your gut (*wait for the affirmative before proceeding further*). Imagine that the extra blood flow is bringing in more oxygen and more nutrition to the areas where you need them most. As a result of this extra blood flow, the lining of your gut, the nerves and the muscles in your gut will become stronger and healthier, and as a result of this your gut will become more and more normal . . . and you will have more and more control over your gut . . . so that your bowel habits will become more and more normal . . . and the pain, the discomfort and the bloating will become less and less frequent, less and less severe, until they will disappear completely.

The imagery training is directed to each area of concern and post-hypnotic suggestions are given:

With practice, you will be able to warm your hand quickly, and you will be able to transfer the warmth easily to wherever you need it. The areas that you can't reach with your hand, you will be able to warm up directly, just by thinking about them. As a result of this you will speed up the healing and, therefore, every day your symptoms will become less and less, until they will disappear completely.

Homework

- Complete the symptom-monitoring form each day.
- Listen to the self-hypnosis CD every day.
- Practise transforming symptoms.
- Practise dissociating each part or the whole body.
- Practise warming up the areas of body that are of concern.
- Increase physical activities.

SESSION 9

In this session the therapist has a joint session with the patient and his or her significant other. The goals of this joint session are to review the week and homework; discuss the rationale for meeting with the patient's significant other; plan joint activities; and assign further homework.

Review of Week and Homework

The same format as for the previous sessions is used to review the last session, the week and homework. The review of the last session is particularly important in this session, as the concept of using self-hypnosis for ameliorating the symptoms was introduced. The therapist needs to check whether the patient finds self-hypnosis useful in the management of symptoms, and which symptom responds to self-hypnosis and which does not respond. It is also important to know how the patient handled the homework. The homework mainly involved practising symptom transformation, dissociation of body parts and warming up areas of body that are of concern. Since these are advanced self-hypnotic procedures for managing symptoms, the therapist needs to be aware of the progress and obstacles. The major goal of these reviews is to maintain close communication with the patient so that the therapist and the patient can work in close collaboration. In addition, the therapist is interested to know the patient's progress with physical activities. Increase in physical activities provides an objective measure of treatment progress.

Discussion of Rationale for Meeting Significant Other

The goals for involving the significant other (domestic partner or spouse) in the treatment of somatisation disorder include:

- To obtain additional information about the patient.
- To gain the support of the significant other for the treatment.
- To alter the behaviour of the significant other that may be reinforcing the patient's symptoms or illness behaviour.
- To utilise the significant other to facilitate some aspects of the treatment (e.g. the significant other can encourage the patient to increase physical activities).

The therapist meets with the significant other in a conjoint session and the rationale for meeting together with the patient and the significant other is to encourage an open dialogue.

The conjoint session(s) revolves around discussions about:

- *Stress management*: The therapist enquires about the impact of stress on the patient's physical symptoms and discusses the rationale for stress management.
- *Impact of illness*: The therapist enquires about the impact of the patient's physical illness on the significant other and suggests that the significant other's involvement in therapy will benefit both parties.
- *Impairment of relationship*: The therapist explores the impact of the patient's illness on the relationship.
- *Withdrawal from activities*: The therapist assesses the impact of reduced activities on the couple.
- *Effect on communication*: The therapist enquires about the effect of the patient's illness on communication.
- *Increasing activities*: Following the discussion, the therapist works collaboratively with the couple to develop a plan for increasing pleasurable conjoint activities and for dealing with some of the issues identified.

Homework

- Complete the symptom-monitoring form each day.
- Listen to the self-hypnosis CD every day.

- Practise transforming symptoms.
- Practise dissociating each part or the whole body.
- Practise warming up the areas of body with concern.
- Increase physical activities.
- Start pleasurable conjoint activities.

SESSIONS 10–13

Patients with somatisation disorder tend to have dysfunctional beliefs about somatic sensations and often about their ability to perform effectively (Woolfolk & Allen, 2007). They can also have non-health-related dysfunctional thinking and these may include perfectionist thoughts, catastrophic thoughts, over-estimating the possibility of negative outcomes, 'should' statements and dichotomous thinking. Woolfolk and Allen (2007) believe these dysfunctional thoughts may reflect the somatiser's core beliefs of being inadequate or unlovable.

The next four sessions focus on cognitive behaviour therapy (CBT). The objects of the CBT sessions are to help the patients identify and restructure the dysfunctional beliefs that may be triggering, exacerbating and maintaining their symptoms. The CBT sessions are structured in the same format as described for depression (see Chapter 3). However, to make the CBT more systematic and structured, the use of the Cognitive Restructuring (ABCDE) form is highly recommended (Appendix B). CBT is particularly helpful with somatisation patients who have comorbid anxiety and depression. As reviewed earlier, as many as 75% of patients with somatisation disorder have comorbid Axis I diagnoses, including major depressive disorder, dysthymia, panic disorder, simple phobia and substance abuse (Katon et al., 1991).

To avoid repetition, and as the reader has become familiar with the format of the initial part of each session, the review of the previous session, the week and the homework will not be described further. The description will instead move on directly to the main theme of each session. In practice, the therapist should review the previous session, progress during the week and homework in every session before moving on to the main agenda of the session.

SESSION 14

Cognitive Restructuring under Hypnosis

As discussed in the context of migraine headache (Chapter 4), insight-oriented or exploratory hypnotic techniques are used within the CH formulation when the patient does not respond to the usual treatment protocol. Cognitive restructuring under hypnosis allows the therapist and the patient to explore intrapersonal dynamics and the unconscious origin or purposes of the symptoms. There are many insight-oriented hypnotic methods (e.g. Brown & Fromm, 1986a). The simplest and most widely used is ideomotor signalling. Chapter 4 provides a script from Hammond (1998, p. 114) that illustrates how ideomotor signalling is introduced to the hypnotised patient. By using the ideomotor signalling technique with somatisation patients, seven key areas can be explored:

- Adaptive function or secondary gain for the symptoms.
- Self-punishment by having the symptoms.
- Inner conflict causing or maintaining the symptoms.
- Imprints or commands transformed into symptoms.
- Somatisation symbolic of past experiences.
- Somatisation adopted as a form of identification.
- Somatisation symbolic of inner pain.

Once the underlying cause of the somatisation symptoms is established, the therapist can help the patient deal with the issue in a satisfactory manner.

SESSION 15

This session is devoted to the second meeting with the significant other. This conjoint session reviews the grounds and prescription of strategies that were covered during the first conjoint session. This conjoint session focus mostly on communication and support.

SESSION 16

Interpersonal Skills Training

Patients with somatisation disorder often have multiple social problems and chaotic lifestyles characterised by poor interpersonal relationships and disruptive or difficult behaviour (see Abbey, 2006). The goal of this session is to help the patient objectively define some of these problems and to adopt a problem-solving strategy to work with these problems. Hypnotherapy can be utilised to build self-esteem (via ego strengthening and imaginal rehearsal), control anger and increase self-efficacy (forward projection). Social skills training, behavioural activation and mindfulness training, as described in Chapter 3, can also be utilised with somatisation disorder.

Follow-ups and Booster Sessions

As somatisation disorder is a chronic condition and not yet curable, regular follow-up visits are essential for successful long-term care.

SUMMARY

The chapter reviewed the aetiology and existing empirical treatments for somatisation disorder and then described *cognitive hypnotherapy* for somatisation disorder, a multi-modal treatment approach that combines cognitive behaviour therapy with hypnosis. The treatment approach described in the chapter can be easily adapted to the treatment of other forms of somatoform conditions. The treatment protocol for somatisation disorder described in the chapter can be easily evaluated to assess the additive effect of hypnotherapy.

CHAPTER 8

COGNITIVE HYPNOTHERAPY IN THE MANAGEMENT OF CHRONIC PRIMARY INSOMNIA

INTRODUCTION

The main goal of this chapter is to describe how clinicians can incorporate sleep therapy with hypnotherapy in the management of primary insomnia (referred as insomnia in the rest of the chapter, unless qualified). Although there are many types of sleep disorders, for our purpose the focus will be on insomnia as it is the most common form of sleep disorder, and it has received most attention in the psychological literature. Insomnia is a common complaint reported by the adult population all over the world (Soldatos *et al.*, 2007). It is also one of the most prevalent health complaints in the general population, in medical practice and in psychiatric practice (Buysse *et al.*, 2005). Despite its high prevalence, insomnia is not well recognised as a disease entity by health professionals. Traditionally, clinicians have taken the view that insomnia is a symptom rather than a disorder and the focus has been on finding and treating the underlying cause. Recent evidence suggests that, although insomnia is commonly associated with other medical and psychiatric conditions, its onset, course and response to treatment are often independent of the comorbid conditions (Buysse *et al.*, 2007). Moreover, psychological and pharmacological treatments for *primary* insomnia are equally efficacious with *secondary* insomnias. Therefore insomnia is currently viewed as a syndrome that merits independent treatment.

The aim of this chapter is to review the aetiology and existing empirical treatments for insomnia and then to describe *cognitive hypnotherapy for primary insomnia*, a multi-modal treatment approach that combines cognitive behaviour therapy with hypnotherapy, based on the work of Graci (Graci, 2005; Graci & Hardie, 2007; Graci & Sexton-Radek, 2006).

DEFINITION AND DESCRIPTION

In clinical practice, chronic insomnia is defined based on the criteria of the Diagnostic and Statistical Manual of Mental Disorders (DSM-IV-TR; American Psychiatric Association, 2000) or the International Classification of Sleep Disorders (ICSD; Diagnostic Classification Steering Committee, 1990). The criteria for the diagnosis include:

- Difficulty falling asleep (*sleep-initiating insomnia*, also known as *sleep-onset insomnia*); nocturnal awakenings and difficulties getting back to sleep (*sleep-maintenance insomnia*); early-morning awakenings (*sleep-offset insomnia*); or a non-refreshing or non-restorative sleep; or a combination of any of the above.
- The difficulties occur at least three times a week for at least one month.
- The insomnia causes clinically significant distress or impairment in social, occupational or other important areas of daytime functioning.

More recently, the American Academy of Sleep Medicine Work Group proposed research-based diagnostic criteria for insomnia disorder (Edinger *et al.*, 2004). This group expanded the symptoms classed under the third criterion to emphasise the social, psychological, occupational and cognitive impact on the person. In addition to meeting the first two criteria listed in DSM-IV-TR and ICSD, this new classification requires the individual to have at least one of the following daytime impairments related to the nighttime sleep difficulty:

- Fatigue/malaise.
- Attention, concentration or memory difficulty.
- Social/vocational dysfunction or poor school performance.
- Mood disturbance/irritability.
- Daytime sleepiness.
- Motivation/energy/initiative reduction.
- Proneness to errors/accidents at work or while driving.
- Tension headaches and/or gastrointestinal symptoms in response to sleep loss.
- Concerns or worries about sleep.

Two of the most common types of insomnia disorders (not including insomnia associated with a medical disorder) are adjustment and psychophysiological sleep disorders. *Adjustment sleep disorder* is a condition in which an individual has experienced a significant life stressor(s), for example the death of a loved one, which interferes with sleep. This type of sleep problem is more commonly associated with a transient sleep disturbance that generally abates within a month. However, when this type of transient insomnia does not attenuate over time, it can progress to chronic insomnia, often accompanied by depression. *Psychophysiological insomnia* is a sleep disorder that results from the presence of heightened physiological arousal in which somatised tension and maladaptive associations (e.g. nervousness, anxiety, ruminative thoughts) interfere with nocturnal sleep.

Insomnia may be primary or secondary and can be comorbid with other medical and psychiatric disorders. *Primary insomnia* is an intrinsic sleep disorder that is characterised by the presence of insomnia for at least one month and is not due to another sleep disorder, a psychiatric condition, a medical problem or substance abuse. *Secondary insomnia* is often associated with other conditions, including sleep disorders, mental or physical disorders, toxicological influence or environmental factors. In these circumstances, insomnia is more properly viewed as a *symptom* (Leger, 2007). Insomnia is considered to be chronic if it lasts more than one to three months (DSM-IV-TR; APA, 2000). Retrospective studies indicate that approximately 40% of severe insomniacs have had the problem for over five years and approximately 80% for over a year (Ohayon *et al.*, 1997). For the treatment of insomnia to be effective, it will be very important to be able to indentify and treat the potential underlying conditions.

PREVALENCE, SOCIODEMOGRAPHICS AND COURSE OF INSOMNIA

Recent point-prevalent studies have estimated 19–21% of the population surveyed to have insomnia (see Leger, 2007). The one-year prevalence of insomnia symptoms in Western nations is approximately 30–40% in the general population and up to 66% in primary care and psychiatric settings (Buysse *et al.*, 2007). The prevalence of primary insomnia as a specific disorder ranges from 5–10% in the general population (Moul *et al.*, 2002). Insomnia complaints increase with age and the annual incidence of insomnia among the elderly is estimated to be 5% (Morin & Gramling, 1989). Women report insomnia more than men (e.g. Mellinger, Balter & Uhlenhuth, 1985). However, older men demonstrate more disrupted sleep on polysomnography (PSG) than do older women (Reynolds *et al.*, 1986). Divorced or separated, widowed, unemployed and individuals with medical and psychiatric conditions report more complaints of insomnia (Spielman, Caruso & Glovinsky, 1987). Counterproductive sleep habits and psychological stresses such as moves, relationship difficulties, occupational and financial problems, and care-giving responsibilities commonly initiate or maintain the insomnia (Kappler & Hohagen, 2003). Although the natural history of insomnia has not been widely studied, follow-up studies of clinical patients and population samples indicate that severe insomnia persists for years and becomes more relentless with time (Mendelson, 1995).

The majority of insomniacs, even severe cases, do not always seek help for treatment. An early Gallup (National Sleep Foundation, 1991) study of insomniacs found that only 5% had visited their doctor for the sleep problem and only 21% had ever taken a prescription medication for the insomnia. The majority of insomniacs deal with their problem by non-medical means such as using non-prescription drugs, watching television, reading or drinking alcohol (Ohayon, 2002).

The consequences of insomnia, which are very substantial, are summarised below (from Buysse *et al.*, 2007):

- It is a risk factor for anxiety, depression and substance abuse.
- In patients with major depressive disorder, insomnia is associated with poor treatment outcomes, suicidal ideation, symptom persistence and relapses.
- In alcohol dependence, insomnia is associated with maintenance and relapses.
- Insomnia is associated with increased medical care utilisation, more absenteeism from work, and increased direct and indirect medical costs. Yapko (2006) cites a study by Stoller (1994) which, over a decade ago, reported the incurring cost of insomnia in USA to be somewhere between $77 billion and $92 billion a year. The figure is likely to be much higher these days.
- It is associated with increased motor vehicle and other accidents.
- Insomnia reduces the quality life to the same magnitude as congestive heart failure and major depressive disorder.

AETIOLOGY OF INSOMNIA

The aetiology of insomnia is unclear (First & Tasman, 2004). The majority of attention in the search for the causes of insomnia has been directed to physiological and psychological causes. Buysse *et al.* (2007) have summarised these two areas of research. The *physiological models* consider insomnia to be a disorder of arousal. *Arousal* is defined as the individual's state of central nervous system (CNS) activity and reactivity, ranging from sleep at one end of the spectrum to excitement at the other (Coull, 1998). Arousal is related to the function of wake-promoting structures in the ascending reticular activating system (ARAS), hypothalamus and basal forebrain, which interact with sleep-promoting brain centres in the anterior hypothalamus and thalamus (Buysse *et al.*, 2007). *Hyperarousal* is characterised by a high level of alertness that may be present tonically or in response to specific situations, such as loud noise, the sleep environment and so on. Buysse *et al.* (2007) provide metabolic, electrophysiological, neuroendocrine and functional neuroanatomic evidence to support their hypothesis that insomniacs have hyperaroused CNS activity. More specifically, these findings suggest that individuals with primary insomnia are hyperaroused during non-rapid eye movement (NREM) sleep and hypoaroused during wakefulness. Although the hyperarousal hypothesis seems promising, without further studies it is difficult to determine whether the hyperarousal results from the insomnia or was pre-existent before the emergence of the sleep problem.

The psychological explanation of insomnia revolves around *cognitive-behavioural models* that view insomnia to be a consequence of such antecedent factors as sleep-related maladaptive habits (thoughts and behaviours) and perceived arousal. Each model, however, differs in its emphasis on the core dysfunction underlying insomnia. Morin (1993) considers cognitive hyperarousal produced by sleep-focused ruminative thoughts, particularly around bedtime, to be central to insomnia. Morin's model is summarised by Buysse *et al.* (2007, pp. 34–5):

Cognitive arousal increases physiological arousal. With repetition, this pairing facilitates conditioning between temporal (e.g., bedtime routines) and environmental (e.g., bed, bedroom) cues and sleeplessness. Resulting sleep disturbance and ruminations ultimately lead to daytime consequences such as mood disturbances and fatigue. Over time, these experiences can alter one's beliefs regarding the ability to sleep and the consequences of sleep difficulties and can lead to the development of maladaptive strategies aimed at maximizing sleep (e.g., spending more time in bed) that further reinforce sleep disturbances and cognitive hyperarousal.

More recently, Harvey (2002) proposed a similar model of insomnia, but the focus is more on the role of attention biases in the maintenance of insomnia (Buysse *et al.*, 2007, pp. 36–7):

The model proposes that cognitive strategies (rather than behavioral strategies) employed by people with insomnia are maladaptive and maintain sleep disturbances. Excessive negative cognitive activity leads to increased physiological hyperarousal, which in turn leads to selective attention to and monitoring of autonomic symptoms and environmental cues indicative of sleeplessness. Such selective attention distorts perceptions regarding sleep deficits and adverse daytime effects. Individuals develop maladaptive safety behavior, such as thought suppression and emotional inhibition, to avoid sleep loss. However, these behaviors further reinforce the negative cognitive activity, physiological arousal, and erroneous beliefs regarding sleep and daytime deficits seen in insomnia.

Spielman, Caruso & Glovinsky (1987) have provided the most comprehensive model of insomnia, integrating biological and psychological factors (diathesis-stress model), and accounting for predisposing, precipitating and perpetuating factors. They assert that insomnia is produced by the interaction between individual predisposing factors (e.g. heightened physiological or cognitive arousal) and external precipitating factors (e.g. life stressors), and maintained by maladaptive coping strategies (e.g. spending more time in bed). The relative importance assumed by these three factors can change over time. A cardinal assumption of this model is that, with time, insomnia can take on a life of its own, and may become independent of the original precipitant. Therefore, regardless of the nature of the precipitating events, additional controlling variables may maintain the sleep problem.

Although both the physiological and the psychological models of insomnia contribute to our understanding and treatment of insomnia, none of the theories explains the complexity of persistent insomnia. Insomnia is a heterogeneous disorder with a variety of symptoms that vary widely in type, intensity, frequency and daytime consequences (Lacks & Morin, 1992). Therefore it is unlikely that a single theory will be able to account for the complexity and variety of the disorder.

TREATMENT OF INSOMNIA

A variety of psychological and pharmacological interventions have been used for the treatment of insomnia. This review will focus on pharmacotherapy, cognitive behaviour therapy and hypnotherapy. Following this review, *cognitive hypnotherapy for primary insomnia*, a multi-faceted approach to treating insomnia based on the work of Graci (Graci, 2005; Graci & Hardie, 2007; Graci & Sexton-Radek, 2006) will be described in the rest of the chapter.

Pharmacological Intervention

Pharmacotherapy is the most frequently used treatment for insomnia. Although benzodiazepine receptor agonists (BzRA) are the only drugs currently approved for the treatment of insomnia (Buysse *et al.*, 2007), physicians frequently use other classes of drugs, particularly anti-depressants, to treat insomnia. Walsh and Schweitzer (1999) reported an exponential increase of 146% in the use of anti-depressants for the treatment of insomnia between 1987 and 1996, whereas the use of BzRA fell by over 50%. This trend has continued and in 2002 the prescriptions for anti-depressants rose to 5.3 million compared to 4.2 million for BzRA (Walsh, 2004). Anti-depressant agents used in the management of insomnia include imipramine, trimipramine and trazadone. These agents have been shown to produce some positive effects both on subjective measures and polysomnographic measures such as sleep deficiency (Hajak *et al.*, 2001; Hohagen *et al.*, 1994; James & Mendelson, 2004). Erman (1998) argues that although the use of anti-depressant medication in the management of insomnia complaints is widespread, there is remarkably little published data to support the safety and efficacy of these drugs. Buysse *et al.* (2007) question the validity of using other drugs such as melatonin, anti-histamines, anti-psychotics and anti-convulsants with insomnia. Several meta-analyses have demonstrated the efficacy of BzRA with chronic insomnia (Holbrook *et al.*, 2000; Nowell *et al.*, 1997; Soldatos, Dikeos & Whitehead, 1999).

As noted in the next section, the effects of BzRA are comparable in magnitude to those of CBT (Smith *et al.*, 2002). However, BzRA, because of its side effects, which include sedation, impaired psychomotor performance, falls and hip fractures, motor vehicle accidents, respiratory depression, tolerance, discontinuance effects and potential abuse (Buysse *et al.*, 2007), has a disadvantage over CBT. Moreover, medication can lead to iatrogenic insomnia and chronic use of sleep medication undermines the development of appropriate self-management skills to cope with insomnia (Morin, 1993). Nonetheless, hypnotic medication is efficacious on a short-term basis, but there are few data available on its efficacy with prolonged use. Medication is a useful adjunct in the treatment of insomnia but should be used cautiously, weighing the initial clinical benefits against its daytime sequelae and long-term effects, especially when more effective, more enduring and less costly non-pharmacological therapy (CBT) is available (Jacobs et al., 2004). Morin (1993) argues that when pharmacotherapy is initiated, there is always a danger of prolonged use, despite the initial intent of relying on the medication only for a limited duration.

Cognitive Behaviour Therapy

The effectiveness of cognitive-behavioural approaches (referred to as cognitive behaviour therapy or CBT in the rest of the chapter) to the treatment of insomnia is well documented and it continues to be a growing area of research (Morin, Mimeault & Gagne, 1999). The goal of CBT in insomnia is to reduce sleep latency and improve sleep consolidation by changing behaviours, habits and maladaptive beliefs that interfere with sleep. CBT for insomnia is a short-term intervention and it involves five components: stimulus-control therapy; sleep-restriction therapy; relaxation training; cognitive restructuring; and sleep hygiene. Each of these components is described in detail later in this chapter.

Three meta-analyses support the efficacy of CBT with chronic insomnia (Montgomery & Dennis, 2003; Morin, Culbert & Schwartz, 1994; Murtagh & Greenwood, 1995). Overall 70–80% of insomnia patients benefited from CBT and the improvements were maintained or enhanced at follow-up. The improvements included significant reduction in sleep-onset latency and wake time after sleep onset, and increase in total sleep time. Three components of CBT – relaxation training, sleep restriction and stimulus control – were found to produce the most robust effects. A fourth meta-analysis (Smith et al., 2002) compared the efficacy of CBT and pharmacotherapy for insomnia. Hypnotic medications were comparable to stimulus-control and sleep-restriction therapies in sleep quality ratings and in the reduction of wake time after sleep onset and number of awakenings. Overall, CBT was associated with greater reductions in sleep-onset latency, whereas hypnotics were associated with greater increases in total sleep time.

Some studies have directly compared the effects of CBT and pharmacotherapy with insomnia. For example, Morin, Mimeault and Gagne (1999), in a randomised trial with elderly patients, found CBT, alone or in combination with pharmacotherapy, to be effective in reducing time awake after sleep onset. Although drug therapy alone was also found to be more effective than placebo, only those patients who continued to use the CBT strategies after the trial maintained the treatment gains at follow-up. Pharmacological treatments, however, produced somewhat faster sleep improvements in the short term. In the intermediate term (four to eight weeks), the behavioural approaches, including hypnosis and relaxation training, showed comparable effects to medication, but in the long term (6–24 months) these psychological interventions produced more favourable outcomes than pharmacotherapy. More recently, Jacobs *et al.* (2004) compared the use of CBT with the popular sleeping pill zolpidem tartrate (Ambien) in the treatment of sleep-onset insomnia. The study clearly indicated the superiority of CBT over zolpidem in reducing sleep-onset latency and increasing sleep efficiency and total sleep time. From these results, the authors concluded that CBT should be the first-line therapy for sleep-initiating insomnia. CBT also proved to be more cost effective and its effects more enduring.

Approximately 70–80% of patients treated with non-pharmacological interventions benefit from CBT (Morin, 2003, 2004; Morin & Azrin, 1987, 1988; Morin, Bastien & Savard, 2003). For patients with chronic primary insomnia, non-pharmacological treatments are likely to reduce sleep onset and/or wake after sleep onset to below 30 minutes with sleep quality and satisfaction scores significantly increasing (Morin, 1999, 2003, 2004; Morin & Azrin, 1987, 1988; Morin, Bastien & Savard, 2003). Three psychological treatments – stimulus-control therapy, progressive muscle relaxation and paradoxical intention – meet the American Psychological Association (APA) criteria for empirically supported behavioural treatments for insomnia. Three other treatments – sleep restriction, biofeedback and multi-faceted cognitive-behavioural therapy – meet APA criteria for 'probably' efficacious treatment. CBT has been found to show significantly more long-lasting improvements following treatment than pharmacological agents in treating chronic primary insomnia (Morin, 1996). This improvement is primarily due to CBT because this therapy targets the underlying problem causing the sleep disturbance and is not a mere 'band-aid approach' like pharmacological interventions. Additionally, termination of pharmacological agents can cause a rebound of the initial sleep difficulties (Graci & Hardie, 2007).

Hypnotherapy

Very little empirical research exists pertaining to the use of hypnotherapy as either a single- or multi-treatment modality for the management of sleep disorders (Graci & Hardie, 2007). Hypnosis as a single-treatment modality has been found to be effective in alleviating insomnia (Bauer & McCanne, 1980; Borkovec & Fowles, 1973; Dement & Vaughan, 2000; Hadley, 1996; Hammond, 1990; Hauri, 1993, 2000; Kryger, 2004; Spiegel & Spiegel, 1990; Stanton, 1990a, 1999; Weaver & Becker, 1996). Both hypnosis and self-hypnosis offer rapid methods for decreasing physiological arousal, managing anxiety, reducing worries and ruminations, facilitating deep relaxation and controlling mental over-activity – all of these being cardinal symptoms of insomnia

(Bauer & McCanne, 1980; Hammond, 1990). Self-hypnosis is considered to be a powerful voluntary relaxation technique (Dement & Vaughan, 2000) that is similar to meditation because it can calm down the mind and the body, preparing the person for sleep (Kryger, 2004). Therefore clinical hypnosis is considered to be a safe and effective method for treating insomnia as it allows the clinician to gain access to the underlying problems (e.g. hyperarousal; Modlin, 2002).

Several trials (Morin, 1999; Morin, Mimeault, & Gagne, 1999), reviews (Lichstein & Riedel, 1994) and meta-analyses (Morin, Culbert & Schwartz, 1994; Murtagh & Greenwood, 1995) have examined the efficacy of relaxation training and hypnosis for treatment of insomnia (Morin, 1999). From their meta-analysis of 59 studies, Morin, Culbert and Schwartz (1994) found that brief psychological interventions for insomnia, averaging five hours, produce reliable changes in sleep onset and time spent awake after an awakening. Similarly, the National Institute of Health (NIH; 1996) Technology Assessment Panel on Integration of Behavioural and Relaxation Approaches into the Treatment of Chronic Pain and Insomnia concluded that hypnosis and biofeedback produce significant changes in some aspects of sleep. However, from the report it was not clear whether the magnitude of improvements in sleep onset and total sleep time were clinically significant.

Graci and Hardie (2007) believe that the inconsistent findings in the studies of hypnosis with insomnia may be related to lack of collaboration with a sleep clinic. They recommend that clinicians trained in hypnotherapy consult with a sleep professional(s) when designing studies to ensure that the population is homogenous in terms of sleep disturbance. Within this context, it is also important to note that somatically based insomnias have not been amenable to hypnotic interventions (Weitzenhoffer, 2000), as Graci and Hardie (2007, p. 289) remind us:

there are many "biologic" based sleep disorders that often mimic psychological/behavioral sleep disorders such as insomnia. For instance, patients with undiagnosed obstructive sleep apnea may complain of difficulty maintaining sleep and experiencing ruminative thoughts centering on lack of sleep. This report could easily lead to an insomnia diagnosis and treatment for insomnia. In this example, treatment most likely will fail because the difficulty with maintaining sleep arises from biologic factors. More specifically, the patient stops breathing during sleep because the pharyngeal airway has narrowed and collapsed, obstructing the patient's airway (the hallmark feature of obstructive sleep apnea), and the body awakens (an evolutionary adaptive response to protect the body) in order to restore breathing. Hypnotherapists must always maintain a conservative approach when treating sleep disturbance. If patients are treated for sleep disturbance and there is no improvement in sleep functioning, referral to a sleep disorder center for evaluation is mandatory. While assessment options are available, a referral to a sleep specialist is strongly preferred (Graci, 2005; Graci & Sexton-Radek, 2005).

However, if psychological or behavioural issues are contributing factors in the biology-based sleep disorders, then hypnotherapy may be efficacious, specifically in reducing somatic and cognitive arousal states. In contrast, psychological insomnias (i.e. those precipitated by anticipatory anxiety and maintained cognitive rumination) are very appropriate for hypnotherapy. Relaxation training and hypnosis have also been found to be effective with late-life insomnia (Morin, Mimeault & Gagne, 1999). As mentioned earlier, in a randomised trial with elderly patients Morin, Mimeault & Gagne (1999) found CBT, alone or in combination with pharmacotherapy, to be effective in reducing time awake after sleep onset. Although the effect of medication and CBT was comparable initially, in the long term (6–24 months) the behavioural approaches, including hypnosis and relaxation, produced more favourable outcomes than pharmacotherapy.

Although there is some evidence that hypnosis is useful as an adjunct to CBT in the management of insomnia, there is an urgent need for more empirically based studies to demonstrate the efficacy of hypnosis in the treatment of insomnia disorders.

COGNITIVE HYPNOTHERAPY FOR INSOMNIA

Since insomnia is a complex disorder, any single-modality treatment is likely to address only one aspect of the sleep problem. It is widely agreed that effective treatment of insomnia must assume a multi-disciplinary approach in which physiological, psychological, behavioural and environmental interventions receive equal emphasis. Better results, although not consistently, are obtained when several strategies are combined (Morin, 1993; Lacks & Morin, 1992). While the earlier studies did not provide a rationale for combining various procedures with insomnia, recent research has used combined and sequential approaches in order to maximise the therapeutic benefits. However, Morin (1993) recommends judicious planning of multi-faceted treatment so that only clinically relevant procedures that target various aspects of the sleep problem are included in the treatment.

With this caveat, Graci (Graci, 2005; Graci & Hardie, 2007; Graci & Sexton-Radek, 2006) has integrated hypnotherapy with CBT, which is considered to be the first-line treatment or the gold standard of psychological treatment for insomnia (Jacobs et al., 2004). CBT is a multi-component intervention for insomnia, consisting of four components, namely education (e.g. sleep hygiene behaviours); stimulus control; sleep-restriction therapies (Manber & Kuo, 2002); and cognitive therapy. Some clinicians also include relaxation training as an adjunct or additional component. Since insomniacs have 'elevated physiologic activation, higher heart rates, body temperature, basal skin resistance, phasic vasoconstriction, and frontalis EMG activation than normal sleepers' (Manber & Kuo, 2002, p. 181), relaxation training is targeted at lowering physiological arousal. Some studies have used relaxation training as a single-component treatment for insomnia (see Morin, Culbert & Schwartz, 1994). The effect has been moderate, which is not surprising given that insomnia is a complex disorder. Relaxation methods have also been useful in facilitating withdrawal from hypnotic medications (Lichstein *et al.*, 1999). As discussed in Chapter 5, hypnosis produces rapid and deeper relaxation and associated syncretic cognition.

Based on these findings, Graci has substituted relaxation training for hypnotherapy within the CBT framework for insomnia. Figure 8.1 illustrates how to incorporate education regarding sleep hygiene, stimulus-control therapy, sleep-restriction strategies and cognitive therapy prior to hypnosis, and how to implement these techniques into hypnotic scripts when appropriate. Although Graci's model has not been subjected to empirical validation, her approach offers an excellent design for assessing the additive effect of hypnosis when combined with CBT, which is considered to be the gold standard for the psychological treatment of insomnia. Graci and Hardie (2007, p. 288) lament that 'very little empirical research exists pertaining to the use of hypnotherapy as either a single or multi-treatment modality for the management of sleep disorders' and as such there

> is an immediate need for more research evaluating the efficacy of hypnotherapy as both a single treatment and multi-treatment modality for managing sleep disturbance. Once this efficacy is established, it will increase the utilization of hypnotherapy and a demand for its services as a treatment of non-biologic sleep disorders.

Like Graci's goal, the aim of this chapter is to inform clinicians how to incorporate sleep therapy with hypnotherapy, with the hope of encouraging outcome studies. The cognitive hypnotherapy approach to insomnia described in this chapter therefore draws heavily on Graci's model.

Cognitive hypnotherapy for chronic insomnia normally requires about ten sessions and it involves six stages: assessment; stimulus-control therapy; sleep-restriction therapy; relaxation training; cognitive restructuring; and sleep hygiene. Each of these stages is described in detail.

Assessment

Deciding which psychological components to use with an individual patient and in what order to apply them is based on a thorough assessment of the patient's presenting problem and the resulting case conceptualisation (see Chapter 2 and Appendices C and D). When conducting the initial assessment

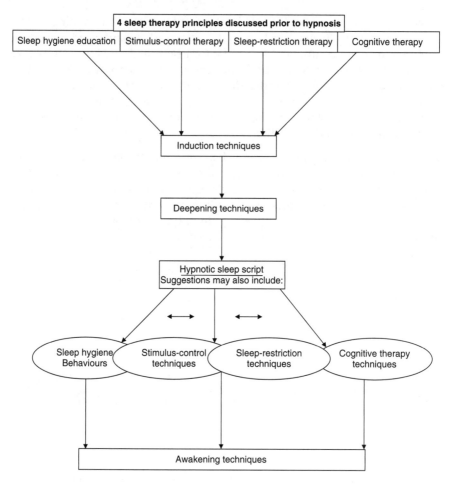

Figure 8.1 Illustration of how to incorporate sleep therapy with hypnotherapy.
Source: Graci, G. M. & Hardie, J. C. (2007). Evidence-based hypnotherapy for the management of sleep disorders. *International Journal of Clinical and Experimental Hypnosis*, 55(3): 288–302.

and formulating the case, Manber and Kuo (2002, p. 181) recommend attaching particular attention to the following factors:

- Sleep habits.
- Circadian tendencies.
- Other sleep disorders, particularly those associated with sleep fragmentation.
- Level of general anxiety and worry and cognitive arousal at bedtime.
- Ability to nap.
- Ability to sleep in environments other than one's bed (e.g. on a couch or away from home).

- Medical and psychiatric comorbid conditions.
- Current use of medications, other than hypnotics, and other substances that could affect sleep.
- Use of hypnotic medications or herbal preparations promising to have hypnotic effect.
- The impact of poor sleep on daytime functioning, particularly on daytime sleepiness.

The clinical history can be substantiated by several tools such as the sleep diary, psychological tests, actigraphy and polysomnography. In addition, a standardised hypnotic suggestibility test is administered to determine appropriateness for hypnosis. As one of the major components of cognitive hypnotherapy for insomnia is hypnotherapy, it is important to assess the patient's level of suggestibility.

Sleep diaries or *sleep logs* are widely employed as a component of the initial evaluation as well as for evaluation of treatment effect. Sleep logs represent a more accurate portrayal of the sleep of insomnia patients than do global, retrospective reports provided by patients during the initial interview. Completion of the logs encourages patients to develop a more objective assessment of their sleep disturbance and, in doing so, have some therapeutic efficacy in their own right (Sataeia, 2002). It is generally recommended that the patient complete the sleep diary daily for at least one to two weeks to obtain a representative profile. Many sleep questionnaires have been developed. The most widely used questionnaire is the Pittsburg Sleep Quality Index (PSQI; Buysse *et al.*, 1989), a 19-item measure of sleep quality and disturbance.

Psychological tests are used mainly for assessing the level of anxiety and depression. It is well documented that insomniacs have increased rates of psychopathology, most often characterised by anxiety, depression and internalisation of emotional conflict, with a tendency to somaticise this conflict (Hauri & Fisher, 1986; Kales *et al.*, 1976). The most commonly used psychometric instruments with insomnia include the Beck Anxiety Inventory (Beck & Steer, 1993a), the Beck Depression Inventory–Revised (Beck, Steer & Brown, 1996), Beck Hopelessness Scale (Beck & Steer, 1993b) and the Spielberger State-Trait Anxiety Scale (Spielberger, Gorsuch & Lushene, 1970).

Actigraphy is the study of sleep by means of a small motion-detection device typically worn on the non-dominant wrist. It is recommended that the actigraphy is conducted for at least three consecutive 24-hour periods (Sataeia, 2002). Actigraphy is a useful assessment tool for insomnia as it is unobtrusive, inexpensive and the data is collected from the patient's usual environment. Although actigraphy tends to overestimate the actual amount of sleep, it correlates strongly with the patterns of sleep monitored by polysomnography (Sadeh & Acebo, 2002).

Polysomnography (PSG), or overnight sleep study, is the gold standard for quantifying sleep and sleep disturbances (Buysse *et al.*, 2007). PSG is not routinely used with chronic insomnia as it confirms the patient's subjective report without indicating a cause for awakenings. However, it can be helpful for evaluating insomnia patients who show no response to first-line treatment, or those who may have symptoms of apnea, periodic limb movements or parasomnias.

Sleep Hygiene

Patients may also contribute to the initiation and maintenance of sleep disturbance. For instance, patients often lack knowledge about foods, drinks, medications and physical activities with psychostimulant properties that can interfere with sleep. Further, patients may know little about stress reduction or relaxation techniques that may promote sleep onset. Patients may overuse 'over-the-counter' or 'herbal remedies' that were designed for short-term use only. These are examples of maladaptive behaviours that interfere with nocturnal sleep and are termed 'poor' sleep hygiene behaviours (Hauri, 1993; Hauri, 2000). Sleep hygiene refers to the organisation of activities (e.g. pre-sleep behaviours) that promote sleep and minimise sleep disturbance. Typically, it incorporates the following behaviours:

• Reduce the intake of nicotine, caffeine and other stimulants.
• Avoid stimulants (if taken) in the afternoon or evening.
• Avoid alcohol near bedtime.
• Keep a regular daytime schedule for work, rest, meals, treatment, exercise and other daily activities.
• Perform strenuous exercises early in the day rather than in the late afternoon or evening.

Table 8.1 illustrates a more comprehensive list of 'adaptive' sleep hygiene behaviours. Insomnia complaints can often be corrected by implementing these 'proper' sleep hygiene behaviours. For instance, some patients are reluctant to avoid napping during the day, or they will unintentionally fall asleep during the day. This unintentional sleep is often a major contributor to the onset and maintenance of insomnia. The goal is to educate the patient so that they can eliminate behaviours that lead to sleep disturbance.

After a brief educational session, the patient initiates the behaviours at home. Subsequent clinic visits require evaluation of the success of these behaviours and discussion of specific barriers to achieving the goals of treatment. All four approaches require that patients monitor their sleep patterns as they initiate these changes, monitoring their sleep/rest/wake times using a sleep self-monitoring form (e.g. sleep diary) or other assessment instrument.

Table 8.1   Adaptive sleep hygiene behaviours.

---

1. Keep a regular time for going to sleep and waking up (even on weekends).
2. Create a bedtime routine – engage in quiet, calming activities.
3. The bedroom is for sleep and intimate activities only.
4. Don't lie down for bed until sleepy.
5. If you don't fall asleep within 15–20 minutes, get out of bed and go into another room and engage in a quiet nonstimulating activity until you are sleepy and then return to bed.
6. Sleep just long enough.
7. Regular exercise during the day can deepen sleep – it should be done 4–6 hours before bedtime.
8. Have a light bedtime snack – avoid heavy foods.
9. Reduce noise and light level.
10. Regulate room temperature.
11. Avoid stimulants – nicotine and food and drinks containing caffeine – 4–6 hours before bedtime and includes chocolate, coffee, and sodas.
12. Avoid alcohol – helps you fall asleep but causes awakenings and poor sleep later.
13. Avoid daytime naps – limit naps to 20 minutes and avoid them after 3 p.m.

Source: Graci, G. M. & Hardie, J. C. (2007). Evidence-based hypnotherapy for the management of sleep disorders. *International Journal of Clinical and Experimental Hypnosis*, 55(3): 288–302. Reprinted by permission.

Stimulus-Control Therapy

The American Academy of Sleep Medicine (Chesson *et al.*, 1999) and a meta-analysis (Morin, Culbert & Schwartz, 1994) of the behavioural interventions for insomnia identified stimulus control as one of the most effective non-pharmacological interventions for insomnia. The technique of stimulus control is based on the principle of classical conditioning, designed to strengthen the bed as a cue for sleep while weakening it as a cue for activities that are incompatible with sleep. The primary objective of stimulus-control therapy is to train the patient to associate the bed with sleeping and sleeping with the bed (Graci & Hardie, 2007). By virtue of fixing the wake-up time, the sleep–wake rhythm is stabilised. A general guideline is to educate patients about the bedroom environment, stressing that the bedroom is for sleep, intimate activities and a safe haven that is conducive to sleep. To achieve these goals, the following instructions are provided:

- Go to bed only when feeling sleepy.
- Use the bed only for sleep. No activity other than sleep, except for sexual activity, is permitted in bed. Other activities such as reading, eating, watching television or completing homework are not be carried out in bed, but in another area of the home.

- Get out of bed if unable to fall asleep within 15 to 20 minutes of retiring at night. When out of bed engage in relaxing and pleasant activities. Return to bed only when sleepy (this may be repeated as often as needed throughout the night).
- Set alarm and wake up at the same time every day, regardless of the amount of sleep achieved during the night.
- Avoid daytime naps.

For the stimulus-control therapy to succeed, the patient needs to be consistent with the instructions. Patients also need to have realistic expectations and the therapist should warn the patients that immediate improvement may not occur, but that it may occur after one or two weeks.

Sleep-Restriction Therapy

Sleep-restriction therapy was developed by Spielman, Caruso & Glovinsky (1987) and based on the homeostasis theory of sleep propensity (Stepanski, 2000). This approach seeks to increase homeostatic sleep drive through partial sleep deprivation and thereby improve sleep ability. This is achieved by creating a mild state of sleep deprivation with the goal of increasing 'sleep pressure' (need and drive to fall asleep) so that patients are able to fall asleep and maintain (i.e. consolidate) their sleep. The patient is initially prescribed a time-in-bed period that is equal in length to the total amount of sleep reported at baseline. For example, if a patient is prescribed to be in bed for seven hours but gets six hours of sleep only, then the patient will be prescribed six hours in bed.

The efficacy of sleep-restriction therapy has been evaluated with older adults (Morin, Culbert & Schwartz, 1994), who found the therapy helpful in reducing time awake after sleep onset. Some variations of this technique have also been found to be successful (Edinger et al., 1992; Friedman et al., 1991; Riedel, Lichstein & Dwyer, 1995). However, as with stimulus-control therapy, the outcome is related to consistent rising time and consistent time spent in bed (Manber & Kuo, 2002). Graci and Hardie (2007) caution hypnotherapists about utilising sleep-restriction therapy without having formal training and experience in this technique. They recommend consulting a sleep specialist if the therapist does not have experience in sleep restriction.

Hypnotherapy for Relaxation and Imagery Training

As mentioned before, insomniacs have elevated tonic arousal. CBT practitioners usually use relaxation or imagery training for lowering arousal, but within the context of cognitive hypnotherapy hypnosis is utilised. In the treatment of insomnia, hypnosis is specifically used for inducing relaxation; demonstrating the power of the mind; ego strengthening; imagery training; teaching self-hypnosis; and offering post-hypnotic suggestions.

Relaxation training

As discussed in previous chapters, one of the important goals of using hypnosis within the cognitive hypnotherapy context is to induce relaxation. Because of their elevated physiological activation, insomia patients derive significant benefit from learning relaxation techniques. Various hypnotic-induction techniques can be utilised to induce relaxation. I use the *relaxation with counting method* adapted from Gibbons (1979; see Alladin, 2007b) for inducing and deepening the hypnotic trance (see Appendix E).

Demonstration of the power of mind

Eye and body catalepsies are hypnotically induced to demonstrate the power of the mind over the body. These demonstrations reduce scepticism over hypnosis, foster positive expectancy and instil confidence in the insomia patients that they can relax and prepare their mind and body for sleep.

Ego strengthening

Ego-strengthening suggestions are offered to insomnia patients to increase confidence in their ability to train their mind and body for sleep. The fostering of *perceived self-efficacy* (Bandura, 1977) counters anticipatory anxiety related to not falling asleep and decreases negative rumination. The hypnosis script in Appendix E provides a list of generalised ego-strengthening suggestions that can be adapted for used with insomnia patients.

Imagery training for sleep

Following the ego strengthening, the patient is provided with an image for promoting further relaxation and preparing the patient for sleep. Although there are many hypnotic scripts provided in the literature (e.g. Hammond, 1990, pp. 253–5; Kroger & Fezler, 1976, pp. 201–5), I have selected two scripts from Graci and Hardie (2007) as they are specially developed within the context of cognitive hypnotherapy.

Hypnotic Scripts for Sleep: Example 1

Before you retire for bed, you will make sure that your bedroom is free of tension and worry. You will prepare yourself for relaxation and slumber by quietly freeing yourself from television or newspapers, as you focus your attention and strength on winding down from your day. Intuitively, you will begin to turn off lights, and quiet your mind. As you get into bed, you will automatically begin to relax. Your breathing will become deeply and profoundly relaxed and methodical. You will notice how you intuitively begin to fall asleep. You can rest assured that your body knows how to fall asleep and stay asleep and rest. You will be surprised at how well you are able

(Continued)

to fall deeply asleep. You will be able to sleep through the night and awake feeling refreshed and rested for the day. Your body will welcome the rest, as it is able to benefit from deep sleep. You will notice how easily you adapt to good restful sleep. You have confidence in knowing that as you sleep, your body is building strength and building its immune system. You will be able to know how profoundly your body is able to benefit from deep, deep, sleep. (Graci & Hardie, 2007, pp. 299–300. Reproduced with permission.)

Hypnotic Scripts for Sleep: Example 2

I want you to imagine walking towards your bedroom and as you are walking you are giving yourself permission to leave all worries, concerns or anything that is troubling you outside of your bedroom. When you awaken in the morning, you can retrieve these worries, concerns or troubles when you walk out of your bedroom. There is no need to bring these with you because your bedroom is a safe haven. It is your personal safety zone. It is here that you can experience comfort, safety and peace.

You notice the bedroom door is getting closer and closer and you are feeling more and more relaxed and peaceful. There is nothing of concern to you as approach your bedroom, and this feeling of relaxation becomes deeper and deeper, especially as you walk into your bedroom. You notice that you are feeling calmer, more secure, and more peaceful as you approach your bed. Your limbs are growing heavier and heavier as you pull back the covers of your bed. As you get into bed, you notice how comfortable you are lying in your bed. Your mind is quiet and you feel calm and relaxed. Your eyelids are beginning to get heavier and heavier and you welcome this feeling.

When you are ready, your eyelids close. You are lying in comfort and you notice that you are free of any emotional or physical discomfort. You don't have any concerns because your mind is very quiet and calm. You are feeling sleepier and sleepier. There is no need to check the clock because your body knows how to fall asleep, how to stay asleep and how to wake up when it is ready to awaken. The clock is unimportant and you will not feel a need to look at it because you are working with your body – nature's original sleep/wake clock. It is important to remember that when your body is ready to sleep, it will sleep. This experience of sleep will be a deep and profound sleep. If you awaken during the night, you will easily return to sleep even if you have gotten up to use the bathroom, because your body knows how to sleep. You feel peaceful and safe and are very, very sleepy. You know that your body knows how to sleep because you have done it since you were a child. And much like a child, you welcome sleep and your body will wake when it has had enough sleep. It is important to sleep just long enough and to keep the same bedtimes and wake times, even during the weekends. Rest assured, you will sleep well. You have the ability to experience deep restorative sleep, just as you have the ability to manage the day-to-day activities of your life right now. When you wake to your alarm in the morning, you will feel refreshed and energetic and ready to start your day. (Graci & Hardie, 2007, pp. 299–300. Reproduced with permission.)

Post-hypnotic suggestions

Before terminating the hypnotic session, post-hypnotic suggestions are given to consolidate the behavioural strategies and the ability to relax and prepare the mind and body for sleep.

Self-hypnosis training

The self-hypnosis component of cognitive hypnotherapy for insomnia is devised to cultivate low physiological reaction, counter negative rumination (negative self-hypnosis), provide continuity between sessions and facilitate transfer of skills to real situations. It is recommended that insomnia patients are trained to self-induce the hypnotic relaxation effectively without the need for external aids such as audiotapes or CDs (Manber & Kuo, 2002).

Cognitive Restructuring

While in bed, chronic insomniacs are cognitively aroused due to 'racing' mind and intrusive thoughts and worries. They tend to ruminate about the details of specific events that occurred during the day. According to Manber and Kuo (2002, p. 180):

> Cognitive arousal is maintained and exacerbated by thoughts and beliefs about sleep that are incompatible with the process of falling asleep. For example, thoughts that reflect high urgency for sleep or amplify the consequences of poor sleep are likely to increase mental arousal and interfere with sleep onset. One example of such thought is, 'I must fall asleep soon, otherwise I will be a mess tomorrow.' Similarly, thoughts that reflect a high need to control sleep lead to frustration and 'performance anxiety' that increase cognitive arousal and impede compliance with the stimulus control instruction to get out of bed when unable to sleep. An example of such thought is, 'If I just stay in bed and try a little longer, then I will fall asleep.'

CBT for insomnia aims to change these maladaptive thoughts and beliefs about sleep. A comprehensive review of CBT implementation with sleep disorders is contained in the work of Morin (Morin, 1996). CBT for insomnia involves the same principles used in cognitive behavioural therapy, except it is directed towards altering dysfunctional beliefs and attitudes about sleep (Lichstein & Morin, 2000). Moreover, maladaptive behaviours are replaced with more adaptive, 'pre-sleep and post-sleep' behaviours. However, the first step in CBT starts patient education. Educating the patient regarding CBT is an essential requirement for managing insomnia. Patients need to learn how to recognise sleep problems, as well as their maladaptive beliefs and behaviours. CBT can be started and conducted in the same format as described in Chapter 3 (also see Alladin, 2007b).

Hypnotherapy can also be integrated with the cognitive restructuring component. Graci and Hardie (2007) have listed three main objectives for integrating these cognitive strategies within the hypnotic scripts for sleep. These are countering the irrational thoughts with rational affirmations; inducing relaxation and deepening hypnotic techniques to increase time spent asleep; and assisting the patient in decreasing both daytime and nighttime heightened states of arousal and somatised tension.

SUMMARY

The chapter reviewed the aetiology and existing empirical literature on applications of hypnotherapy in the treatment of sleep disturbance.

There is an immediate need for more research evaluating the efficacy of hypnotherapy as both a single-treatment and multi-treatment modality for managing sleep disturbance. Once this efficacy is established, it will increase the utilisation of hypnotherapy and a demand for its services as a treatment of non-biological sleep disorders.

Although behavioural treatment approaches for sleep disturbance are initially more time consuming and more expensive than hypnotic medications, there are long-lasting benefits associated with behavioural treatments. For instance, over the course of total physician visits and prescriptions, it may be more cost effective for patients to engage in behavioural treatments. Current research findings support the use of behavioural approaches for treating 'non-biological' (i.e. behavioural) sleep disorders such as insomnia because these approaches target and resolve the underlying problem(s) associated with sleep disturbance, whereas pharmaceutical agents are a 'band-aid' approach to treatment. Emphasis must be placed on combining CBT and hypnotherapy as treatment approaches for sleep disorders.

In the meantime, it may be beneficial for hypnotherapists to gain specialist training in the evaluation and management of behavioural sleep disorders. This specialist training should teach clinicians how to incorporate sleep therapy treatment(s) into hypnotic scripts. Currently, the utilisation of hypnosis as either a single- or multi-treatment modality is limited to a very small subset of behavioural sleep disorders. There is an immediate need for more research evaluating the efficacy of hypnotherapy as a single- or multi-treatment modality for the management of sleep disorders. Once this efficacy is established, it will increase the utilisation of hypnotherapy and a demand for its services as a treatment for non-biological sleep disorders.

CHAPTER 9

COGNITIVE HYPNOTHERAPY IN THE MANAGEMENT OF SEXUAL DYSFUNCTIONS

INTRODUCTION

Sexual dysfunctions are characterised by disturbance in sexual desire and in the psychophysiological changes that characterise the sexual response cycle and cause marked distress and interpersonal difficulty (DSM-IV-TR; American Psychiatric Association, 2000). DSM-IV-TR lists three types of sexual dysfunctions: sexual desire disorders, sexual arousal disorders and orgasmic disorders. This chapter will focus on sexual arousal disorder, namely *male erectile disorder* (ED). With the 'Viagra revolution', the understanding and treatment of ED have changed dramatically in the past 10 years. The goal of this chapter is to review the aetiology and existing empirical treatments for ED and then to describe cognitive hypnotherapy for erectile dysfunction, a multi-modal treatment approach that combines sex therapy and medication (phosphodiesterase type-5 inhibitors; Cialis, Viagra and Levitra) with hypnotherapy in the management of ED. The multi-factor treatment protocol can be easily adapted to the treatment of other sexual dysfunctions. The chapter also discusses innovative ways of delivering treatment for ED within the context of sexual medicine. The detailed description of cognitive hypnotherapy for erectile dysfunction can be evaluated easily and from such an evaluation the additive effect of hypnosis to sex therapy for ED will be determined.

MALE ERECTILE DISORDER

Description and Classification

The essential feature of male erectile disorder (which will be referred to as erectile dysfunction or ED) is a persistent or recurrent inability to attain, or to maintain until completion of the sexual activity, an adequate erection

(DSM-IV-TR, 2000). For a diagnosis to be made the disturbance must cause marked distress or interpersonal difficulty and it must not be due to a psychiatric disorder, medical condition or substance abuse. Different patterns of ED can occur:

1. Inability to obtain an erection from the outset of a sexual experience.
2. A full erection is attained, but tumescence is lost at penetration.
3. A full erection is maintained at penetration, but tumescence is lost before or during thrusting.
4. An erection is experienced only during self-masturbation or on awakening.
5. Loss of erection during masturbation (rare occurrence).

ED is a very common sexual problem in men, affecting more than half of all men above the age of 50, including single and married men, irrespective of class. It can cause significant emotional distress and affect quality of life and relationship with partner. ED is associated with a variety of medical and psychological risk factors, and recent epidemiological studies have suggested that ED may be an early marker for cardiovascular disorders, diabetes mellitus and metabolic syndromes (e.g. Rosen et al., 2005; Thompson et al., 2005). These studies identified age, cardiovascular disease and depression as strong predictors of ED. The National Health and Social Life Survey (Laumann, Paik & Rosen, 1999) conducted in the United States found 7% of men under the age of 30 and 18% of men older than 50 to experience ED (defined as difficulty achieving or maintaining erection). The survey also found ED to be significantly related to overall health, emotional stress and history of lower urinary tract symptoms. Although distress and treatment seeking have usually been higher in younger and middle-aged men, recently there had been a dramatic increase in the number of men of all ages seeking oral therapies (PDE-5 inhibitors). It is estimated that there are currently 25–30 million men worldwide taking PDE-5 (phosphodiesterase type-5) inhibitors (Cialis, Viagra and Levitra) and an additional 50 million or more may be potential candidates for treatment (Rosen, 2007). The 'Viagra revolution' has encouraged many millions of men with ED to acknowledge their sexual problem and to seek medical treatment. Some writers (e.g. Bancroft, 2002) have, however, expressed concern about the potential risks associated with the 'medicalisation' of male sexuality and the entrepreneurial role of the pharmaceutical industry in this area. In addition, concerns have also been expressed about the 'false dichotomisation' of sexual dysfunction into organic and psychogenic classifications (Wincze & Carey, 2001) and an integrated model of treatment is recommended (e.g. Perelman, 2005).

ED is subclassified into organic or psychogenic, based on the absence or presence of specific organic factors, such as vascular, hormonal or neurogenic conditions. In the absence of these organic conditions, a psychogenic diagnosis of ED has been traditionally allocated. In other words, the psychogenic diagnosis was made by exclusion of organic causation. Lizza and Rosen (1999) proposed an expanded classification of psychogenic ED by incorporating clinical features (e.g. generalised vs situational ED) and the hypothesised aetiological mechanisms of central excitation or inhibition (see Table 9.1). This new classification broadened the scope and depth of psychological treatment for ED.

Table 9.1   Classification of psychogenic erectile dysfunction. Adapted from Rosen, C. R. (2007). Erectile dysfunction: Integration of medical and psychological approaches. In S. R. Leiblum (ed.), *Principles and Practice of Sex Therapy* (4th edn) (pp. 277–310). New York: Guilford Press.

I. Generalised type
  A. Generalised unresponsiveness
    1. Primary lack of sexual arousability
    2. Aging-related decline in sexual arousability
  B. Generalised inhibition
    1. Chronic disorder of sexual intimacy

II. Situational type
  A. Partner related
    1. Lack of arousability in specific relationship
    2. Lack of arousability due to sexual object preference
    3. High central inhibition due to partner conflict or threat
  B. Performance related
    1. Associated with other sexual dysfunction(s) (e.g. rapid ejaculation)
    2. Situational performance anxiety (e.g. fear of failure)
  C. Psychological distress or adjustment related
    1. Associated with negative mood state (e.g. depression) or major life stress (e.g. death of partner)

Masters and Johnson (1970) suggested that ED should also be subdivided into either *primary* (life-long) or *secondary* (acquired) type. Primary psychogenic ED, which is rare, refers to a life-long inability to achieve successful sexual performance, usually associated with a chronic pattern of sexual or interpersonal inhibition. Secondary psychogenic ED occurs after a period of satisfactory sexual performance (Rosen, 2007). Psychogenic ED can also be secondary to substance abuse, another psychiatric disorder (e.g. depression, generalised anxiety disorder) or another sexual problem.

AETIOLOGY OF ERECTILE DYSFUNCTION

Erection is a consequence of a sequence of responses involving the brain, spinal cord, peripheral nerves and local vasculature (Bancroft, 1989). In addition, awareness of a lack of erectile response can adversely affect this system by means of psychological mechanisms, as reviewed above. Therefore it is logical that a variety of factors can intervene at different points in this complex system, all producing failure of erection, and often more than one mechanism may be involved. The predominant theoretical hypotheses concerning the pathogenesis of ED can be grouped into psychogenic, organic and mixed approaches (Perelman, 2005).

Psychogenic Causes

During the first half of the 20th century, the main causes of ED were attributed to psychogenic factors. Freud highlighted deep-seated anxiety and internal conflicts as the root of sexual dysfunctions (Reynolds, 1981). In the genesis of ED, psychodynamic theories emphasise the role of underlying unconscious conflicts and hypothesise that ED is a manifestation of a generalised personality problem. Unresolved Oedipal conflicts are believed to produce feelings of guilt and fear about sex and, most importantly, result in unconscious castration anxiety. There is no evidence that specific psychological traits or styles are associated with ED, although anxiety and depression may manifest as sexual dysfunction (Perelman, 2005). Moreover, situational factors such as stress, environmental stimuli and relationship problems may contribute to or even cause ED. Kaplan (1974) suggested that ED may be better conceptualised as the physiological concomitant of anxiety rather than as the defence against it. This anxiety, she argued, need not be due to castration fears or an unresolved Oedipal conflict, but may be the result of sexual arousal being associated with negative contingencies (shame, fear of punishment or of physical illness) during a child's formative years. Similarly, *performance anxiety* (fear of inadequate performance) was identified by Masters and Johnson (1970), and also by Kaplan (1974), as the prime cause of ED. Some men have such unrealistically high expectations of their performance that they have to constantly monitor that performance. This monitoring behaviour causes anxiety, which can affect sexual arousal. Cognitive-behavioural theories emphasise the importance of being focused on sexual stimuli for arousal and erection to occur. Erection is impaired if a man instead focuses on non-sexual thoughts, such as work problems or the idea that he has to succeed at sex (Ellis, 1980). Marital therapists have emphasised that sexual problems are often a manifestation of underlying couple dynamics (Segraves, 1982).

Although none of the psychogenic theories explains the full complexity of ED, they all emphasise the role of anxiety in erectile dysfunction. Bancroft (1999) provides some understanding of the role of anxiety and other psychogenic factors in ED in his description of the delicate balance between central excitatory and inhibiting mechanisms. Other investigators and clinicians have described the role of cognition in initiating anxiety and maintaining sexual arousal difficulties. For example, Rosen (2001) and Zilbergeld (1992) have shown how alterations in perceptual and attentional processes can directly lead to variation in erection. Moreover, Masters and Johnson (1970) have demonstrated how 'spectatoring' during intercourse (focusing attention away from arousing stimulus and preoccupied with negative cognitions) has a dampening effect on erectile capacity and response.

Organic Causes

Despite the large literature indicative of psychogenic aetiologies, there is significant evidence of the role of organic factors in the causation of ED. Specific organic factors such as vascular, hormonal, neurogenic or mechanical can determine ED. If these factors are present to a significant degree and if the patient's history indicates a temporal association between the onset of the erectile dysfunction and the patient's medical condition, an organic diagnosis is suggested (Rosen, 2007). Although ED has multi-factorial causes, several chronic diseases such as atherosclerosis, heart disease, hypertension and diabetes have been identified to be associated with ED (Feldman *et al.*, 1994). From the men presenting with ED, 18% have been found also to suffer from undiagnosed hypertension, 16% from diabetes, 15% from benign prostatic hyperplasia, 5% from ischaemic heart disease, 4% from prostate cancer and 1% from depression (Curkendall *et al.*, 2001). Also as noted before, there is a strong correlation between age and erectile failure in clinical populations. This may reflect the greater likelihood of pathological factors, such as arterial disease, in older men. In the last 10 years with the progressive shift in diagnostic sophistication, advances in surgical techniques and predominantly pharmaceutical treatments, ED is seen as an organic disorder by most clinicians and the general public.

Mixed Causes

The current approach to the pathogenesis of ED embraces a 'mixed' paradigm, wherein the importance of both organic and psychological factors is appreciated for their role in predisposing, precipitating, maintaining and reversing erectile dysfunction (Perelman, 2005). This rebalancing of perspective is catalysed by the consensus of opinions voiced by the mental health professionals that psychological factors are critical to the understanding of sexual function and dysfunction (Althof, 1998; Leiblum & Rosen, 2000; McCarthy, 1998; Perelman, 2003). While sexual pharmaceuticals are highly efficacious, rewarding sexual function is only experienced in a satisfactory relationship. Perelman (2005, p. 434) states:

> ED, like other sexual dysfunctions, is best understood as being caused by an interaction of organic and psychogenic factors. There is a strong likelihood of biologic variability in the arousal threshold. Although the exact nature of a biologic predisposition is not known, it is reasonable to conclude that the 'threshold' for erectile onset and latency may have a distribution curve like numerous other human variables.

This view is similar to theories regarding biologically predisposed thresholds for ejaculation described by Perelman (2001) and Waldinger (2002, 2005). Determining whether the exact physiologic mechanism(s) of such a 'threshold' are central, peripheral or some combination, requires further research. However, this pattern of susceptibility presumably interacts with a variety of sexual circumstances and intra- and interpersonal dynamics, in addition to environmental and medical risk factors, resulting in a manifest dysfunction.

Moreover, the biological set point for erectile latency is affected by multiple organic and psychogenic factors in varying combinations over the course of a man's life cycle. The 'mixed' approach to understanding ED is very well illustrated by the study conducted by LoPiccolo (1992). LoPiccolo studied 63 men with ED, who were thoroughly investigated both organically and psychologically. He found 10 men to have a purely psychogenic etiology, 3 men a purely organic etiology and the majority (50 out of 63) displayed a mixture of factors. Interestingly, one third of the men (19 out of 63) had 'mild organic impairments' but 'significant psychological problems'. LoPiccolo's findings suggest that even if a factor that is of *potential* aetiological significance is found (biological or psychological), it is not necessarily *the* factor. In other words, the detection of some possible aetiological factor does not mean that the cause has been fully explained (Maurice, 1999). Such a factor may be coincidental and of no actual aetiological significance. Furthermore, when any one organic factor occurs in isolation, it may serve to make erections more vulnerable to emotional disturbances and sympathetic over-activity, facilitating the vicious circle of performance anxiety that maintains ED (Buvat *et al.*, 1990). In addition, regardless of the aetiology, men with ED have performance anxiety, which affects their tumescence during sex.

TREATMENT OF ERECTILE DYSFUNCTION

With the Viagra revolution, the approach to the treatment of ED has changed significantly in the past 10 years. In the 1970s and 1980s the first-line treatment for ED was sex therapy, revolutionised by the work of Masters and Johnson and Kaplan, and the treatment was mainly provided by sex therapists and mental health workers. The current trend is the pharmacological treatment of ED, predominantly carried out by family physicians and urologists. In this section, psychological, hypnotic, medical and combined medical and sex therapy approaches to the treatment of ED will be reviewed.

Psychological Approaches

Rosen (2007) identifies five approaches to the psychological management of psychogenic ED. These approaches include anxiety reduction and desensitisation; cognitive behavioural interventions; increased sexual stimulation;

interpersonal assertiveness and couple communication training; and relapse-prevention training. These approaches will be described in detail later in this chapter. From their review of the evidence-based psychological treatments for ED, Segraves and Althof (2002) concluded that both life-long and acquired ED patients achieved significant gains initially and over the long term following participation in sex therapy. Men with acquired ED tended to do better than those with primary erectile dysfunction. Masters and Johnson (1970) reported initial failure rates of 41% for primary ED and 26% for secondary ED, and long-term failure rates of 41% and 31% for primary and secondary ED respectively.

In an excellent review of the well-controlled investigations of psychological therapies for ED, Mohr and Beutler (1990) noted that the results were not as impressive as those reported by Masters and Johnson (1970); nonetheless, two-thirds of the patients improved and the treatment gains were maintained at follow-ups ranging from six weeks to six years. However, all the long-term follow-up studies noted a tendency for men to suffer relapses. Hawton, Catalan and Fagg (1992) found positive treatment outcome to be associated with better pre-treatment communication and general sexual adjustment, especially the female partner's interest in and enjoyment of sex, the absence of psychiatric history in women, and the couple's willingness to complete home-work. From these findings it would appear the combination of medication and sex therapy involving the partner may enhance the treatment outcome.

Hypnotherapy for Erectile Dysfunction

Although hypnotherapy for ED comes under psychological intervention, it is reviewed separately here to highlight hypnotic approaches to treatment. Many clinicians and authors (e.g. Araoz, 1985, 2005; Crasilneck, 1982; Hammond, 1990; Lemke, 2005) have written about the usefulness of hypnotherapy in the management of sexual dysfunctions, but as yet there is no controlled trial of hypnotherapy with any specific sexual disorder. Crasilneck (1979, 1982) has reported a large number of case studies and follow-ups of patients with ED treated with hypnosis. Due to lack of objective pre- and post-measures it is difficult to draw conclusions about the effectiveness of hypnosis with ED. An assortment of hypnotic techniques for ED can be gleaned from the literature, including anxiety management, ego strengthening, ego integration, imagery training, sensitivity training, reframing, regression, and unconscious explor-ation and reprocessing. Although most writers stress the adjunctive nature of hypnosis, a detailed description of how these hypnotic techniques are integ-rated with other forms of therapy is not provided. For example, Yapko (2003, p. 443) states that 'hypnosis and sex therapy are two highly compatible and easily integrated approaches to the treatment of sexual dysfunction', but there is no description or treatment protocol for such an integration with ED avail-able from the literature. The purpose of this chapter is to provide a conceptual framework of multi-modal therapy for ED within which hypnotic techniques can be easily assimilated.

Figure 9.1 provides a schematic representation of utilising hypnosis as an adjunct to sex therapy with ED patients. Zilbergeld and Hammond (1988)

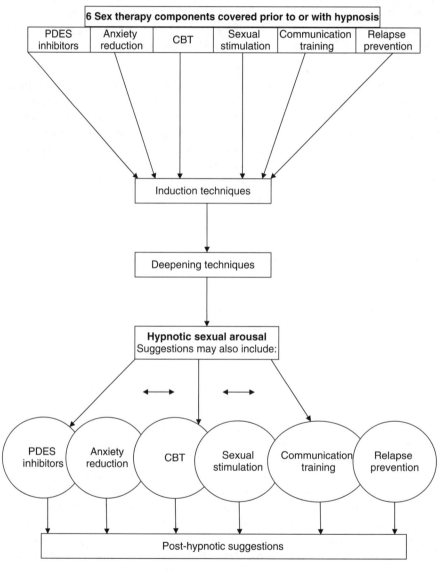

Figure 9.1   Illustration of how to incorporate sex therapy with hypnotherapy. Based on Graci, G. M. & Hardie, J. C. (2007). Evidence-based hypnotherapy for the management of sleep disorders. *International Journal of Clinical and Experimental Hypnosis*, 55(3): 288–302.

provide several reasons for utilising hypnosis as an adjunct to sex therapy. As these reasons provide the rationale for integrating hypnosis with sex therapy, they are summarised below:

- Hypnosis has an additive effect when combined with other forms of therapy. The therapist does not have to change their theoretical orientation to accommodate hypnosis within their preferred mode of therapy to gain 'a group of methods that can enhance the results of whatever he or she already does' (Zilbergeld & Hammond, 1988, p. 196).
- Hypnosis provides several methods of uncovering unconscious or forgotten causes of sexual dysfunction. Although modern sex therapy focuses on 'here and now', Masters and Johnson (1970) used a two-tier model of *current* (e.g. performance anxiety, spectatoring) and *historical* (e.g. religious orthodoxy, psychosexual trauma) causes to conceptualise the aetiology of human sexual dysfunctions (Davison *et al.*, 2005). Hypnosis can facilitate the recovery of historical information in cases where current factors do not adequately explain the causes of ED and the patient is not responding to traditional sex therapy.
- Hypnosis facilitates 'goal' or 'result imagery'.
- Hypnosis enhances 'process' imagery or 'mental rehearsal'.
- Hypnosis helps to alter the *structure* and *content* of the patient's mental representations.
- Hypnosis induces relaxation rapidly and this response is consolidated and generalised to various situations via self-hypnosis.

Medical Treatments

In this section, the review will focus on pharmacotherapy and miscellaneous medical procedures such as intracavernosal injection, intraurethral alprostadil, vacuum constriction device therapy and surgery.

Pharmacotherapy

The most common and the most popular pharmacotherapy for ED is oral medication. Currently, there are three highly efficacious PDE-5 inhibitors, FDA (Food and Drugs Administration) approved treatments for ED: sildenafil (Viagra), vardenafil (Levitra) and tadalafil (Cialis). These three PDE-5 inhibitors are used worldwide and they are reported to be safe, well tolerated and effective in restoring erections in about 75% of the men using the drugs (Rosen, 2007). With proper advice and a cooperative sex partner, simple cases of ED respond well to the medication. However, these drugs may prove to be ineffective in the presence of relationship difficulties, desire deficits, partner sexual dysfunctions or other medical conditions (Rosen, 2007). The successful outcome in clinical trials obscures the fact that participants in the trials were screened out for depression and relationship problems. Nowadays, in a busy primary care practice, most physicians will initiate treatment with PDE-5 regardless of the aetiology (Perelman, 2005) and without a comprehensive assessment of medical, psychological and relationship issues contributing to the genesis of ED. Leiblum (2007, p. 218), in her editorial comments on Rosen's chapter (Rosen, 2007), summarides the concerns:

> Determining whether the erectile problems are situational or generalized, lifelong or acquired is important as well as interviewing the man alone and with his partner. Evaluation of *patient factors* such as performance anxiety or sexual inhibition, *partner factors* such as low self-esteem or dysfunction, *relationship quality and satisfaction*, and *contextual issues* such as financial or extended family stresses sheds light on variables that may need to be addressed in treatment.

> Increased genital tactile stimulation is often a critical ingredient in achieving good erections and this becomes especially important when treating older men. Often, a female partner is unaware of the physiological necessity of direct stimulation and may misattribute a man's lack of erection to sexual disinterest or her loss of sexual appeal. At the same time, menopausal or sexual desire and arousal problems may interfere with a partner's sexual responsivity or receptivity. It is for this reason that it is so important to assess individually and together the patient with ED and his partner.

When a PDE-5 inhibitor is used within the context described by Leiblum (2007), not only will the medication be perceived as a powerful remedy, but it will also serve as an extremely helpful adjunct to the comprehensive treatment of erectile disorders. On the other hand, there are some disadvantages and risks to using PDE-5 inhibitors with ED, and these are summarised below:

- They present special risks to selected subpopulations. Concomitant nitrate use is strongly contra-indicated with all three PDE-5 inhibitors.
- Although they are not contra-indicated with high-risk cardiac conditions such as angina and recent heart attack, sexual activity may be risky. So these patients should not be prescribed any of the three PDE-5 inhibitors.
- They are contra-indicated with sickle-cell disease and with patients using other eretogenic agents such as intracorporal injection (may cause *priapism* – prolonged erection).
- Patients with ophthamological disorders should be carefully evaluated before prescribing PDE-5 inhibitors, as these drugs have an effect on the phosphodiesterase enzymes in the eye.
- Over 25% of patients with ED do not respond to any of the PDE-5 inhibitors.
- The drugs do not address key individual and couple issues that may be the cause or the maintaining factors.
- A substantial proportion of men with ED discontinue with the medication. A large study (N = 25,000, from eight countries) found that only 16% of patients with SD continued with the medication (Rosen *et al.*, 2004).
- The success rate of PDE-5 inhibitors is lower in ED patients with chronic sexual or marital conflict, lack of desire in both partners and significant psychiatric illness in either partner (Leiblum, 2002; Perelman, 2005). In these cases a combination of medication and sex or marital intervention is recommended.

- The use and effectiveness of these drugs are over-publicised, providing a narrow or medicalised view of ED.
- The medicalisation of sex therapy perpetuates the 'false dichotomisation' of sexual dysfunctions into organic and psychogenic classifications.

Miscellaneous medical procedures

These procedures involve intracavernosal injection, intraurethral alprostadil, vacuum constriction device therapy and surgery. Prior to the advent of PDE-5 inhibitors, these medical and surgical options were available for the treatment of ED. Since the introduction of PDE-5 inhibitors, these procedures have been less widely used and nowadays they are considered to be 'second-line' treatments for ED. For a detailed presentation and discussion of each method, readers are referred to the 2nd International Consultation on Sexual Medicine (Lue *et al.*, 2004).

Combined Medical and Sex Therapy

Although PDE-5 inhibitors are considered the first-line treatment for ED, from the above reviews it would appear that many clinicians have been advocating a multi-modal approach to therapy consisting of pharmacological and sex therapy interventions. Rosen (2007, p. 297) provides several reasons for such integration:

> There are several reasons for this, including growing awareness of the limitations of pharmacological therapy for individuals or couples with psychological barriers or conflicts. In some cases, prescription of a PDE5 inhibitor may underscore or exacerbate a couple's underlying conflicts or reveal a lack of desire in one or both partners. Sexual problems in the partner or other couple issues may be accentuated following successful (or unsuccessful) use of sildenafil. Although this concern applies equally in the case of any medical or surgical treatment for ED (Althof, 1998), in light of the sheer numbers of men taking PDE5 inhibitors (more than 20 million at the time of writing) and the widespread use of the drugs, the role of concomitant psychological or interpersonal problems has been highlighted dramatically. Rather than rendering sex therapy obsolete or unnecessary, the introduction of PDE5 inhibitors has led to a redefining of the role and importance of psychological interventions in ED. This is particularly relevant nowadays, in view of high rates of discontinuation and dropout from medical therapy (Rosen *et al.*, 2004).

A very recent study (Banner, Rodney & Anderson, 2007) compared the effectiveness of an integrative treatment protocol (ITP) consisting of sildenafil and cognitive behaviour sex therapy (CBST) with sildenafil alone. The subjects consisted of 53 men (couples) with psychogenic ED who were randomly allocated to either ITP or sildenafil. After four weeks of combined treatment, 48% of men met criteria for success on erectile function and 65.5% for satisfaction compared to men on sildenafil alone with 29% and 37.5% success rates, respectively. After the first four weeks of treatment, the sildenafil group also received CBST for four weeks and the results were compared to the first mixed group. This study clearly indicates the higher rate of clinical success with combined psychological and pharmacological treatment. Perelman (2005) has proposed two models of integrated care for ED that can be adopted within the framework of sexual medicine. These two models of care delivery can be labelled independent practice and collaborative practice.

- *Independent practice model.* Primary care physicians (PCPs) or urologists practise independently but integrate sex counselling with pharmaceutical armamentarium to treat sexual dysfunction.
- *Collaborative practice model.* In this model the PCPs or the urologists, armed with the pharmaceutical armamentarium, collaborate with sex therapists within a coordinated multi-disciplinary treatment approach. The clinical combinations are determined by the presenting symptoms and the varying expertise of these healthcare professionals.

For these two models to work, Perelman (2005, p. 442) has listed several criteria that need to be met:

- The clinician first consulted by the patient will determine his or her own desire, interest, training and competence to treat ED.
- A biopsychosocial approach to aetiology, assessment and treatment will be adopted.
- The clinician in consideration of the two previous criteria, in collaboration with the patient, will determine who initiates the treatment as well as how and when to refer.
- The independent or the collaborative model will be determined by the psychosocial complexity of the case.
- The treating clinician will diagnose the patient as suffering from mild, moderate or severe psychosocial obstacles. This characterisation will be determined by assessment of all the available information and the assessment should continue throughout the therapy (taking a case-formulation approach).
- The consulted clinician would continue treatment and make referrals based on progress obtained.
- Hypnosis can facilitate sex therapy in the absence of a partner.

The cognitive hypnotherapy approach described in the next section adopts the collaborative model, as in most cases the ED patient is referred to the sex therapist after an unsuccessful trial of PDE-5 inhibitors.

COGNITIVE HYPNOTHERAPY FOR ERECTILE DYSFUNCTION

Cognitive hypnotherapy (CH) combines sex therapy with hypnotherapy within the framework of sexual medicine. This multi-modal approach to treating ED can be delivered solo, either by primary care physicians (PCP) or by urologists depending on the complexity of the case and the interest and competence of the treating clinician. Or the mixed treatment can be offered collaboratively by the PCP or the urologist and the sex therapist. In practice, the combined treatment is normally delivered within the collaborative practice model. Usually the patient is referred to a sex therapist or a mental health professional following an initial trial of a PDE-5 inhibitor, or while the patient is on it. As the majority of the sex therapists or mental health professionals practising sex therapy and hypnotherapy are non-physicians, the collaborative approach is the most widely used model of care delivery for the ED patients.

As we saw earlier, CH for ED involves six components: medication; anxiety reduction and desensitisation; cognitive behavioural interventions; increased sexual stimulation; interpersonal assertiveness and couple communication training; and relapse-prevention training. Figure 9.1 earlier in the chapter illustrates how to incorporate sex therapy and sexual medicine with hypnotherapy. Hypnotherapy serves the dual purpose of enhancing and consolidating the effect of each of the six components. The description of CH will illustrate how hypnotherapy is integrated with each component as an adjunct. Although there is no controlled trial of hypnotherapy with sexual dysfunctions, as reviewed in previous chapters several reviews, meta-analyses and trials have demonstrated the additive effect of hypnotherapy when combined with cognitive behaviour therapy (CBT) in the management of various emotional disorders (e.g. Alladin & Alibhai, 2007; Bryant *et al.*, 2005; Kirsch, Montgomery & Sapirstein, 1995; Schoenberger, (2000). It is expected that hypnotherapy as an adjunct to sex therapy (including medication) will enhance the treatment effect. However, this hypothesis can be reliably tested by controlled trials. Nonetheless, the CH protocol for ED as described in this chapter provides a design for evaluating the additive effect of hypnotherapy with ED. Before describing the six components of CH for ED, the assessment procedure is discussed.

Assessment

The evaluation of ED is complex and often requires considerable collaboration with other health professionals. As with other disorders covered in this book, the medical and the psychosexual assessments of ED are carried out within the context of case formulation (see Appendices C and D). Given the strong evidence of the association between ED and various medical risk factors (e.g. diabetes, coronary artery disease), a comprehensive medical history, physical examination and selected laboratory testing for all men with ED are recommended by the recent guidelines published by the 2nd International Consultation on Sexual Dysfunction in Men and Women (Lue *et al.*, 2004). Although this screening is not different from a routine physical examination, special emphasis is placed on genitourinary, endocrine, vascular and neurologic systems (Rosen, 2007). The assessment should also review patient factors, such as performance anxiety or sexual inhibition; partner issues, such as low self-esteem or sexual performance problems; quality of the overall relationship; and sexual and contextual variables, such as financial stress and family dysfunction (Althof *et al.*, 2005). The clinician should also briefly screen for obvious psychopathology that may significantly interfere with the initiation of treatment (Perelman, 2005).

Medication

The referring physician is usually responsible for the prescription and monitoring of PDE-5 inhibitors. However, the physician should offer patients choices about their preference for treatment. Perelman (2005) points out that the provision of an unbiased and balanced description of treatment options, including information about pharmacokinetics, efficacy studies and the clinician's own experience, results in the patient attaching greater importance to the clinician's opinions. Incorporation of the patient's preference in treatment promotes a therapeutic alliance, improves compliance, and minimises psychosocial obstacles. Perelman (2005) advises physicians to take advantage of this information to increase treatment efficacy. The physician should also be sensitive about addressing the patient's concern about the safety and long-term side effects of the medication.

Anxiety Reduction and Desensitisation

Anxiety-reduction techniques have historically been a central feature of the psychological treatment of ED. For example, Wolpe (1958) and Lazarus (1965) emphasised the importance of systematic desensitisation in overcoming performance anxiety and inhibitions typically associated with ED. They also recommended the use of relaxation techniques and avoidance of intercourse during the early phases of treatment. But it was Masters and Johnson (1970) who developed the 'sensate focus' exercises, a form of in vivo desensitisation to overcome or neutralise the effects of performance anxiety in men with ED. As the sensate focus is still considered central to the psychological management of ED, it is described in detail here (summarised from Bancroft, 1989). Sensate focus consists of three stages: sensate focus one (SF1), sensate focus two (SF2) and sensate focus three (SF3).

Sensate Focus One (SF1)

SF1 is designed to eliminate performance anxiety, develop feelings of trust in the relationship, gain a sense of self-protection and acquire self-assertion. The couple are instructed to take it in turn to caress and touch each other when unclothed, comfortable and securely private. However, there will be no genital touching or intercourse. The person doing the touching or caressing should be

doing it for his or her own sake; that is, enjoying the touching rather than trying to please the partner (i.e. self-asserting). The person being touched should
not reciprocate, except to indicate if he or she is finding anything unpleasant,
however slight (i.e. self-protecting); then the person doing the touching will
stop or change what is being done. After about 20 minutes the couple change
places and the other person becomes the active toucher. This alternating pattern applies also to the initiating process; that is, the couple take turns to be
the first to start the exercise at every session.

Prior to starting the sensate focusing, the couple are given a clear rationale for
doing the exercises. The main reason behind SF1 is to learn to touch for one's
own pleasure; that is, the exercises allow those participating:

- To check that each person feels comfortable being sexually assertive and does not
  have to give pleasure first before being able to experience it.
- To discover or rediscover that touching can be pleasurable in itself.
- To remove a sense of obligation to respond on the part of the recipient, e.g. 'She is
  trying to arouse me, why aren't I getting an erection?' This relief from performance
  pressure often allows the person being touched to enjoy the experience even more.

The couple are advised to practise SF1 about three times a week. It takes
about one to three weeks, depending on the complexity of the case, to achieve
the goals related to SF1. The therapist reviews progress and addresses any
concerns that arise.

Sensate Focus Two (SF2)

Once the couple are able to relax and begin to enjoy the pleasuring exercises,
they graduate to SF2. This stage differs from SF1 only in that the person being
touched is asked to give positive as well as negative feedback. In other words,
the person is able to freely communicate what is enjoyable as well as what is
unpleasant. The touching partner can then act accordingly. About one to two
weeks (three times a week) are needed to achieve the goals of SF2.

Sensate Focus Three (SF3)

When the couple are able deal with the exercises involved in SF2, they are
instructed to move on to SF3. In this stage genital touching is allowed and
if full erection is achieved intercourse is allowed. Patients with ED who are
on PDE-5 inhibitors are instructed to take the medication 30 minutes before
the initiation of an SF3 exercise. ED patients with a prescription for PDE-
5 inhibitors are instructed not to take the medication while their therapy is
at SF1 and SF2 phases. The goal of SF3 is simply to enjoy the experience of
touching and being touched. If full erection is achieved intercourse is allowed,
but it should occur at the end of the SF3 exercises. Although touching of the
genitals is allowed, one person should not try to arouse or masturbate the

partner. During intromission, the ED patient is encouraged to focus on the feeling of being 'inside' rather than focusing on performance. The subsequent sessions are tailored to suit the needs of the couple.

Hypnotherapy for Relaxation and Imagery Training

The reduction of anxiety, in vivo desensitisation and SF exercises can be enhanced with the aid of hypnosis. As anxiety seems to be central to ED, hypnosis can be utilised to induce relaxation; to demonstrate the power of the mind; in ego strengthening; in imagery training; to teach self-hypnosis; and to offer post-hypnotic suggestions.

Relaxation training

As mentioned in previous chapters, one of the important goals of using hypnosis within the cognitive hypnotherapy context is to induce relaxation. Zilbergeld and Hammond (1988) have made the observation that although sex therapists emphasise the role of anxiety in ED, they do not train their patients to relax. It is also ironic that sex therapists inhibit sexual intercourse during SF1 and SF2 stages, but do not teach their patients skills to cope with the sexual prohibition. Patients can learn these skills very easily via hypnosis.

Various hypnotic induction techniques can be utilised to produce deep relaxation. I routinely use the relaxation with counting method adapted from Gibbons (1979; see Alladin, 2007b) for inducing and deepening the hypnotic trance (see Appendix E). By learning to relax, ED patients are able to reduce anxiety and enhance feelings of self-efficacy, well-being and sense of control (Bernstein, Borkovec & Hazlett-Stevens, 2000). These experiences promote positive expectancy and a strong therapeutic alliance.

Demonstration of the power of the mind

Eye and body catalepsies are hypnotically induced to demonstrate the power of the mind over the body. These demonstrations ratify the power of hypnotic trance, foster positive expectancy and instil confidence in ED patients that they can have control over their sexual dysfunction.

Ego strengthening

Ego-strengthening suggestions are offered to ED patients to increase confidence in their ability to overcome their symptoms. The fostering of *perceived self-efficacy* (Bandura, 1977) counters performance anxiety and negative cognitions related to their dysfunction. The hypnosis script in Appendix E provides a list of generalised ego-strengthening suggestions that can be adapted for use with ED patients.

Imagery training for arousal

Following ego strengthening, the patient is provided with an image for promoting relaxation, getting involved in the SF exercises and getting aroused. Hammond (1990, pp. 358–9) provides a hypnotic script for helping the ED patient avoid spectatoring and get involved and absorbed in the SF exercises. He also provides a script for inducing arousal and promoting erection (Hammond, 1990, p. 354). Hammond calls it the *Master Control Room Technique*, which involves the ED patient imagine entering a control room in the hypothalamus and regulating sexual desire and erection.

> In this technique, the patient imagines entering a control room in the hypothalamus, where there is a panel regulating sexual desire on which is a dial or lever that may be set from 0 to 10. The patient is told that 0 represents the level of no desire, while 10 is very high sexual interest. The patient tells the therapist what number the dial is set on (most typically 1 or 2). Suggestions are then given to imagine gradually moving the dial upward, one number at a time. Between numbers, suggestions are offered that hormones are being released and that the patient is beginning to feel increasing sexual desire. Many patients are surprised to find themselves feeling arousal during this experience. The therapist then negotiates with the patient the number that the sexual desire should remain set on. Interestingly, several patients have returned a week or two later not only to report daily sexual activity, but also to convey their partners' request that it would be fine if we turned the dial down a couple of numbers! (Zilbergeld & Hammond, 1988, pp. 204–5)

Here is another imagery script, *Erectile Imagery*, from Saral (2003, pp. 272–3) that can become part of the hypnotic suggestions for regressing the patient to a time when he was experiencing full erection. This regressive technique can revivify the good memories that may help to rekindle and recapture positive sexual and affectional feelings. As discussed in Chapter 5, hypnosis can be a more powerful technique than imagery training.

> Imagine your most joyful and satisfying erection experience. Recall all the sensory memories associated with that experience. Bring alive all of the sensory experiences at that moment. Recall if you were touching someone or something, if someone was touching you, and if so, where and how. Were you wearing any clothes or were you naked? How did the touch of your own body feel? Were you alone, or was there someone with you? If alone, what were you visualizing? Recall the sounds that may have been occurring at that time – music, talk, moaning, sighing, blowing wind. Remember also the fragrances and smells that were in the air. Were you indoors or outdoors? What was your body position? Were you sitting, standing, or lying down?
>
> Recall your most joyous and fulfilling sexual encounter. How did the erection start? How flaccid or hard was your penis? What made the erection get harder? How long did the erection last? How did the experience end? Now that you

know that you have the ability to create and maintain an erection, I want you to recall a time when you had the most exciting and satisfying intercourse with a partner, maintaining your full erection.

Posthypnotic suggestions

Before terminating the hypnotic session, post-hypnotic suggestions are given to consolidate the relaxation training, self-hypnosis, lessening of performance anxiety and spectatoring, and increase in arousal and erection.

Self-hypnosis training

The self-hypnosis component of cognitive hypnotherapy for ED is devised to reduce performance anxiety, increase self-confidence, counter negative rumination (negative self-hypnosis) and facilitate transfer of skills to real situations.

Cognitive Behaviour Therapy

Based on psychophysiological studies of males with ED, Barlow and associates (Barlow, Sakheim & Beck, 1983; Cranston-Cuebas & Barlow, 1990) have suggested that it is not anxiety per se that is responsible for the psychological component of erectile dysfunction, but the associated effects of cognitive distraction. Thus the physiological concomitants of anxiety appear to be less important than the effects of performance demand or cognitive distraction in males with ED (Rosen, 2007). Therefore it is important for sex therapy to focus on the cognitive aspects of performance anxiety. Relaxation-based approaches often fail to address the cognitive aspects of ED. For example, LoPiccolo (1992) argued that SF may represent a form of paradoxical intervention. While the sex therapist assigns SF with the intention of relieving performance anxiety, many patients may not experience reduction in anxiety; rather, they may experience 'metaperformance anxiety', that is, anxiety about not performing despite the injunction not to feel pressure to perform. Rosen (2007, p. 291) argues:

> According to this perspective, it is insufficient to assign sensate focus or relaxation exercises in the face of highly internalized performance demands. Rather, the focus of therapy should be on confronting the source of these performance demands via cognitive or psychoeducational interventions.

Based on the above findings and recommendations, some clinicians routinely integrate cognitive interventions with sex therapy for ED. Cognitive behaviour therapy (CBT) is usually used to challenge unrealistic sexual expectations, misconceptions regarding the basic mechanisms and processes of erectile function, and the causes of ED. Zilbergeld (1992) has noted that men frequently subscribe to a 'fantasy model of sex', in which male performance is viewed as the cornerstone of every sexual experience, and a firm erection is seen as the sine qua non of a satisfying sexual encounter. According to this view sexual performance difficulties are often interpreted as loss of masculinity or declining sexual interest in the partner.

The CBT is conducted in the same format as described with other disorders. To make the cognitive restructuring more systematic, use of the Cognitive Restructuring (ABCDE) form is recommended (Appendix B). Some of the hypnotic techniques mentioned before, namely ego strengthening, imagery training, self-hypnosis and post-hypnotic suggestions, can be used to alter the negative self-talk or rumination. Yapko (2006) provides a hypnotic script for altering negative rumination. Although the script is for insomnia, it can be adapted for ED patients (Yapko, 2006, pp. 150–3).

Increased Sexual Stimulation

Zilbergeld (1992) and others have noted that ED is most psychologically distressing to individuals or couples who have limited sexual scripts and very few alternatives to sexual intercourse. Performance demands and fear of failure increase significantly in individuals or couples who have never explored or do not know of any other techniques, besides penile-vaginal intercourse. In these individuals there is a complete cessation of all sexual activities once the man is unable to achieve a firm or lasting erection. This can lead to diminished sexual desire in one or both partners, often resulting in distancing and conflict in the relationship. This 'vicious cycle' can further increase the performance demands. LoPiccolo (1992) has also emphasised the critical role of the female partner's attitude towards non-intercourse forms of sexual stimulation. According to this author, a patient's knowledge that his partner's sexual gratification does not just depend on him having an erection reduces performance anxiety. The patient with ED finds it reassuring to know that his partner finds their love making and manual or oral stimulation highly pleasurable, although it does not involve penile-vaginal intercourse.

To break the vicious cycle, Rosen and colleagues (e.g. Rosen, Leiblum & Spector, 1994) advocate the use of 'sexual scripting' in sex therapy for ED. I use an adapted version of sexual scripting that involves detailed assessment of the couple's performative (current) and ideal (private) scripts and modification or replacement of the sexual script based on mutual trust and respect. Modification or replacement of the sexual script allows increased opportunities for sexual stimulation. New or modified sexual scripting can be enhanced by hypnotic imagery training.

Interpersonal Assertiveness and Couple Communication Training

As sexuality usually involves a couple, interpersonal and relationship issues play a major role in most cases of ED. Relationship conflicts (e.g. Masters & Johnson, 1970) and communication difficulties (Hawton, Catalan & Fagg,

1992) can precipitate, exacerbate and maintain ED. Rosen and colleagues (e.g. Rosen, Leiblum & Spector, 1994) have identified three major dimensions of couple conflict that are frequently encountered in cases of ED that need to be addressed in the course of sex therapy. These dimensions comprise status and dominance issues (e.g. due to loss of employment, loss of self-esteem, depression); loss of intimacy and trust (e.g. due to an extramarital affair, a new career, a child being born); and loss of sexual attraction (e.g. due to illness, surgery, weight gain). Resolution of these issues may require additional counselling and couple or marital therapy. Hypnosis can be used to enhance self-esteem via ego strengthening and self-hypnosis. While working with conflict issues, problems related to communication can also be addressed.

Relapse-Prevention Training

There is a high rate of drop-out and relapse from both medical and psychological treatment of ED. Moreover, ED is recognised to be a progressive disease in terms of underlying organic pathology, which may attenuate the manifestation of the dysfunction (Perelman, 2005). However, it is only recently that clinicians have advocated the use of relapse prevention in the treatment of ED (e.g. McCarthy, 2001). Several strategies can be utilised to prevent relapse and these include occasional SF1 or SF2 exercises; rehearsal of coping with negative sexual response, e.g. not achieving a desired level of erection when expected to; increasing sexual scripts – widening the range of sexual stimulation; self-hypnosis; imagery practice; monitoring and addressing conflicts in the relationship; regular use of medication; and regular scheduling of appointments with the therapist or treating physician. Hypnosis can also be utilised, for example rehearsing some of the above techniques when in trance, to enhance relapse prevention. Alladin (2007b; see also Chapter 3) has described several techniques, including mindfulness training, for preventing relapse in depression. Some of these strategies can be easily adapted for intervention with ED.

SUMMARY

This chapter reviewed the aetiology and existing empirical treatments for ED and then described a multi-modal treatment approach for treating ED that combines hypnotherapy, sex therapy and medication (PDE-5 inhibitors: Cialis, Viagra and Levitra). With the 'Viagra revolution', the understanding and treatment of ED have changed dramatically in the past 10 years. The chapter described two models of providing sex therapy to ED patients within the context of the Viagra revolution. Although hypnosis has been used with sexual dysfunctions for over half a century, there is a controlled trial of hypnosis with sexual disorders. The chapter described an innovative and conceptual model for integrating hypnosis with modern sex therapy. The model provides a design for evaluating the additive effect of hypnosis in sex therapy.

CHAPTER 10

FUTURE DIRECTIONS

Although many writers and clinicians advocate that hypnotherapy is very effective in the treatment of a wide range of disorders, very little empirical research exists in support of this claim. The current empirical state of and the future of hypnotherapy can be summarised by quoting Graci and Hardie's (2007, p. 288) observation about the empirical status of insomnia:

> There is a plethora of research suggesting that combining cognitive behavioral therapy with hypnosis is therapeutic for a variety of psychological, behavioral, and medical disorders. Yet, very little empirical research exists pertaining to the use of hypnotherapy as either a single or multi-treatment modality for the management of sleep disorders. The existing literature is limited to a very small subset of 'non-biologic' sleep disorders, specifically the insomnia disorders... There is an immediate need for more research evaluating the efficacy of hypnotherapy as both a single treatment and multi-treatment modality for managing sleep disturbance. Once this efficacy is established, it will increase the utilization of hypnotherapy and a demand for its services as a treatment of non-biologic sleep disorders.

However, the empirical evidence for the usefulness of hypnosis is better than insomnia with certain conditions, particularly when hypnosis is combined with cognitive behaviour therapy (CBT). For example, the adunctive effectiveness of hypnosis has been empirically validated with chronic pain (Elkins, Jensen & Patterson, 2007), acute stress disorder (Bryant *et al.*, 2005), depression (Alladin & Alibhai, 2007), somatisation disorder (Moene *et al.*, 2003) and public speaking anxiety (Schoenberger *et al.*, 1997). For the latest empirical status of clinical hypnosis with various medical and psychiatric disorders, see the special issues on evidence-based practice in clinical hypnosis in the *International Journal of Clinical and Experimental Hypnosis* (Alladin, guest editor, 2007a,b). Considering modern hypnosis has been around for over a quarter of a century, the relative empirical foundation of clinical hypnosis is not very solid and hypnotherapy is far from being recognised as mainstream psychotherapy. As Graci and Hardie (2007) indicate, in order to increase the credibility and utilisation of clinical hypnosis, the empirical basis of hypnotherapy needs to be widely established.

The goal of writing *Cognitive Hypnotherapy: An Integrated Approach to the Treatment of Emotional Disorders* was to describe and encourage evidence-based clinical practice and research in hypnotherapy. This book, like Lynn and Kirsch (2006), is an attempt to guide clinicians on how to assimilate hypnosis as an adjunct with CBT in the management of various emotional disorders. However, the book goes beyond this.

First, it lays down a solid theoretical foundation for combining hypnosis with CBT in the management of emotional disorders. Cognitive hypnotherapy is formally conceptualised as an assimilative model of psychotherapy, for which it meets the criteria (Lampropoulos, 2001; Stricker & Gold, 2006). The assimilative approach to psychotherapy is the latest integrative psychotherapy model described in the literature. Assimilative integration is considered to be the best model for integrating both theory and empirical findings to achieve maximum flexibility and effectiveness under a guiding theoretical framework (Lampropoulos, 2001).

Second, the book provides a case-formulation approach to clinical practice. Such a model of practice allows the assimilation of techniques based on empirical findings rather than using techniques haphazardly in a hit-and-miss fashion. Evidence suggests that matching treatment to particular patient characteristics increases outcome (Beutler, Clarkin & Bongar, 2000).

Third, each chapter pertaining to a particular emotional disorder offers a detailed, step-by-step treatment protocol. The treatment protocol, based on the latest empirical evidence, provides an *additive design* for studying the additive effect of hypnosis. The treatment protocols are specifically designed in a structured way to test for the clinical usefulness of adding a hypnotherapy component to the CBT. An *additive design* involves a strategy in which the treatment to be tested is added to another treatment to determine whether the treatment added produces an incremental improvement over the first treatment (Allen *et al.*, 2006). It is hoped that the detailed and structured protocol will providence guidance for treatment and encourage evaluation of the adjunctive techniques.

Fourth, the book provides a template for integrating other forms of psychotherapy with hypnotherapy. In the cognitive hypnotherapy model, CBT is chosen as the host psychotherapy for assimilation because CBT meets the criteria for a good scientific theory, it is empirically validated and it constitutes a unifying theory of psychotherapy and psychopathology (Alford & Beck, 1997). Theory is essential to clinical practice; without theory the practice of psychotherapy becomes a purely technical exercise, devoid of any scientific basis.

Although cognitive hypnotherapy meets the criteria for an assimilative model of psychotherapy, it requires further empirical validation. Without empirical validation it is not possible to establish whether importation of hypnotic techniques into CBT have a positive impact on therapy, especially when the techniques are decontextualised and placed in a new framework. It is only through empirical validation that ineffective and idiosyncratic assimilation can be avoided. Moreover, empirical validation is also important for the re-evaluation of the assimilative model itself. The book offers several structured and well-described cognitive hypnotherapy protocols that can be easily validated.

The trials in those protocols that have already been validated, for example for depression and somatisation disorder, need to replicated and subjected to *second-generation studies*; that is, studies using dismantling design to evaluate the relative effectiveness of the imported techniques (Alladin & Alibhai, 2007). These investigators imported several hypnotic techniques into CBT for depression, including hypnotic relaxation, ego strengthening, expansion of awareness, positive mood induction, post-hypnotic suggestions and self-hypnosis. Without further studies (second-generation studies), there is no way of knowing which techniques were effective and which were superfluous. First-generation studies involve assessing the additive effect of CBT, or comparing a single-modality hypnotherapy with another well-established therapy. For example, hypnotic reprocessing therapy (see Chapter 5) can be compared with exposure therapy in the treatment of PTSD as a first-generation study.

However, cognitive hypnotherapy as an assimilate model of psychotherapy is not to be seen as a finished product but as an evolving process. Although it is important to evaluate and validate assimilative integrative therapies empirically, it is also important to bear in mind that 'psychotherapy integration is synonymous with psychotherapeutic creativity and originality' and thus 'many advances occur in the consulting room of individual therapists who cannot submit their work to large-scale research investigations' (Gold & Stricker, 2006, p. 13). In other words, these non-publishers, but competent clinicians, have a lot to offer to clinical practice. Often their work can be very creative and innovative, providing several hypotheses that can be tested by the investigators. Moreover, beyond blending techniques, clinicians should also attempt to integrate patients' insights and feedback into their assimilative therapies.

Therefore, in closing I have several wishes for the future:

- I would like to see experienced clinicians and investigators write serious books about hypnosis; that is, books that are empirically based or innovative, rather than listing the usefulness of hypnosis.
- In research papers and treatment handbooks, it is important to examine the complexity of psychological disorders, paying particular attention to recent progress in aetiology, existing empirical treatments and comorbid disorders. The treatment protocol should be clearly described so that the techniques can be replicated and evaluated. It is important not to give the readers that depression can be treated

by ego strengthening, or PTSD treated by regression or abreaction. Multi-faceted psychotherapy, often including medication, is required to treat these complex disorders.

- It is hoped that some of the treatment protocols described in the book are evaluated and that both first-generation and second-generation studies are conducted.
- If we do all these, maybe cognitive hypnotherapy as an assimilative form of psychotherapy, will be recognised as a superior mainstream psychotherapy in the future.

CAB FORM FOR MONITORING IRRATIONAL BELIEFS/THOUGHTS/IMAGES/DAYDREAMS RELATED TO EVENTS/SITUATIONS

Date	C = Emotions	A = Facts or events	B = Automatic thoughts about A
	1. Specify sad/anxious/angry etc. 2. Rate degree of emotion 0–100	Describe: 1. Actual event that activated unpleasant emotion/reaction 2. Images, daydreams, recollection leading to unpleasant emotion	1. Write automatic thoughts that preceded emotions/reactions 2. Rate belief in automatic thoughts 0–100%
Jan. 04/06	*Anxious (100) Depressed (75) Unhappy (100) Miserable (90)*	*Thinking of going to birthday party*	*I won't enjoy it (100) I can't cope with it (100) Everyone will hate me (90) I will spoil it for everyone(90) I can never be happy again so what's the point of going (100)*

COGNITIVE RESTRUCTURING (ABCDE) FORM (OVERLEAF)

Date	A Activating event	B Irrational beliefs	C Consequences	D Disputation	E Effect of disputation
	Describe actual event, stream of thoughts, daydream etc. leading to unpleasant feelings	Write automatic thoughts and images that came in your mind. Rate beliefs or images 0–100%	1. **Emotion:** Specify sad, anxious or angry. Rate feelings 1–100% 2. **Physiological:** Palpitations, pain, dizzy, sweat etc. 3. **Behavioural:** Avoidance, in bed 4. **Conclusion:** Reaching conclusions, self-affirmation	Challenge the automatic thoughts and images. Rate belief in rational response/image 0–100%	1. **Emotion:** Re-rate your emotion 1–100% 2. **Physiological:** Changes in bodily reactions (i.e. less shaking, less tense etc.) 3. **Behavioural:** Action taken after disputation 4. **Conclusion:** Reappraise your conclusion and initial decision. Future beliefs in similar situation

Date	A Activating event	B Irrational beliefs	C Consequences	D Disputation	E Effect of disputation

COGNITIVE HYPNOTHERAPY CASE FORMULATION AND TREATMENT PLAN

Identifying Information:

Today's date:
Name:
Age:
Gender:
Marital status:
Ethnicity:
Occupational status:
Living situation:
Referred by:

1. Problem List:
(List all major symptoms and problems in functioning.)

Psychological/psychiatric symptoms:
Medical problems:
Interpersonal difficulties:
Occupational problems:
Financial difficulties:
Housing problems:
Legal issues:
Leisure problems:

2. Diagnosis:

Axis I:
Axis II:
Axis III:
Axis IV:
Axis V:

3. Working Hypothesis:
(Hypothesise the underlying mechanism producing the listed problems.)

Assess schemas related to:
Self:
Other:
World:
Future:
Recurrent core beliefs
Rumination/Negative self-hypnosis:
Hypnotic suggestibility:

4. Precipitant/Activating Situations:
(List triggers for current problems and establish connection between under-lying mechanism and triggers of current problems.)

Triggers:
Are triggers congruent with self-schemas/rumination/self-hypnosis:

5. Origins of core beliefs:
(Establish origin of core beliefs from childhood's experience.)

Early adverse negative life-events:
Genetic predisposition:
History of treatment (include response):

6. Summary of Working Hypothesis
    1.
    2.
    3.

7. Treatment Plan:
    1.
    2.
    3.
    4.

Modality:
Frequency:
Interventions:
Adjunct Therapies:
Obstacles:

8. Strengths and Assets:
(Based on the formulation, predict obstacles to treatment that may arise.)

1.
2.
3.

APPENDIX D

COGNITIVE HYPNOTHERAPY CASE FORMULATION AND TREATMENT PLAN FOR JACKIE

Identifying Information:

Today's date: *May 10, 2004*
Name: *Jackie*
Age: *36 years old*
Gender: *Female*
Marital status: *Married*
Ethnicity: *White Caucasian*
Occupational status: *Home maker*
Living situation: *Lives with her husband and two sons, aged 12 and 10 years*
Referred by: *Dr Mind, Psychiatrist*

1. Problem List:

(List all major symptoms and problems in functioning.)

Psychological/psychiatric symptoms:

Depressed, lacking energy and motivation, disturbed sleep, loss of libido, tired, difficulty with concentration, and feels guilty most of the time. At times she feels suicidal, but has no intent or plan. She feels angry and fearful about the world. She always feels a sense of inner tension, can't unwind or relax and has recurrent tension headaches.

Interpersonal difficulties:

Socially she is withdrawn. She avoids friends, although she has some good friends, and social events because she feels she is not good enough. She also believes she is ugly and unattractive and, therefore, she does not want anyone to notice how 'horrible' she looks.

Occupational problems:

She used to work in a bank before she had her first son. She has not worked since her son was born (12 years ago). Since her husband has a demanding job as senior police officer, she decided to become a full-time home-maker. She like being at home and looking after her family. However, she feels guilty believing that she is not doing a good job and is not a worthy wife and mother.

Medical problems:

None, except for recurrent tension headaches, which appears to be secondary to her anxiety and depression.

Financial difficulties:

None

Housing problems:

None

Legal issues:

None

Leisure problems:

She avoids going out because she believes she is ugly and hence she will become conspicuous to others. She also feels unsafe venturing out of her home. However, she is not agoraphobic, she mainly avoids social situations. She spends her leisure time watching chat shows and the food channels on television.

2. Diagnosis:

Axis I: *Major Depressive Disorder, Recurrent, Moderate*
Axis II: *Obsessive-compulsive personality traits*
Axis III: *None*
Axis IV: *Socially withdrawn*
Axis V: *GAF score = 50*

3. Working Hypothesis:
(Hypothesise the underlying mechanism producing the listed problems.)
Assess schemas related to:
Self:

'I am no good, I am a failure.'
'I am a useless wife and mother; I can't do anything right.'
'I am ugly and unattractive, no one will like me; everyone, especially my friends, think I am horrible looking.'
'I have no confidence, I am inferior.'

Other:

'You can't trust anyone, people are bad and hurtful, they always want to undermine you and put you down.'

World:

'The world is a scary place; no one is there to protect you.' 'I hate this world; I wish the world were safer.'

Future:

'I am confused about the future. It sounds bleak and uncertain.' 'I see my family getting fed up of me and leaving me.' 'I am scared I will end up in the psych unit.'

Recurrent core beliefs:

'I am no good; I am useless; I am a failure; I am ugly and horrible.'

Rumination/Negative self-hypnosis:

She ruminates with the belief that she is useless and ugly. The ruminations lead to further cognitive distortions and exacerbation of her anxiety and depressive symptoms. Such experience results in the validation of her anxious and depressive realities (self-affirmations or post-hypnotic suggestions).

Hypnotic suggestibility:

She scored maximum on the Barer Suggestibility Scale. Jackie reports she has a very good imagination. However, the focus of her imagination seems to be mainly on negative thinking.

4. **Precipitant/Activating Situations**
(List triggers for current problems and establish connection between underlying mechanism and triggers of current problems.)

Triggers:

Whenever she has to attend a social function or whenever she experiences feelings of anxiety or depression. On occasions when she is getting undressed or having a shower.

Are triggers congruent with self-schemas/rumination/self-hypnosis:

The triggers activate her self-schema of being inferior, a failure and ugly.

5. **Origins of core beliefs**
(Establish origin of core beliefs from childhood's experience.)

Early adverse negative life-events:

She was brought up in a cold and hostile environment. Her parents did not show much love or affection to her. Her father was a successful farmer but very harsh, rigid, angry and aggressive. He believed in hard work and he had little time for *people with emotional problems. His belief was that only bored and weak people get depressed. He wanted his children to succeed academically as he did not want them to become farmers. He believed in physical punishment. On many occasions Jackie was physically punished by her father and she was not allowed to express her opinions to her parents. She was constantly undermined by her father as she was not doing well at school. Her father strongly believed that children should be disciplined and physically punished for wrong doing and that parents should be heard. She described her mum as being very passive, cold and detached as she herself came from a farming family, and therefore her husband's behaviours were considered normal to her. Jackie was very scared of her father and never confronted him. She chose to back down whenever there was conflict with her mum or dad. The most traumatic childhood memory was when Jackie failed her Grade 10 exam in math. Her father was furious and threw away all her books and clothes out of the window and called her 'stupid' and 'useless'. Jackie was so frightened that she believed her father was going to kill her. She was extremely distressed that she had to collect her books and clothes, one by one, from the field covered with snow. She felt very deeply hurt and humiliated. Gradually Jackie came to believe that it was her fault since she is useless.*

Genetic predisposition:

Jackie's paternal uncle and grandmother had a history of major depressive disorder. Jackie always lacked confidence and thought negatively about herself. These got worse during her teenage years, especially when she became very conscious of her body. She described herself as being chubby when she was a teenager and became convinced that she is ugly and unattractive. She hated looking at her body when she undressed or while having a shower.

History of treatment(include response):

Although Jackie felt anxious and depressed since she was a teenager, she had her first episode of major depressive disorder eight years ago. Since then she has been having recurrent episodes of major depression. She was followed up by a psychiatrist for three years and then discharged to the care of her family physician, who monitors her anti-depressant medication. However, she has never been free of residual symptoms and her symptoms get worse when stressed out, and hence her family physician referred her for psychotherapy.

6. Summary of Working Hypothesis:

Whenever Jackie is invited to a social function, she feels anxious and depressed. The anxiety is triggered by her belief that, because she lacks confidence, she will not be able to deal with the social situation and may lose control. The fact that she is not able to control her fear and her anxiety, and lacks confidence, revives her underlying self-schema that she inferior, no good and useless. The feeling of inadequacy and incompetence leads to depressive affect. In turn this incites rumination about her symptoms, resulting in the circular feedback of the depressive affect. She copes by avoiding social situations which further reinforce her underlying self-schemas.

Her depression is also triggered by situations, such as undressing or having a shower, where she becomes conscious of her body image. These situations elicit the self-schema that she is ugly and useless.

7. **Strengths and Assets:**

Stable family life; financial security; and good social skills.

8. **Treatment Plan**

Goals (Measures):

1. *Reduce anxiety symptoms; monitor anxiety level with BAI.*
2. *Reduce depressive symptoms; monitor improvement in depression with BDI-II and the logging of activities.*
3. *Reduce frequency and intensity of headaches; measured by logging frequency and intensity of headaches.*
4. *Increase attendance at social functions; measured directly by keeping count of attendance.*
5. *Increase time spent with friends; measured via number of contacts.*
6. *To register at the local gym and start going to the gym regularly; measured by counting the frequency of going to the gym per week.*

Modality:

Individual cognitive hypnotherapy.

Frequency:

Weekly for 16 weeks.

Interventions:

Teach the formulation (to provide rationale for interventions). Activity scheduling (housework, socialising, going to gym). Cognitive restructuring (RET-Worksheet, behavioural experiments). Hypnotherapy for anxiety and depression management. Schema change interventions.

Adjunct Therapies:

Taking anti-depressant medication; medication may be reviewed by her Family Physician if she shows significant improvement with cognitive hypnotherapy. If she does not improve, she may be referred to a psychiatrist.

Obstacles:

Fixed beliefs that she is no good and useless; husband is very dominant and, at times, intolerant of her depressive symptoms.

HYPNOTIC INDUCTION AND EGO STRENGTHENING: COUNTING WITH RELAXATION METHOD

This script (adapted from Alladin, 2007b) provides the main content of the first hypnotherapy session. It consists of hypnotic induction, deepening, creating a pleasant state of mind, ego strengthening and termination of the trance.

INDUCTION

Close your eyes and make yourself as comfortable as you can. Now I am going to count ONE to TEN . . . As I count . . . with every count you will become more and more relaxed . . . so that when I reach the count of 10 . . . at the count of 10 you will be resting in a deep trance.

ONE: Just continue to breathe gently . . . in and out . . . and as you concentrate on my voice you begin to relax . . . relaxing very deeply as you continue to listen to my voice.

TWO: You begin to feel a heavy and relaxing feeling coming over you as you continue to listen to my voice. . . . And as you continue to breathe in and out . . . you will begin to feel your arms relaxing . . . your legs relaxing . . . and your entire body relaxing completely.

THREE: You begin to feel that heavy and relaxing feeling beginning to increase . . . more and more . . . and you are beginning to relax . . . more and more . . . relaxing deeper and deeper all the time as you continue to listen to my voice.

FOUR: You can feel that heavy and relaxing feeling increasing...more and more as you continue to listen to my voice.... And as I continue to count, with every count...that heavy and relaxing feeling will continue to increase more and more...until they causes you to drift into a deep and pleasant trance.

FIVE: Just notice...progressively you are becoming more and more relaxed...more and more at ease...more and more comfortable...so that when I reach the count of TEN you will be resting in a deep trance.

SIX: Just listen to my voice as I continue to count...and by the time I get to the count of TEN...you will be resting in a deep and pleasant trance.

SEVEN: You are beginning to drift slowly into a deep...deep trance.

EIGHT: Just notice you are becoming more and more comfortable...more and more at ease...more and more deeply relaxed...so that when I reach the count of TEN, you will be resting in a deep trance.

NINE: And every time you breathe in and out...you are drifting slowly into a deep and pleasant trance...drifting slowly...into a deep and pleasant trance.

TEN: Drifting slowly into a deep trance as you continue to listen to my voice...as you continue to breathe in and out...drifting deeper...and deeper...down...and down...into a deep and pleasant trance.

DEEPENING THE TRANCE

You are in such a deep hypnotic trance now...that your mind and your body feel calm and peaceful...And now I am going to help you to feel even more relaxed...In order to do this I am going to count ONE to FIVE...When I reach the count of FIVE...at the count of FIVE...you will be resting in a deep...deep...very deep trance.

ONE: Just let yourself go...just let yourself relax.

TWO: Not doing anything...not trying anything...just letting go...no efforts...effortless.

THREE: Becoming heavier and heavier...or lighter and lighter...sinking deeper and deeper into a deep trance.

FOUR: At the same time feeling detached...very, very detached...your whole body feeling completely detached...drifting into a deeper and deeper trance.

FIVE: Letting yourself drift into a deeper and deeper trance...drifting deeper and deeper all the time as you continue to listen to my voice.

CREATING A PLEASANT STATE OF MIND

You have now become so deeply relaxed ... and you are in such a deep ... deep trance ... that your mind and your body feel completely relaxed ... completely at ease. And you begin to feel a beautiful sensation of peace and relaxation ... tranquility and calm ... flowing through your mind and body ... giving you such a pleasant feeling ... such a beautiful sensation ... that you feel completely relaxed ... completely at ease ... Your mind and your body feel completely relaxed ... and perfectly at ease ... feeling peaceful ... calm ... comfortable ... completely relaxed ... totally relaxed ... drifting into a deeper and deeper trance as you continue to listen to my voice.

EGO-STRENGTHENING SUGGESTIONS

Just continue to enjoy these beautiful feelings ... and as you continue to enjoy this feeling of deep relaxation ... I am going to repeat some helpful and positive suggestions to you ... and since you are very relaxed and in such a deep hypnotic trance ... your mind has become so sensitive ... so receptive to what I say ... so that every suggestion that I give you ... will sink so deeply into the unconscious part of your mind ... that they will begin to cause such a lasting impression there ... that nothing will eradicate them ... These suggestions from within your unconscious mind will help you resolve your difficulties ... They will help you with your thinking ... that is, they will help you to think more clearly, more objectively, more realistically, and more positively ... They will help you with your feelings ... that is, they will make you to feel less anxious, less upset, less depressed ... They will also help you with your actions and your behaviours ... that is, they will help you to do more and more things that are helpful to you, and you will do less and less things that are not helpful to you.

You are now so deeply relaxed, you are in such deep hypnotic trance ... that everything that I say will happen to you ... for your own good ... will happen more and more ... And every feeling that I tell you that you will experience ... you will begin experience more and more ... These same things will happen to you more and more often as you listen to your tape ... And the same things will begin to happen to you just as strongly ... just as powerfully ... when you are at home ... or at work or at school ... or in any situation that you may find yourself in.

You are now so deeply relaxed ... you are in such a deep hypnotic trance ... that you are going to feel physically stronger and fitter in every way. At the end of the session ... and every time you listen to your tape ... you will feel more alert ... more wide awake ... more energetic ... Every day as you learn to relax ... you will become much less easily tired ... much less easily fatigued . . . much less easily discouraged . . . much less easily upset . . . much less easily depressed.

Therefore every day as you learn to relax . . . your mind and your body will feel physically stronger and healthier . . . your nerves will become stronger and steadier . . . your mind will become calmer and clearer . . . you will feel more composed . . . more relaxed . . . and able to let go . . . You will begin to develop the tendency to ruminate less . . . to catastrophise less . . . therefore, you will become less worried . . . less anxious and less apprehensive . . . less easily upset . . . less easily depressed.

As you become more relaxed, less anxious and less worried every day . . . you will begin to take more and more interest in whatever you are doing . . . in whatever is going on around you . . . that your mind will become completely distracted away from yourself . . . You will no longer think nearly so much about yourself . . . you will no longer dwell nearly so much on yourself and your difficulties . . . and you will become much less conscious of yourself . . . much less preoccupied with yourself and your difficulties . . . much less preoccupied with your own feelings . . . and much less preoccupied with what you think others think of you.

As you become less preoccupied with yourself, less conscious of yourself . . . you will be able to think more clearly . . . you will be able to concentrate more easily . . . You will be able to give your whole undivided attention to whatever you are doing . . . to the complete exclusion of everything else . . . Even if some thoughts cross your mind, you will be able to concentrate on the task without being distracted . . . As a result of this, your memory will begin to improve . . . so that you begin to see things in their true perspective . . . without magnifying your difficulties . . . without ever allowing them to get out of proportion . . . In other words, from now on . . . whenever you have a problem, you will examine it objectively and realistically . . . and decide what you can and cannot do about it . . . If you cannot resolve the problem . . . you will accept it and come to terms with it . . . But if the problem can be resolved . . . then you will make a plan . . . or come up with some strategies to overcome it however long it may take . . . Therefore from now on . . . whenever you have a problem you will become less emotionally upset and less overwhelmed by it . . . From now on you will begin to examine your difficulties like a scientist, that is, taking everything into consideration and then coming up with a plan . . . As a result of this new attitude . . . you will become emotionally less upset . . . less anxious . . . less agitated . . . and less depressed.

Every day . . . you will begin to feel all these things happening . . . more and more rapidly . . . more and more powerfully . . . more and more completely . . . so that . . . you will feel much happier . . . much more contented . . . much more optimistic in every way . . . And you will gradually become much more able to rely on . . . to depend on yourself . . . your own efforts...your own judgement...your own opinions...In fact...you will begin to feel much less need...to rely on...or to depend...on...other people.

TERMINATION

Now...for the next few moments just let yourself relax completely...and continue to feel this beautiful sensation of peace...and relaxation...tranquility ...and calm...flowing through your entire body...giving you such a pleasant...such a soothing sensation...that you feel so good...so at ease...that you feel a sense of well-being.

In a moment...when I count from ONE to SEVEN you will open your eyes...and will be alert...without feeling tired...without feeling drowsy... You will feel much better for this deep and pleasant hypnotic experience...You will feel completely relaxed both mentally and physically...and you will feel confident both in yourself and the future.

Now I am going to count ONE to SEVEN...ONE...TWO...THREE... FOUR...FIVE...SIX...SEVEN...Open your eyes...feeling relaxed, refreshed and a sense of well-being.

REFERENCES

Abbey, S. E. (2006). Somatization and somatoform disorders. In J. L. Levenson (ed.), *Textbook of Psychosomatic Medicine* (pp. 271–96). Washington, DC: American Psychiatric Publishing.

Abramson, L. Y., Alloy, L. B., Hankin, B. L., Haeffel, G. J., MacCoon, D. G. & Gibb, B. E. (2002). Cognitive-vulnerability-stress models of depression in a self-regulatory and psychobiological context. In I. H. Gotlib & C. L. Hammen (eds), *Handbook of Depression* (pp. 268–94). New York: Guilford Press.

Absolon, C. M., Cottrell, D., Eldridge, S. M. *et al.* (1997). Psychological disturbance in atopic eczema: The extent of the problem in school aged children. *British Journal of Dermatology*, 137: 241–5.

Adelman, L. C., Adelman, J. U. & Von Seggern, R. (2002). *Cost-effectiveness of Antiepileptic Drugs in Migraine Prophylaxis*. Greensboro, NC: Headache Wellness Center.

Adler, R. H., Zamboni, P., Hofer, T. & Hemmeler, W. (1997). How not to miss a somatic needle in a haystack of chronic pain. *Journal of Psychosomatic Research*, 42: 499–505.

Alford, B. A. & Beck, A. T. (1997). *The Integrative Power of Cognitive Therapy*. New York: Guilford.

Alladin, A. (1989). Cognitive-hypnotherapy for depression. In D. Waxman, D. Pederson, I. Wilkie & P. Mellett (eds), *Hypnosis: The 4th European Congress at Oxford* (pp. 175–82). London: Whurr.

Alladin, A. (1992a). Hypnosis with depression. *American Journal of Preventive Psychiatry and Neurology*, 3(3): 13–18.

Alladin, A. (1992b). Depression as a dissociative state. *Hypnos: Swedish Journal of Hypnosis in Psychotherapy and Psychosomatic Medicine*, 19: 243–53.

Alladin, A. (1994). Cognitive hypnotherapy with depression. *Journal of Cognitive Psychotherapy: An International Quarterly*, 8(4): 275–88.

Alladin, A. (2006a). Cognitive hypnotherapy for treating depression. In R. Chapman (ed.), *The Clinical Use of Hypnosis with Cognitive Behavior Therapy: A Practitioner's Casebook* (pp. 139–87). New York: Springer.

Alladin, A. (2006b). Experiential cognitive hypnotherapy: Strategies for relapse prevention in depression. In M. Yapko (ed.) *Hypnosis and Treating Depression: Advances in Clinical Practice* (pp. 281–313). London: Routledge.

Alladin, A. (Guest Editor) (2007a). Special Issue: Evidence-Based Practice in Clinical Hypnosis – Part I. *International Journal of Clinical and Experimental Hypnosis*, 55(2): 115–249.

Alladin, A. (2007b). *Handbook of Cognitive Hypnotherapy for Depression: An Evidence-Based Approach*. Philadelphia: Lippincott Williams & Wilkins.

Alladin, A. (2008). *Hypnotherapy Explained*. Oxford: Radcliffe.

Alladin, A. & Alibhai, A. (2007). Cognitive-hypnotherapy for depression: An empirical investigation. *International Journal of Clinical and Experimental Hypnosis*, 55: 147–66.

Alladin, A. & Heap, M. (1991). Hypnosis and depression. In M. Heap & W. Dryden (eds), *Hypnotherapy: A Handbook* (pp. 49–67). Milton Keynes: Open University Press.

Allen, J. G. (2001). *Traumatic Relationships and Serious Mental Disorders*. Chichester: John Wiley & Sons Ltd.

Allen, L. A., Woolfolk, R. L., Escobar, J. I., Gara, M. A. & Hamer, R. M. (2006). Cognitive-behavioral therapy for somatization disorder: A randomized controlled trial. *Archives of Internal Medicine*, 166: 1512–18.

Allen, L. A., Woolfolk, R. L., Lehrer, P. M., Gara, M. A. & Escobar, J. I. (2001). Cognitive behavior therapy for somatization: A pilot study. *Journal of Behaviour Therapy and Experimental Psychiatry*, 32: 53–62.

Allen, R. P. (2004). *Scripts Strategies in Hypnotherapy: The Complete Works*. Norwalk, CT: Crown House.

Alman, B. (2001). Self-care: Approaches from self-hypnosis for utilizing your unconscious (inner) potentials. In B. Geary & J. Zeig (eds), *The Handbook of Ericksonian Psychotherapy* (pp. 522–40). Phoenix, AZ: Milton H. Erickson Foundation Press.

Althof, S. E. (1998). New roles for mental health clinicians in the treatment of erectile dysfunction. *Journal of Sex Education and Therapy*, 23: 229–31.

Althof, S. E., Leiblum, S. R., Chevret-Measson, M. *et al.* (2005). Psychological and interpersonal dimensions of sexual function and dysfunction. *Journal of Sexual Medicine*, 2: 793–818.

Ament, P. & Milgram, H. (1967) Effects of suggestion on pruritus with cutaneous lesions in chronic myelogenous leukemia. *New York State Journal of Medicine*, 67: 833–5.

American Psychiatric Association (2000). *Diagnostic and Statistical Manual of Mental Disorders* (4th edn, text rev.). Washington, DC: American Psychiatric Association.

Anderson, J. A. D., Basker, M. A. & Dalton, R. (1975). Migraine and hypnotherapy. *International Journal of Clinical and Experimental Hypnosis*, 23(1): 48–58.

Andreychuk, T. & Skriver, C. (1975). Hypnosis and biofeedback in the treatment of migraine headache. *International Journal of Clinical and Experimental Hypnosis*, 23(3): 172–83.

Angst, J. & Preizig, M. (1996). Course of a clinical cohort of unipolar, bipolar and schizoaffective patients: Results of a prospective study from 1959 to 1985. *Schweizer Archiv für Neurologie und Psychiatrie*, 146: 1–16.

Araoz, D. L. (1981). Negative self-hypnosis. *Journal of Contemporary Psychotherapy*, 12: 45–52.

Araoz, D. L. (1985). *The New Hypnosis*. New York: Brunner/Mazel.

Araoz, D. L. (2005). Hypnosis in human sexuality problems. *American Journal of Clinical Hypnosis*, 47: 229–42.

Arnold, L. M. (2005). Dermatology. In J. L. Levenson (ed.), *Textbook of Psychosomatic Medicine* (pp. 629–46). Washington, DC: American Psychiatric Publishing.

Arnold, L. M., Keck, P. E. & Welge, J. A. (2000). Antidepressant treatment of fibromyalgia: A meta-analysis and review. *Psychosomatics*, 41: 104–13.

Asmundson, G. J., Taylor, S., Sevgur, S. & Cox, B. J. (2001). Health anxiety: Classification and clinical features. In G. J. G. Asmundson, S. Taylor & B. J. Cox (eds), *Health*

Anxiety: Clinical and Research Perspectives on Hypochondriasis and Related Conditions (pp. 3–21). Toronto: John Wiley & Sons Ltd.

Asmundson, G. J. G., Stapleton, J. A. & Taylor, S. (2004). Are avoidance and numbing distinct PTSD symptom clusters? *Journal of Traumatic Stress*, 17: 467–75.

Bakal, D. A. (1982). *The Psychology of Chronic Headache*. New York: Springer.

Baldwin, M. W., Fehr, B., Keedian, E., Seidel, M. & Thompson, D. W. (1993). An exploration of the relational schemata underlying attachment styles: Self-report and lexical decision approaches. *Personality and Social Psychology Bulletin*, 19: 746–54.

Ballenger, J. C., Davidson, J. R., Lecrubier, Y. *et al.* (2000). Consensus statement on posttraumatic stress disorder from the International Consensus Group on Depression and Anxiety. *Journal of Clinical Psychiatry*, 61(Suppl. 5): 60–6.

Bancroft, J. (1989). *Human Sexuality and Its Problems* (2nd edn). Oxford: Churchill Livingstone.

Bancroft, J. (1999). Central inhibition of sexual response in the male: A theoretical perspective. *Neuroscience and Biobehavioral Reviews*, 23: 763–84.

Bancroft, J. (2002). The medicalization of female sexual dysfunction: The need for caution. *Archives of Sexual Behavior*, 31: 451–5.

Bandura, A. (1977). Self-efficacy: Toward a unifying theory of behavioural change. *Psychological Review*, 84: 191–215.

Banner, L. L. & Anderson, R. U. (2007). Integrated sildenafil and cognitive-behavior sex therapy for psychogenic erectile dysfunction: A pilot study. *Journal of Sexual Medicine*, 4: 1117–25.

Barabasz, A. & Watkins, J. G. (2005). *Hypnotherapeutic Techniques* (2nd edn). Hove: Brunner-Routledge.

Barber, T. X. & Wilson, S. C. (1978/79). The Barber suggestibility scale and the creative imagination scale: Experimental and clinical applications. *American Journal of Clinical Hypnosis*, 21: 85.

Barlow, D. H. (2002). *Anxiety and Its Disorders: The Nature and Treatment of Anxiety and Panic* (2nd edn). New York: Guilford Press.

Barlow, D. H. & Durand, V. M. (2005). *Abnormal Psychology: An Integrative Approach* (4th edn). Stamford, CT: Thomson Wadsworth.

Barlow, D. H., Durand, V. M. & Stewart, S. H. (2006). *Abnormal Psychology: An Integrative Approach*. Toronto: Thomson Nelson.

Barlow, D. H., Sakheim, D. K. & Beck, A. T. (1983). Anxiety increases sexual arousal. *Journal of Abnormal Psychology*, 92: 49–54.

Barrios, A. A. (1973). Posthypnotic suggestion in high-order conditioning: A methodological and experimental analysis. *International Journal of Clinical and Experimental Hypnosis*, 21: 32–50.

Barsky, A. J., Wyshak, G. & Klerman, G. L. (1992). Psychaitric comorbidity in DSM-III-R hypochondriasis. *Archives of General Psychiatry*, 49: 101–8.

Basker, M. A. (1979). A hypnobehavioural method of treating agoraphobia by the clenched fist method of Calvert Stein. *Australian Journal of Clinical Hypnosis*, 7: 27–34.

Bauer, K. E. & McCanne, T. R. (1980). An hypnotic technique for treating insomnia. *International Journal of Clinical and Experimental Hypnosis*, 28: 1–5.

Beck, A. (1976). *Cognitive Therapy and Emotional Disorders*. New York: International University Press.

Beck, A. T. (1967). *Depression: Clinical, Experimental and Theoretical Aspects*. New York, Hoeber.

Beck, A.T. & Steer, R.A. (1993a). *Beck Anxiety Inventory*. San Antonio, TX: Harcourt Brace.

Beck, A. T. & Steer, R. A. (1993b). *Beck Hopelessness Scale*. San Antonio, TX: Harcourt Brace.

Beck, A. T. & Steer, R. A. (1993c). *Manual for the Beck Anxiety Inventory*. San Antonio, TX: Psychological Corporation/Harcourt Brace.

Beck, A. T., Emery, G. & Greenberg, R. L. (1985). *Anxiety Disorders and Phobias: A Cognitive Perspective*. New York: Basic Books.

Beck, A. T., Steer, R. A. & Brown, K. B. (1996). *Beck Depression Inventory – Revised*. San Antonio, TX: Psychological Corporation/Harcourt Brace.

Beck, A. T., Brown, G., Steer, R. A., Eidelson, J. I. & Riskind, J. H. (1987). Differentiating anxiety and depression: A test of the cognitive-content-specificity hypothesis. *Journal of Abnormal Psychology*, 96: 179–83.

Beck, A. T., Rush, A. J., Shaw, B. F. & Emery, G. (1979). *Cognitive Therapy of Depression*. New York: Guilford Press.

Beck, J. (1995). *Cognitive Therapy: Basics and Beyond*. New York: Guilford Press.

Beckham, E. E., Leber, W. R., Watkins, J. T., Boyer, J. L. & Cook, J. B. (1986). Development of an instrument to measure Beck's cognitive triad: The Cognitive Triad Inventory. *Journal of Consulting and Clinical Psychology*, 54: 566–7.

Bergin, A. E. & Garfield, S. L. (1994). Overview, trends, and future issues. In A. E. Bergin & S. L. Garfield (eds), *Handbook of Psychotherapy and Behavior Change* (4th edn, pp. 821–30). New York: John Wiley & Sons Ltd.

Bernstein, D. A., Borkovec, T. D. & Hazlett-Stevens, H. (2000). *New Directions in Progressive Relaxation Training: A Guidebook for Helping Professions*. Westport, CT: Praeger.

Beutler, L. E., Alomohamed, S., Moleiro, C. & Romanelli, R. (2002). Systematic treatment selection and prescriptive therapy. In F. W. Kaslow (ed. in chief) & J. Lebow (vol. ed.), *Comprehensive Handbook of Psychotherapy: Vol. 4. Integrative/Eclectic* (pp. 255–72). New York: John Wiley & Sons Ltd.

Beutler, L. E., Clarkin, J. E. & Bongar, B. (2000). *Guidelines for the Systematic Treatment of the Depressed Patient*. New York: Oxford University Press.

Blanchard, E. B., Appelbaum, K. A., Guarnieri, P., Morrill, B. & Dentinger, M. P. (1987). Five year prospective follow-up on the treatment of chronic headache with biofeedback and/or relaxation. *Headache*, 27: 580–3.

Bliss, E. L. (1984). Hysteria and hypnosis. *Journal of Nervous and Mental Disorders*, 172: 203–6.

Bolay, H., Reuter, U., Dunn, A. K. *et al.* (2002). Intrinsic brain activity triggers trigeminal meningeal afferents in a migraine model. *Natural Medicines*, 8: 136–42.

Borkovec, T. D. & Fowles, D. C. (1973). Controlled investigation of the effects of progressive and hypnotic relaxation on insomnia. *Journal of Abnormal Psychology*, 82: 153–8.

Boutin, G. (1978). The treatment of test anxiety by rational stage directed hypnotherapy. *American Journal of Clinical Hypnosis*, 21: 52.

Boutin, G. E. & Tosi, D. J. (1983). Modification of irrational ideas and test anxiety through rational stage directed hypnotherapy RSDH. *Journal of Clinical Psychology*, 39: 382–91.

Bower, G. (1981). Mood and memory. *American Psychologist*, 36: 129–48.

Bowlby, J. (1982). *Attachment and Loss. Vol. 1: Attachment* (2nd edn). New York: Basib Books.

Bowlby, J. (1988). *A Secure Base: Parent-Child Attachment and Healthy Human Development*. New York: Basic Books.

Brewin, C. R. & Holmes, E. A. (2003). Psychological theories of posttraumatic stress disorder. *Clinical Psychology Review*, 23: 339–76.

Brewin, C. R., Dalgleish, T. Y. & Joseph, S. (1996). A dual representation theory of posttraumatic stress disorder. *Psychological Review*, 103: 670–86.

Briere, J. & Scott, C. (2006). *Principles of Trauma Therapy: A Guide to Symptoms, Evaluations, and Treatment*. Thousand Oaks, CA: Sage.

Brom, D., Kleber, R. J. & Defare, P. B. (1989). Brief psychotherapy for posttraumatic stress disorder. *Journal of Consulting and Clinical Psychology*, 87: 607–12.

Brown, D. P. & Fromm, E. (1986a). *Hypnotherapy and Hypnoanalysis*. Hillsdale, NJ: Lawrence Erlbaum.

Brown, D. P. & Fromm, E. (1986b). *Hypnotherapy and Behavioural Medicine*, Hillsdale, NJ: Lawrence Erlbaum.

Brown, D. P. & Fromm, E. (1990). Enhancing affective experience and its expression. In D. C. Hammond (ed.), *Hypnotic Suggestions and Metaphors* (pp. 322–4). New York: W. W. Norton.

Brown, R. J. (2004). Psychological mechanisms of medically unexplained symptoms: An integrative conceptual model. *Psychological Bulletin*, 130: 793–812.

Brown, R. J., Schrag, A. & Trimble, M. R. (2005). Dissociation, childhood interpersonal trauma, and family functioning in patients with somatization disorder. *American Journal of Psychiatry*, 162, 899–905.

Brown, S. & Shalita, A. (1998). Acne vulgaris. *The Lancet*, 351: 1871–6.

Bryant, R.A., Guthrie, R. M. & Moulds, M. L. (2001). Hypnotizability in acute stress disorder. *American Journal of Psychiatry*, 158: 600–04.

Bryant, R., Moulds, M., Gutherie, R. & Nixon, R. (2005). The additive benefit of hypnosis and cognitive-behavioral therapy in treating acute stress disorder. *Journal of Consulting and Clinical Psychology*, 73: 334–40.

Bryant, R. A., Moulds, M. L., Nixon, R. D. *et al.* (2005). Hypnotherapy and cognitive behaviour therapy of acute stress disorder: A 3-year follow-up. *Behavioral and Research Therapy*, 44: 1331–5.

Burns, D. D. (1999). *Feeling Good: The New Mood Therapy*. New York: Avon Books.

Burrows, G. D. & Boughton, S. G. (2001). Hypnosis and depression. In G. D. Burrows, R. O. Stanley & P. B. Bloom (eds), *International Handbook of Clinical Hypnosis* (pp. 129–42). Chichester: John Wiley & Sons Ltd.

Buske-Kirshbaum, A., Geiben, A. & Hellhammer, D. (2001). Psychobiological aspects of atopic dermatitis: An overview. *Psychotherapy and Psychosomatics*, 70: 6–16.

Buvat, J., Buvat-Herbaut, M., Lemaire, A., Marcolin, G. & Quittelier, E. (1990). Recent developments in the clinical assessment and diagnosis of erectile dysfunction. *American Review of Sexual Research*, 1: 265–308.

Buysse, D. J., Germain, A., Moul, D. & Nofzinger, E. A. (2007). Insomnia. In D. J. Buysse (ed.), *Sleep Disorders and Psychiatry*. Washington, DC: American Psychiatric Publishing.

Buysse, D. J., Reynolds, C. F., Monk, T. H. *et al.* (1989). The Pittsburgh Sleep Quality Index: A new instrument for psychiatric practice and research. *Psychiatry Research*, 28: 193–213.

Cady, R. K. & Schreiber, C. P. (2004). Sinus headache: A clinical conundrum. *Otolaryngology Clinics of North America*, 37(2): 267–88.

Cady, R. K., Schreiber, C. P., Farmer, K. U. & Sheftell, F. D. (2002). Primary headaches: A convergence hypothesis. *Headache*, 42: 204–16.

Cardeña, E. (2000). Hypnosis in the treatment of trauma: A promising but not fully supported, efficacious intervention. *International Journal of Clinical and Experimental Hypnosis*, 48: 225–38.

Cardeña, E., Butler, L. D. & Spiegel, D. (2003). Stress disorders. In G. Stricker & T. Widiger, (eds) *Handbook of Psychology. Vol. 8* (pp. 229–49). New York: John Wiley & Sons Ltd.

Cardeña, E., Maldonado, J., van der Hart, O. & Spiegel, D. (2000). Hypnosis. In E. B. Foa, T. M. Keane & M. J. Friedman (eds), *Effective Treatments for PTSD* (pp. 247–79). New York: Guilford.

Chambless, D. & Hollon, S. D. (1998). Defining empirically supported therapies. *Journal of Consulting and Clinical Psychology*, 66: 7–18.

Chapman, R. A. (2006a). Case conceptualization model for integration of cognitive behaviour therapy and hypnosis. In R. A. Chapman (ed.), *The Clinical Use of Hypnosis in Cognitive Behavior Therapy: A Practitioner's Casebook* (pp. 71–98). New York: Springer.

Chapman, R. A. (2006b). Introduction to cognitive behavior therapy and hypnosis. In R. A. Chapman (ed.), *The Clinical Use of Hypnosis with Cognitive Behavior Therapy: A Practitioner's Casebook* (pp. 3–24). New York: Springer.

Chard, K. M. (2005). An evaluation of cognitive processing therapy for the treatment of posttraumatic stress disorder related to childhood sexual abuse. *Journal of Consulting and Clinical Psychology*, 73: 965–71.

Chaves, J. F. (1996). Hypnotic strategies for somatoform disorders. In S. J. Lynn, I. Kirsch & J. W. Rhue (eds), *Casebook of Clinical Hypnosis* (pp. 131–51). Washington, DC: American Psychological Association.

Chesson, A. L., McDowell Anderson, W., Littner, M. *et al.* (1999). Practice parameters for nonpharmacologic treatments of chronic insomnia. *Sleep*, 22: 1128–33.

Chiu, A., Chon, S. Y. & Kimball, A.B. (2003). The response of skin disease to stress: Changes in the severity of acne vulgaris as affected by examination stress. *Archives of Dermatology*, 139: 897–900.

Christophers, E. & Mrowietz, U. (1999). Epidermis: Disorders of persistent inflammation, cell kinetics and differentiation. In I. M. Friedberg, A. Z. Eisen, K. Wolff *et al.* (eds.), *Fitzpatrick's Dermatology in General Medicine*, 5th edn (pp. 495–521). New York: McGraw-Hill.

Chu, J. A. & Dill, D. L. (1990). Dissociative symptoms in relation to childhood physical and sexual abuse. *American Journal of Psychiatry*, 147: 887–92.

Clark, M. R. & Chodynicki, M. P. (2005). Pain. In J. L. Levenson (ed.), *Textbook of Psychosomatic Medicine* (pp. 827–67). Washington, DC: American Psychiatric Publishing.

Clarke, J. C. & Jackson, J. A. (1983). *Hypnosis and Behavior Therapy: The Treatment of Anxiety and Phobias*. New York: Springer.

Cloninger, C. R. (1993). Somatoform and dissociative disorders. In G. Winokur & P. J. Clayton (eds), *Medical Basis of Psychiatry*, 2nd edn (pp. 169–92). Philadelphia: W. B. Saunders.

Corove, M. B. & Gleaves, D. H. (2001). Body dysmorphic disorder: A review of conceptualizations, assessments, and treatment strategies. *Clinical Psychology Review*, 21: 949–70.

Cotterill, J. A. (1981). Dermatological non-disease: A common and potentially fatal disturbance of cutaneous body image. *British Journal of Dermatology*, 142: 611–19.

Coull, J. T. (1998). Neural correlates of attention and arousal: Insights from electrophysiology, functional neuroimaging and psychopharmacology. *Progress in Neurobiology*, 55: 343–61.

Cranston-Cuebas, M. A. & Barlow, D. H. (1990). Cognitive and affective contributions to sexual functioning. *Annual Review of Sex Research*, 1: 119–61.

Crasilneck, H. B. (1979). The use of hypnosis in the control of psychogenic impotency: The second follow-up study of 100 consecutive males. *American Journal of Clinical Hypnosis*, 7: 147–53.

Crasilneck, H. B. (1982). The use of hypnotherapy in the treatment of psychogenic impotency: The third follow-up study of 100 consecutive males. *American Journal of Clinical Hypnosis*, 25: 52–61.

Curkendall, S. M., Jones, J. K., Glasser, D. *et al.* (2001). Incidence of medically detected erectile dysfunction and related diseases before and after Viagra (sildenafil citrate). *European urology*, 37(Suppl. 2): 81.

Daud, I. R., Garralda, M. E., David, T. J. *et al.* (1993). Psychosocial adjustment in preschool children with atopic eczema. *Archives of Diseases in Children*, 69: 670–76.

Davidson, J. R. T., Rothbaum, B. O., van der Kolk, B. A., Sikes, C. R. & Farfel, G. M. (2001). Multi-center, double-blind comparison of sertraline and placebo in the treatment of posttraumatic stress disorder. *Archives of General Psychiatry*, 58: 485–92.

Davison, G. C., Neale, J. M., Blankstein, K. R. & Flett, G. L. (2005). Abnormal Psychology (2nd edn). Mississauga, ON: John Wiley & Sons Canada, Ltd.

De Jong, J. T. V. M., Komproe, I. H., van Ommeran, M. *et al.* (2001). Life events and posttraumatic stress disorder in 4 postconflict settings. *Journal of the American Medical Association*, 286: 555–62.

Deckersbach, T., Wilhelm, S., Keuthen, N. J. *et al.* (2002). Cognitive-behaviour therapy for self-injurious skin picking. *Behaviour Modification*, 26: 361–77.

Dement, W. & Vaughan, C. (2000). *The Promise of Sleep*. New York: Random House.

Dengrove, E. (1973). The use of hypnosis in behaviour therapy. *International Journal of Clinical and Experimental Hypnosis*, 21: 13–17.

DePiano, F. A. & Salzberg, H. C. (1981). Hypnosis as an aid to recall of meaningful information presented under three types of arousal. *International Journal of Clinical and Experimental Hypnosis*, 29: 283–400.

DePiano, F. A. & Salzberg, H. C. (eds.) (1986). *Clinical Applications of Hypnosis*. Norwood, NJ: Ablex.

Diagnostic Classification Steering Committee (1990). *International Classification of Sleep Disorders: Diagnostic and Coding Manual*. Rochester, MN: American Sleep Disorders Association.

Dollard, J. & Miller, N. E. (1950). *Personality and Psychotherapy*. New York: McGraw-Hill.

Dowd, E. T. (2000). *Cognitive Hypnotherapy*. Northvale, NJ: Jason Aronson.

Dowson, A. J., Lipscombe, S., Sender, J., Rees, T. & Watson, D. (2002) New guidelines for the management of migraine in primary care. *Current Medical Research Opinion*, 18: 414–39.

Dozois, D. J. A. & Westra, H. A. (2004). The nature of anxiety and depression: Implications for prevention. In D. J. A. Dozois & K. S. Dobson (eds), *The Prevention of Anxiety and Depression: Theory, Research, and Practice* (pp. 9–41). Washington, DC: American Psychological Association.

Edgette, J. H. & Edgette, J. S. (1995). *The Handbook of Hypnotic Phenomena in Psychotherapy*. New York: Brunner/Mazel.

Edinger, J. D., Bonnet, M. H., Bootzin, R. R. *et al.* (2004). Derivation of research diagnostic criteria for insomnia: Report of an American Academy of Sleep Medicine Work Group. *Sleep*, 27: 1567–96.

Edinger, J. D., Hoelscher, T. J., Marsh, G. R. *et al.* (1992). A cognitive-behavioral therapy for sleep-maintenance insomnia in older adults. *Psychology of Aging*, 7: 282–9.

Ehlers, A. & Steil, R. (1995). Maintenance of intrusive memories in posttraumatic stress disorder: A cognitive approach. *Behavioural and Cognitive Psychotherapy*, 23: 217–49.

Ehlers, A., Stangier, U. & Gieler, U. (1995). Treatment of atopic dermatitis: A comparison of psychological and dermatological approaches to relapse prevention. *Journal of Consulting and Clinical Psychology*, 63: 624–35.

Eimer, B. N. & Freeman, A. (1998). *Pain Management Psychotherapy: A Practical Guide.* New York: John Wiley & Sons Inc.

Elkins, G., Jensen, M. & Patterson, D. R. (2007). Hypnotherapy for the management of chronic pain. *International Journal of Clinical and Experimental Hypnosis*, 55: 275–87.

Ellis, A. (1980). Treatment of erectile dysfunction. In S. R. Leiblum & L. A. Pervin (eds), *Principles and Practice of Sex Therapy*. New York: Guilford Press.

Ellis, A. (1986). Anxiety about anxiety: The use of hypnosis with rational-emotive therapy. In E. T. Dowd & J. M. Haley (eds), *Case Studies in Hypnotherapy* (pp. 3–11). New York: Guilford Press.

Ellis, A. (1993). Rational-emotive therapy and hypnosis. In J. W. Rhue, S. J. Lynn & I. Kirsch (eds), *Handbook of Clinical Hypnosis* (pp. 173–86). Washington, DC: American Psychological Association.

Ellis, A. (1996). Using hypnosis in rational-emotive behaviour therapy in the case of Ellen. In S. J. Lynn, I. Kirsch & J. W. Rhue (eds), *Casebook of Clinical Hypnosis* (pp. 335–47). Washington, DC: American Psychological Association.

Erickson, M. H. & Rossi, E. (1979). *Hypnotherapy: An Exploratory Casebook.* New York: Irvington.

Erman, M. K. (1998). Insomnia. In J. S. Poceta & M. M. Mitler (eds), *Sleep Disorders: Diagnosis and Treatment*. Totowa, NJ: Humana Press.

Farber, E. M. (1995). Therapeutic perspectives in psoriasis. *International Journal of Dermatology*, 34: 456–60.

Farber, E. M. & Nall, L. (1974). The natural history of psoriasis in 5600 patients. *Dermatologica*, 148: 1–18.

Fava, G. A., Perini, G. I., Santonasto, P. & Fornasa, C. V. (1980). Life events and psychological distress in dermatologic disorders: Psoriasis, chronic urticaria and fungal infections. *British Journal Medical Psychology*, 53: 277–82.

Feldman, H. A., Goldstein, I., Hatzichristou, D. G. *et al.* (1994). Impotence and its medical and psychosocial correlates: Results of the Massachusetts Male Aging Study. *Journal of Urology*, 151: 54–61.

Feuerstein, M. & Gainer, J. (1982). Chronic headache: Etiology and management. In D. M. Doleys, R. L. Meredith & A. R. Ciminero (eds), *Behavioral Medicine: Assessment and Treatment Strategies*. New York: Plenum.

Finer, B. (1974). Clinical use of hypnosis in pain management. In J. Bonica (ed.), *Advances in Neurology* (pp. 573–9). New York: Raven Press.

First, M. B. & Tasman, A. (2004). *DSM-IV-TR Mental Disorders: Diagnosis, Etiology, and Treatment*. Chichester: John Wiley & Sons Ltd.

First, M. B., Spitzer, R. L., Gibbon, M. & Williams, J. B. W. (1997). *Structured Clinical Interview for DSM-IV Axis I disorders (SCID-I)*. Washington, DC: American Psychiatric Press.

Flammer, E. & Alladin, A. (2007). The efficacy of hypnotherapy in the treatment of psychosomatic disorders: Meta-analytical evidence. *International Journal of Clinical and Experimental Hypnosis*, 55: 251–74.

Foa, E. & Rothbaum, B. O. (1998). *Treating the Trauma of Rape: Cognitive-Behavioral Therapy for PTSD*. New York: Guilford Press.

Foa, E., Steketee, G. & Rothbaum, B. O. (1989). Behavioral/cognitive conceptualizations of post-traumatic stress disorder. *Behavior Therapy*, 20: 155–76.

Foa, E. B., Davidson, J. R. & Frances, A. (1999). Treatment of PTSD: The NIH expert consensus guideline series. *Journal of Clinical Psychiatry*, 60(Suppl. 16): 4–76.

Foa, E. B., Zinbarg, R. & Rothbaum, B. O. (1992). Uncontrollability and unpredictability in post-traumatic stress disorder: An animal model. *Psychological Bulletin*, 112: 218–38.

Foa, E. B., Riggs, D. S., Massie, E. D. & Yarczower, M. (1995). The impact of fear activation and anger on the efficacy of exposure treatment for posttraumatic stress disorder. *Behavior Therapy*, 26: 487–99.

Foa, E. B., Hembree, E. A., Cahill, S. P. *et al.* (2005). Randomized trial of prolonged exposure for posttraumatic stress disorder with and without cognitive restructuring: Outcome at academic and community clinics. *Journal of Consulting and Clinical Psychology*, 73: 953–64.

Ford, C. V. (1995). Dimensions of somatization and hypochondriasis. Special Issue: Malingering and conversion reactions. *Neurological Clinics*, 13: 241–53.

Fortune, D. G., Main, C. J., O'Sullivan, T. M. *et al.* (1977). Assessing illness-related stress in psoriasis: The psychometric properties of the psoriasis life stress inventory. *Journal of Psychosomatic Research*, 42: 467–75.

Fortune, D. G., Richards, H. L., Kirby, B. *et al.* (2002). A cognitive-behavioural symptom management programme as an adjunct in psoriasis therapy. *British Journal of Dermatology*, 146: 458–65.

Frankel, J. D. (1994). Dissociation in hysteria and hypnosis: A concept aggrandized. In S. J. Lynn & J. W. Rhue (eds), *Dissociation: Clinical and Theoretical Perspectives* (pp. 80–94). New York: Guilford Press.

Freeman, C. (1989). Psychological and drug therapies for post-traumatic stress disorder. *Psychiatry*, 5: 231–7.

Freinhar, J. P. (1984). Delusions of parasitosis. *Psychosomatics*, 25: 47–53.

French, T. M. (1933). Interrelations between psychoanalysis and the experimental work of Pavlov. *American Journal of Psychiatry*, 89: 1165–203.

Freud, A. (1967). Comments on trauma. In S. S. Furst (ed.), *Psychic Trauma* (pp. 235–45). New York: Basic Books.

Friedman, L., Bliwise, D. L., Yesavage, J. A. & Salom, S. R. (1991). A preliminary study comparing sleep restriction and relaxation treatments for insomnia with older adults. *Journal of Gerontology and Psychological Science*, 46: 1–8.

Fromm, E. & Nash, M. R. (1996). *Psychoanalysis and Hypnosis*. Madison, CT: International University Press.

Garg, A., Chren, M. M., Sands, L. P. *et al.* (2001). Psychological stress perturbs epidermal permeability barrier homeostasis. *Archives of Dermatology*, 137: 53–9.

Gaston, L., Crombez, J., Lassonde, M. *et al.* (1991). Psychological stress and psoriasis: Experimental and prospective correlational studies. *Acta Dermatology and Venereology*, 156: 37–43.

Germer, C. K. (2005). Mindfulness: What is it? What does it matter? In C. K. Germer, R. D. Siegel & P. R. Fulton (eds), *Mindfulness and Psychotherapy* (pp. 3–27). New York: Guilford Press.

Gibbons, D. E. (1979). *Applied Hypnosis and Hyperempiria*. New York, Plenum Press.

Gieler, U., Niemeier, V., Kupfer, J. & Brosig, B. (2003). Psychophysiological aspects of atopic dermatitis. In J. Y. M. Koo & C. S. Lee (eds), *Psychocutaneous Medicine* (pp. 97–117). New York: Marcel Dekker.

Giffin, N. J., Ruggiero, L., Lipton, R. B. *et al.* (2003). Premonitory symptoms in migraine: An electronic diary study. *Neurology*, 60: 935–40.

Gillham, J. E., Shatte, A. J. & Freres, D. R. (2000). Preventing depression: A review of cognitive-behavioral and family interventions. *Applied and Preventive Psychology*, 9: 63–88.

Ginsburg, I. H., Prystowsky, J. H., Kornfeld, D. S. *et al.* (1993). Role of emotional factors in adults with atopic dermatitis. *International Journal of Dermatology*, 32: 656–60.

Gold, J. R. & Stricker, G. (2001). Relational psychoanalysis as a foundation for assimilative integration. *Journal of Psychotherapy Integration*, 11: 47–63.

Gold, J. R. & Stricker, G. (2006). Introduction: An overview of psychotherapy integration. In G. Stricker & J. Gold (eds), *A Casebook of Psychotherapy Integration*. Washington, DC: American Psychological Association.

Gold, S. (2000). *Not Trauma Alone*. New York: Taylor & Francis.

Goldapple, K., Segal, Z., Garson, C. *et al.* (2004). Modulation of cortical-limbic pathways in major depression: Treatment-specific effects of cognitive behavior therapy. *Archives of General Psychiatry*, 61: 34–41.

Golden, W. L. (1986). An integration of Ericksonian and cognitive-behavioral hypnotherapy in the treatment of anxiety disorders. In E. T. Dowd & J. M. Haley (eds), *Case Studies in Hypnotherapy* (pp. 3–11). New York: Guilford Press.

Golden, W. L. (1994). Cognitive-behavioral hypnotherapy for anxiety disorders. *Journal of Cognitive Hypnotherapy*, 8: 265–74.

Golden, W. L. (2006). Hypnotherapy for anxiety, phobias and psychophysiological disorders. In R.Chapman (ed.), *The Clinical Use of Hypnosis with Cognitive Behavior Therapy: A Practitioner's Casebook* (pp. 101–37). New York: Springer.

Golden, W. L., Dowd, E. T. & Friedberg, F. (1987). *Hypnotherapy: A Modern Approach*. New York: Pergamon Press.

Goldstein, A. & Hilgard, E. R. (1975). Failure of the opiate antagonist naloxone to modify hypnotic analgesia. *Proceedings of the National Academy of Science USA*, 72: 2041–3.

Gonsalkorale, W. M. (2006). Gut-directed hypnotherapy: The Manchester approach for treatment of irritable bowel syndrome. *International Journal of Clinical and Experimental Hypnosis*, 54: 27–50.

Gotlib, I. H. & Goodman, S. H. (1999). Children of parents with depression. In W. K. Silverman & T. H. Ollendick (eds), *Developmental Issues in the Clinical Treatment of Children* (pp. 415–32). Boston: Allyn & Bacon.

Gotlib, I. H. & Hammen, C. L. (2002). Introduction. In I. H. Gotlib & C. L. Hammen (eds), *Handbook of Depression* (pp. 1–20). New York: Guilford Press.

Graci, G. (2005). Pathogenesis and management of cancer-related insomnia. *Journal of Supportive Oncology*. 3: 349–59.

Graci, G. & Sexton-Radek, K. (2006). Treating sleep disorders using cognitive behavioral therapy and hypnosis. In R. A. Chapman (ed.), *The Clinical Use of Hypnosis in Cognitive Behavior Therapy: A Practitioner's Casebook*, pp. 295–331. New York: Springer.

Graci, G. M. & Hardie, J. C. (2007). Evidenced-based hypnotherapy for the management of sleep disorders. *International Journal of Clinical and Experimental Hypnosis*, 55: 288–302.

Green, J. & Sinclair, R. D. (2001). Perceptions of acne vulgaris in final year medical student written examination answers. *Australas Journal of Dermatology*, 42: 98–101.

Grunert, B. K., Smucker, M. R., Weiss, J. M. & Rusch, M. D. (2003). When prolonged exposure falls: Adding an imagery-based cognitive restructuring component in the treatment of industrial accident victims suffering from PTSD. *Cognitive and Behavioral Practice*, 10: 333–46.

Gupta, M. A. & Gupta, A. K. (1995). Chronic idiopathic urticaria associated with panic disorder: A syndrome responsive to selective serotonin reuptake inhibitor antidepressants? *Cutis*, 56: 53–4.

Gupta, M. A. & Gupta, A. K. (1996). Psychodermatology: An update. *Journal of American Academy of Dermatology*, 34: 1030–46.

Gupta, M. A. & Gupta, A. K. (1998). Depression and suicidal ideation in dermatology patients with acne, alopecia areata, atopic dermatitis and psoriasis. *British Journal of Dermatology*, 139: 846–50.

Gupta, M. A. & Gupta, A. K. (2003). Depression and dermatological disorders. In J. Y. M. Koo & C. S. Lee (eds), *Psychocutaneous Medicine* (pp. 233–49). New York: Marcel Dekker.

Gupta, M. A., Gupta, A. K. & Haberman, H. F. (1987). The self-inflicted dermatoses: A critical review. *General Hospital Psychiatry*, 11: 166–73.

Gupta, M. A., Gupta, A. K. & Watteel, G. N. (1997). Stress and alopecia areata: A psychodermatologic study. *Acta Dermatology and Venereology*, 77: 296–8.

Gupta, M. A., Gupta, A. K., Schork, N. J. *et al.* (1990). Psychiatric aspects of the treatment of mild to moderate facial acne: Some preliminary observations. *International Journal of Dermatology*, 29: 719–21.

Gupta, M. A., Gupta, A. K., Schork, N. J. *et al.* (1994). Depression modulates pruritis perception: A study of pruritus in psoriasis, atopic dermatitis, and chronic idiopathic urticaria. *Psychosomatic Medicine*, 56: 36–40.

Guze, S. B. (1993). Genetics of Briquet's syndrome and somatization disorder. A review of family, adoption, and twin studies. *Annals of Clinical Psychiatry*, 5: 225–30.

Hadley, J. (1996). Sleep. In J. Hadley & C. Staudacher (eds), *Hypnosis for Change*. New York: MJF Books.

Hajak, G., Rodenbeck, A., Voderholzer, U. *et al.* (2001). Doxepin in the treatment of primary insomnia: A placebo-controlled, double-blind, polysomnographic study. *Journal of Clinical Psychiatry*, 62: 453–63.

Halgin, R. P. & Whitbourne, S. K. (2006). *Abnormal Psychology: Clinical Perspectives on Psychological Disorders*, 4th edn. New York: McGraw-Hill.

Halligan, P. W., Athwal, B. S., Oakley, D. A. & Frackowiak, R. S. J. (2000). Imaging hypnotic paralysis: Implications for conversion hysteria. *The Lancet*, 355: 986–7.

Hamann, K. & Avnstorp, C. (1982). Delusions of infestation treated by pimozide: A double-blind crossover clinical study. *Acta Dermatology and Venereology*, 62: 55–8.

Hammond, D. C. (ed.) (1990). *Handbook of Hypnotic Suggestions and Metaphors*. New York: W.W. Norton.

Hammond, D. C. (ed.) (1998). *Hypnotic Induction and Suggestions*. Chicago: American Society of Clinical Hypnosis.

Hammond, D. C. (2007). Review of the efficacy of clinical hypnosis with headaches and migraines. *International Journal of Clinical and Experimental Hypnosis*, 55: 207–19.

Hargreaves, R. J. & Shepheard, S. L. (1999). Pathophysiology of migraine – new insights. *Canadian Journal of Neurological Science*, 26(Suppl 3): S12–19.

Harrington, A. (ed.) (1997) *The Placebo Effect*. Cambridge, MA: Harvard University Press.

Harrison, P. V. & Stepanek, P. (1991). Hypnotherapy for alopecia areata (letter). *British Journal of Dermatology*, 124: 509–10.

Hartland, J. (1971). *Medical and Dental Hypnosis*, 2nd edn. London: Bailliere Tindall.

Harvey, A. G. (2002). A cognitive model of insomnia. *Behaviour Research and Therapy*, 40: 869–93.

Hashiro, M. & Okumura, M. (1997). Anxiety, depression and psychosomatic symptoms in patients with atopic dermatitis: Comparison with normal controls and among groups of different degrees of severity. *Journal of Dermatological Science*, 14: 63–7.

Hauri, P. J. (1993). Consulting about insomnia: A method and some preliminary data. *Journal of Sleep Research and Sleep Medicine*, 16: 344–50.

Hauri, P. J. (2000). The many faces of insomnia. In D. I. Mostofsky & D. H. Barlow (eds), *The Management of Stress and Anxiety in Medical Disorders*, pp. 143–59. Needham Heights, MA: Allyn & Bacon.

Hauri, P. J. & Fisher, J. (1986). Persistent psychophysiologic (learned) insomnia. *Sleep*, 9: 38–53.

Haustein, U. (1990). Adrenergic urticaria and adrenergic pruritus. *Acta Dermatology and Venereology*, 70: 82–4.

Hawton, K., Catalan, J. & Fagg, J. (1992). Sex therapy for erectile dysfunction: Characteristics of couples, treatment outcome, and prognosis factors. *Archives of Sexual Behavior*, 71: 161–75.

Headache Classification Committee of the International Headache Society: ICHD-II Abbreviated Pocket Version (2004). *Cephalalgia*, 24(Suppl 1): 1–160.

Heap, M. & Aravind, K. K. (2002). *Hartland's Medical and Dental Hypnosis*, 4th edn. London: Churchill Livingstone.

Herman, J. L., Perry, J. C. & van der Kolk, B. A. (1989). Childhood trauma in borderline personality disorder. *American Journal of Psychiatry*, 146: 490–95.

Hilgard, E. R. (1977). *Divided Consciousness: Multiple Controls in Human Thought and Action*. New York: John Wiley & Sons Inc.

Hohagen, F., Montero, R. F., Weiss, E. *et al.* (1994). Treatment of primary insomnia with trimipramine: An alternative to benzodiazepine hypnotics? *European Archives of Psychiatry and Clinical Neuroscience*, 244: 65–72.

Holbrook, A. M., Crowther, R., Lotter, A. *et al.* (2000). Meta-analysis of benzodiazepine use in the treatment of insomnia. *Canadian Medical Association Journal*, 162: 225–33.

Hollander, M. B. (1959). Excoriated acne controlled by post-hypnotic suggestion. *American Journal of Clinical Hypnosis*, 1: 122–3.

Hollon, S. D. & Shelton, M. (1991). Contributions of cognitive psychology to assessment and treatment of depression. In P. R. Martin (ed.), *Handbook of Behavior Therapy and Psychological Science: An Integrated Approach* (Vol. 164, pp. 169–95). New York: Pergamon Press.

Hollon, S. D., Haman, K. L. & Brown, L. L. (2002). Cognitive-behavioral treatment of depression. In I. H. Gotlib & C. C. Hammen (eds), *Handbook of Depression* (pp. 383–403). New York: Guilford Press.

Holroyd, K. A. (2006). Behavioral and educational approaches to the management of migraine: Clinical and public health applications. In R. B. Lipton & M. E. Bigal (eds), *Migraine and Other Headache Disorders* (pp. 261–72). New York: Taylor & Francis.

Holroyd, K. A. & Andrasik, F. (1982). A cognitive-behavioral approach to recurrent tension and migraine headache. In P. C. Kendall (ed.), *Advances in Cognitive-Behavioral Research and Therapy* (Vol. 1). New York: Academic Press.

Hughes, H., Brown, B. W., Lawlis, G. F. *et al.* (1983). Treatment of acne vulgaris by biofeedback relaxation and cognitive imagery. *Journal of Psychosomatic Research*, 27: 185–91.

Husid, M. S. & Rapoport, A. M. (2006). Principles of headache management. In R. B. Lipton & M. E. Bigal (eds), *Migraine and Other Headache Disorders* (pp. 241–59). New York: Taylor & Francis.

Jacobs, G., Pace-Schott, E., Stickgold, R. & Otto, M. (2004). Cognitive behavior therapy and pharmacotherapy for insomnia: A randomized controlled trial and direct comparison. *Archives of Internal Medicine*, 164(Sept. 27): 1888–96.

Jailwala, J., Imperiale, T. F. & Kroenke, K. (2000). Pharmacologic treatment of the irritable bowel syndrome: A systematic review of randomized, controlled trials. *Annals of Internal Medicine*, 133: 136–47.

James, S. P. & Mendelson, W. B. (2004). The use of trazadone as a hypnotic: A critical review. *Journal of Clinical Psychiatry*, 65: 752–5.

Janet, P. (1889). *L'Automatisme Psychologique*. Paris: Felix Alcan.

Jaycox, L. H., Zoellner, L. A. & Foa, E. B. (2002). Cognitive-behavior therapy for PTSD in rape survivors. *Journal of Clinical Psychology*, 58: 891–906.

Jick, S. S., Kremers, H. M. & Vasilakis-Scaramozza, C. (2000). Isotretinoin use and risk of depression, psychotic symptoms, suicide, and attempted suicide. *Archives of Dermatology*, 136: 1231–36.

Kales, A., Caldwell, A. B., Preston, T. A. *et al.* (1976). Personality patterns in insomnia: Theoretical implications. *Archives of General Psychiatry*, 33: 1128–34.

Kaplan, H. S. (1974). *The New Sex Therapy*. New York: Brunner/Mazel.

Kappler, C. & Hohagen, F. (2003). Psychosocial aspects of insomnia: Results of a study in general practice. *European Archives of Psychiatry and Clinical Neuroscience*, 253: 49–52.

Kardiner, A. & Spiegel, H. (1947). *War Stress and Neurotic Illness*. New York: Paul Hoeber.

Katon, W., Lin, E., Von Korff, M. *et al.* (1991). Somatization: A spectrum of severity. *American Journal of Psychiatry*, 148: 34–40.

Kazdin, A. E. (1984). Integartion of psychodynamic and behavioral psychotherapies: Conceptual versus empirical synthesis. In H. Arkowitz & S. B. Messer (eds), *Psychoanalytic Therapy and Behavior Therapy: Is Integration Possible?* (pp. 139–70). New York: Plenum.

Keane, T. M. & Barlow, D. H. (2002). Posttraumatic stress disorder. In D. H. Barlow (ed.), *Anxiety and Its Disorders: The Nature and Treatment of Anxiety and Panic*, 2nd edn (pp. 418–53). New York: Guilford Press.

Keane, T. M., Fairbank, J. A., Caddell, J. M., Zimering, R. T. & Bender, M. E. (1985). A behavioral approach to assessing and treating post-traumatic stress disorder in Vietnam veterans. In C. Figley (ed.), *Trauma and Its Wake. Vol. I: The Study and Treatment of Post-traumatic Stress Disorder* (pp. 257–94). New York: Brunner/Mazel.

Keane, T. M., Solomon, S. & Maser, J. (1996). *NIMH-National Center for PTSD Assessment Standardization Conference*. Paper presented at the 12th annual meeting of the International Society for Traumatic Stress Studies, Nov., San Francisco, CA.

Kendall, P. C., Howard, B. L. & Hays, R. C. (1989). Self-referent speech and psychopathology: The balance of positive and negative thinking. *Cognitive Therapy and Research*, 13: 583–98.

Kessler, R., Sonnega, A., Bromet, E., Hughes, M. & Nelson, C. (1995). Post-traumatic stress disorder in the National Comorbidity Survey. *Archives of General Psychiatry*, 52: 1048–60.

Kessler, R. C. (2002). Epidemiology of depression. In I. H. Gotlib & C. C. Hammen (eds), *Handbook of Depression* (pp. 23–42). New York: Guilford Press.

Kessler, R. C., McGongale, K. A., Zhao, S. *et al.* (1994). Lifetime and 12-month prevalence of DSM-III-R psychiatric disorders in the United States: Results from the National Comorbidity Survey. *Archives of General Psychiatry*, 51: 8–19.

Kilpatrick, D. G. (1983). Rape victims: Detection, assessment, and treatment. *The Clinical Psychologist*, 36: 92–5.

Kilpatrick, D. G., Saunders, B. E., Amick-McMullan, A. *et al.* (1989). Victim and crime factors associated with the development of crime-related posttraumatic stress disorder. *Behavior Therapy*, 20: 199–214.

King, S. A. (1994). Pain disorders. In R. E. Hales, S. C. Yudofsky & J. A. Talbot (eds), *The American Psychiatric Press Textbook of Psychiatry*, 2nd edn (pp. 591–622). Washington, DC: American Psychiatric Press.

Kirsch, I. (1985). Response expectancy as a determinant of experience and behavior. *American Psychologist*, 40: 1189–202.

Kirsch, I. (1993). Cognitive-behavioral hypnotherapy. In J. W. Rhue, S. J. Lynn & I. Kirsch (eds), *Handbook of Clinical Hypnosis* (pp. 151–71). Washington, DC: American Psychological Association.

Kirsch, I. (1999). *How Expectancies Shape Experience*. Washington, DC: American Psychological Association.

Kirsch, I. (2000). Are drugs and placebo effects in depression additive? *Biological Psychiatry*, 47: 733–5.

Kirsch, I., Montgomery, G. & Sapirstein, G. (1995). Hypnosis as an adjunct to cognitive-behavioral psychotherapy: A meta-analysis. *Journal of Consulting and Clinical Psychology*, 63: 214–20.

Klein, K. B. (1988). Controlled treatment trials in the irritable bowel syndrome: A critique. *Gastroenterology*, 95: 232–41.

Kodama, A., Horikawa, T., Suzuki, T. *et al.* (1999). Effects of stress on atopic dermatitis: Investigations in patients after the great Hanshin earthquake. *Journal of Allergy and Clinical Immunology*, 104: 173–6.

Koo, J. Y. M. & Lee, C. S. (2003). General approach to evaluating psychodermatological disorders. In J. Y. M. Koo & C. S. Lee (eds), *Psychocutaneous Medicine* (pp. 1–12). New York: Marcel Dekker.

Koo, J. Y. M. & Smith, L. L. (1991). Psychologic aspects of acne. *Pediatric Dermatology*, 8: 185–8.

Koo, J. Y. M., Lee, C. S., Kesterbaum, T. *et al.* (2003). International consensus on care of psychodermatological patients. In J. Y. M. Koo & C. S. Lee (eds), *Psychocutaneous Medicine* (pp. 31–40). New York: Marcel Dekker.

Kosslyn, S. M., Thompson, W. L., Costantini-Ferrando, M. F., Alpert, N. M. & Spiegel, D. (2000). Hypnotic visual illusion alters color processing in the brain. *American Journal of Psychiatry*, 157: 1279–84.

Kroger, W. S. & Fezler, W. D. (1976). *Hypnosis and Behavior Modification: Imagery Conditioning*. Philadelphia: J. B. Lippincott.

Kryger, M. (2004). *A Woman's Guide to Sleep Disorders*. New York: McGraw-Hill.

Krymchantowski, A. & Tepper, S. J. (2006). Nonspecific migraine acute treatment. In R. B. Lipton & M. E. Bigal (eds), *Migraine and Other Headache Disorders* (pp. 273–88). New York: Taylor & Francis.

Kubany, E. S. & Watson, S. B. (2002). Cognitive trauma therapy for formerly battered women with PTSD: Conceptual bases and treatment outlines. *Cognitive and Behavioral Practice*, 2: 27–61.

Lacks, P. & Morin, C. M. (1992). Recent advances in the assessment and treatment of insomnia. *Journal of Consulting and Clinical Psychology*, 60: 586–94.

Lake, A. E. (2001). Behavioral and nonpharmacologic treatments of headache. *Medical Clinics of North America*, 85: 1055–75.

Lampropoulos, G. K. (2001). Bridging technical eclecticism and theoretical integration: Assimilative integration. *Journal of Psychotherapy Integration*, 11: 5–19.

Lankton, S. (1980). *Practical Magic*. Cupertino, CA: Meta Publications.

Lasek, R. J. & Chren, M. M. (1998). Acne vulgaris and the quality of life of adult dermatology patients. *Archives of Dermatology*, 134: 454–8.

Laumann, E. O., Paik, A. & Rosen, R. C. (1999). The epidemiology of erectile dysfunction: Results from the National Health and Social Life Survey. *International Journal of Impotence Research*, 11(Suppl.): S60–64.

Lazarus, A. A. (1965). The treatment of a sexually inadequate man. In L. P. Ullmann & L. Krasner (eds), *Case Studies in Behavior Modification* (pp. 243–60). New York: Holt, Rinehart & Winston.

Lazarus, A. A. (1973). 'Hypnosis' as a facilitator in behaviour therapy. *International Journal of Clinical and Experimental Hypnosis*, 6: 83–9.

Lazarus, A. A. (1992). Multimodal therapy: Technical eclecticism with minimal integration. In J. C. Norcross & M. R. Goldfried (eds), *Handbook of Psychotherapy Integration* (pp. 231–63). New York: Basic Books.

Lazarus, A. A. (1999). A multimodal framework for clinical hypnosis. In I. Kirsch, A. Capafons, E. Cardeña-Buelna & S. Amigo (eds), *Clinical Hypnosis and Self-Regulation* (pp. 181–210). Washington, DC: American Psychological Association.

Lazarus, A. A. (2002). The multimodal assessment treatment method. In F. W. Kaslow (ed. in chief) & J. Lebow (vol. ed.), *Comprehensive Handbook of Psychotherapy: Vol. 4. Integrative/Eclectic* (pp. 241–54). New York: John Wiley & Sons Inc.

Lazarus, A. A. & Messer, S. B. (1991). Does chaos prevail? An exchange on technical eclecticism and assimilative integration. *Journal of Psychotherapy Integration*, 1: 143–58.

Leahy, R. L. (2003). *Cognitive Therapy Techniques: A Practitioner's Guide*. New York: Guilford Press.

Ledley, D. R., Marx, B. P. & Heimberg, R. G. (2005). *Making Cognitive-Behavioral Therapy Work: Clinical Process for New Practitioners*. New York: Guilford Press.

Lee, E. & Koo, J. Y. M. (2003). Psychological aspects of acne. In J. Y. M. Koo & C. S. Lee (eds), *Psychocutaneous Medicine* (pp. 339–50). New York: Marcel Dekker.

Leger, D. (2007). Insomnia: Impact on work, economics, and quality of life. In D. Leger & S. R. Pandi-Perumal (eds), *Sleep Disorders: Their Impact on Public Health*. Oxford: Informa Healthcare.

Leiblum, S. R. (2002). After sildenafil: Bridging the gap between pharmacologic treatment and satisfying sexual relationships. *Journal of Clinical Psychiatry*, 63(Suppl. 5): 17–22.

Leiblum, S. R. (ed.) (2007) *Erectile Disorders: Assessment and Management*. New York: Guilford Press.

Leiblum, S. R. & Rosen, R. C. (2000). *Principles and Practice of Sex Therapy*. New York: Guilford Press.

Lemke, W. (2005). Utilizing hypnosis and ego-state therapy to facilitate healthy adaptive differentiation in the treatment of sexual disorders. *American Journal of Clinical Hypnosis*, 47: 179–89.

Lewinshon, P. M. & Gotlib, I. H. (1995). Behavioural therapy and treatment of depression. In E. E. Beckham & W. R. Leber (eds), *Handbook of Depression*, 2nd edn, pp. 352–75. New York: Guilford Press.

Ley, R. G. & Freeman, R. J. (1984). Imagery, cerebral laterality, and the healing process. In A. A. Sheikh (ed.), *Imagination and Healing* (pp. 51–68). New York: Baywood.

Lichstein, K. L. & Morin, C. M. (eds) (2000). *Treatment of Late-Life Insomnia*. Thousand Oaks, CA: Sage.

Lichstein, K. L., & Riedel, B. W. (1994). Behavioral assessment and treatment of insomnia: A review with an emphasis on clinical application. *Behavioral Therapy*, 25: 659–88.

Lichstein, K. L., Peterson, B. A., Riedel, B. W. *et al.* (1999). Relaxation to assist sleep medication withdrawal. *Behavior Modification*, 23: 379–402.

Lieberzon, I., Taylor, S. F., Amdur, R. *et al.* (1999). Brain activation in PTSD in response to trauma-related stimuli. *Biological Psychiatry*, 45: 817–26.

Lindemann, E. (1944). Symptomatology and management of acute grief. *American Journal of Psychiatry*, 101: 141–8.

Linden, J. H. (2007). Hypnosis in childhood trauma. In W. C. Wester, II & L. I. Sugarman (eds), *Therapeutic Hypnosis with Children and Adolescents* (pp. 135–59). Bethel, CT: Crown House.

Linton, S. J. (1994). Chronic back pain: Integrating psychological and physical therapy – an overview. *Behavioral Medicine*, 20: 101–04.

Lipton, R. B. & Bigal, M. E. (2006). The epidemiology and impact of migraine. In R. B. Lipton & M. E. Bigal (eds), *Migraine and Other Headache Disorders* (pp. 23–36). New York: Taylor & Francis.

Lipton, R. B., Bigal, M. E., Rush, S. *et al.* (2004). Migraine practice among neurologists. *Neurology*, 62: 1926–31.

Lipton, R. B., Diamond, D., Freitag, F. *et al.* (2005). Migraine prevention patterns in a community sample: Results from the American Migraine Prevalence and Prevention (AMPP) study. *Headache*, 45: 792.

Lipton, R. B., Diamond, S., Reed, M., Diamond, M. L. & Stewart, W. F. (2001). Migraine diagnosis and treatment: Results from the American Migraine Study II. *Headache*, 41: 638–45.

Lipton, R. B., Stewart, W. F., Cady, R. *et al.* (2000) Sumatriptan for the range of headaches in migraine sufferers: Results of the Spectrum Study. *Headache*, 40(10): 783–91.

Lipton, R. B., Stewart, W. F., Stone, A. M., Lainez, M. J. & Sawyer, J. P. (2000) Stratified care vs step care strategies for migraine: The Disability in Strategies of Care (DISC) Study: A randomized trial. *Journal of the American Medical Association*, 284: 2599–605.

Lizza, E. F. & Rosen, R. C. (1999). Definition and classification of erectile dysfunction: Report of the Nomenclature Committee of the International Society of Impotence Research. *International Journal of Impotence Research*, 11: 141.

Looper, K. J. & Kirmayer, L. J. (2002). Behavioural medicine approaches to somatoform disorders. *Journal of Consulting and Clinical Psychology*, 70: 810–27.

LoPiccolo, J. (1992). Postmodern sex therapy for erectile failure. In R. C. Rosen & S. R. Leiblum (eds) *Erectile Disorders: Assessment and Treatment* (pp. 171–97). New York: Guilford Press.

Ludwig, A. M. (1972). Hysteria: A neurobiological theory. *Archives of General Psychiatry*, 27: 771–7.

Lue, T., Giuliano, F., Montorsi, F. *et al.* (2004). Summary of the recommendations on sexual dysfunctions in men. *Journal of Sexual Medicine*, 1: 6–23.

Lynn, S. J. & Cardeña, E. (2007). Hypnosis and the treatment of posttraumatic conditions: An evidence-based approach. *International Journal of Clinical and Experimental Hypnosis*, 55: 167–88.

Lynn, S. J. & Kirsch, I. (2006). *Essentials of Clinical Hypnosis: An Evidence-Based Approach.* Washington, DC: American Psychological Association.

Lynn, S. J., Das, L. S., Hallquist, M. N. & Williams, J. C. (2006). Mindfulness, acceptance, and hypnosis: Cognitive and clinical perspectives. *International Journal of Clinical and Experimental Hypnosis*, 54: 143–66.

Lynn, S. J., Kirsch, I., Barabasz, A., Cardeña, E. & Patterson, D. (2000). Hypnosis as an empirically supported clinical intervention: The state of the evidence and a look to the future. *International Journal of Clinical and Experimental Hypnosis*, 48: 239–58.

Lyubomirsky, S. & Tkach, C. (2004). The consequences of dysphoric rumination. In C. Papageorgiou & A. Wells (eds), *Depressive Rumination: Nature Theory and Treatment* (pp. 21–41). Chichester: John Wiley & Sons Ltd.

Maldonado, J. R. (1996a). Physiological correlates of conversion disorders. Paper presented at the 149th annual meeting of the American Psychiatric Association, New York.

Maldonado, J. R. (1996b). Psychological and physiological factors in the production of conversion disorder. Paper presented at the Society for Clinical and Experimental Hypnosis annual meeting, Tampa, Fl.

Maldonado, J. R. & Spiegel, D. (2003). Hypnosis. In R. E. Hales & S. C. Yudofsky (eds), *Textbook of Psychiatry*, 4th edn (pp. 1285–331). New York: American Psychiatric Association.

Manber, R. & Kuo, T. (2002). Cognitive-behavioral therapies for insomnia. In T. L. Lee-Chiong, M. J. Satela & M. A. Carskadon (eds), *Sleep Medicine*, pp. 177–85. Philadelphia: Hanley and Belfus.

Marcel, A. J. (1983). Conscious and unconscious perception: An approach to the relations between phenomenal experience and perceptual processes. *Cognitive Psychology*, 15: 238–300.

Marshall, J. C., Halligan, P. W., Fink, G. R., Wade, D. T. & Frackowiak, R. S. J. (1997). The functional anatomy of a hysterical paralysis. *Cognition*, 64: B1–8.

Marshall, R. D., Schneier, F. R., Fallon, B. A. *et al.* (1998). An open trial of paroxetine in patients with noncombat related, chronic posttraumatic stress disorder. *Journal of Clinical Psychopharmacology*, 18: 10–18.

Masters, W. H. & Johnson, V. E. (1970). *Human Sexual Inadequacy.* Boston: Little, Brown.

Mathew, N. T. & Tfelt-Hansen, P. (2006). General pharmacologic approach to migraine management. In J. Olesen, P. J. Goadsby, N. M. Ramadan, P. Tfelt-Hansen & K. M. A. Welch (eds), *The Headaches*, 3rd edn (pp. 433–40). Philadelphia: Lippincott Willaims & Wilkins.

Maurice, W. L. (1999). *Sexual Medicine in Primary Care.* St. Louis, MI: Mosby.

Mayou, R., Kirmayer, L., Simon, G. & Sharpe, M. (2005). Somatoform disorders: Time for a new approach in DSM-IV. *American Journal of Psychiatry*, 162: 847–55.

McCarthy, B. W. (1998). Integrating sildenafil into cognitive-behavioral couples sex therapy. *Journal of Sex Education and Therapy*, 23: 302–8.

McCarthy, B. W. (2001). Relapse prevention strategies and techniques with erectile dysfunction. *Journal of Sex and Marital Therapy*, 27: 1–8.

McGrath, P. J., Penzien, D. & Rains, J. C. (2006). Psychological and behavioral treatments of migraine. In J. Olesen, P. J. Goadsby, N. M. Ramadan, P. Tfelt-Hansen & K. M. A. Welch (eds), *The Headaches*, 3rd edn (pp. 441–8). Philadelphia: Lippincott Willaims & Wilkins.

McKnight, D. L., Nelson, R. O., Hayes, S. C. & Jarrett, R. B. (1984). Importance of treating individually assessed response classes in the amelioration of depression. *Behavior Therapy*, 15: 315–35.

Meadows, E. A. & Foa, E. B. (1998). Intrusion, arousal, and avoidance: Sexual trauma survivors. In V. M. Follette, J. I. Ruzek & F. R. Abueg (eds), *Cognitive-Behavioral Therapies for Trauma* (pp. 100–23). New York: Guilford Press.

Meichenbaum, D. & Fong, G. T. (1993). How individuals control their own minds: A constructive narrative perspective. In D. M. Wegner & J. W. Pennebaker (eds), *Handbook of Mental Control* (pp. 473–90). New York: Prentice Hall.

Meichenbaum, D. (1994). *A Clinical Handbook/Practical Therapist Manual for Assessing and Treating Adults with Post-traumatic Stress Disorder (PTSD)*. Clearwater, FL: Institute Press.

Mellinger, G. D., Balter, M. B. & Uhlenhuth, E. H. (1985). Insomnia and its treatment. Prevalence and correlates. *Archives of General Psychiatry*, 42: 225–32.

Melzack, R. & Wall, P. D. (1983). *The Challenge of Pain*. New York: Basic Books.

Mendelson, W. B. (1995). Long-term follow-up of chronic insomnia. *Sleep*, 18: 698–701.

Messer, S. (1989). Integrationism and eclecticism in counselling and psychotherapy: Cautionary notes. *British Journal of Guidance and Counselling*, 19: 275–85.

Messer, S. (1992). A critical examination of belief structures in integrative and eclectic psychotherapy. In J. C. Norcross & M. R. Goldfried (eds) *Handbook of Psychotherapy Integration* (pp. 130–68). New York: Basic Books.

Modlin, T. (2002). Sleep disorders and hypnosis: To cope or cure? *Sleep and Hypnosis*, 4: 39–46.

Moene, F. C., Spinhoven, P., Hoogduin, C. A. L. & Van Dyck, R. (2003). A randomized controlled clinical trial of a hypnosis-based treatment for patients with conversion disorder, motor type. *International Journal of Experimental and Clinical Hypnosis*, 51: 29–50.

Mohr, D. C. & Beutler, L. E. (1990). Erectile dysfunction: A review of diagnostic and treatment procedures. *Clinical Psychology Review*, 10: 123–50.

Montgomery, G. H., DuHamel, K. N. & Redd, W. H. (2000). A meta-analysis of hypnotically induced analgesia: How effective is hypnosis? *International Journal of Clinical and Experimental Hypnosis*, 48(2): 138–53.

Montgomery, P. & Dennis, J. (2003). Cognitive behavioral interventions for sleep problems in adults aged 60+. *Cochrane Database Systematic Review (1)*: CD003161.

Moore, J. D. & Bona, J. R. (2001). Depression and dysthymia. *Medical Clinics of North America*, 85(3): 631–44.

Morgan, C. A., Grillon, C., Lubin, H. & Southwick, S. M. (1997). Startle reflex abnormalities in women with sexual assault-related posttraumatic stress disorder. *American Journal of Psychiatry*, 154: 1076–80.

Morgan, C. A., Grillon, C., Lubin, H. *et al.* (1996). Exaggerated acoustic startle reflex in Gulf War veterans with posttraumatic stress disorder. *American Journal of Psychiatry*, 153: 64–8.

Morin, C. (1993). *Insomnia: Psychological Assessment and Management.* New York: Guilford Press.

Morin, C. M. (1996). *Insomnia: Psychological Assessment and Management: Treatment Manual for Practitioners.* New York: Guilford Press.

Morin, C. M. (1999). Empirically supported psychological treatments: A natural extension of the scientist–practitioner paradigm. *Canadian Psychology*, 40: 312–15.

Morin, C. M. (2003). Measuring outcomes in randomized clinical trials of insomnia treatments. *Sleep Medicine Reviews*, 7: 263–79.

Morin, C. M. (2004). Insomnia treatment: Taking a broader perspective on efficacy and cost-effectiveness issues. *Sleep Medicine Reviews*, 8: 3–6.

Morin, C.M. & Azrin, N. H. (1987). Stimulus control and imagery training in treating sleep-maintenance insomnia. *Journal of Consulting and Clinical Psychology*, 55: 260–62.

Morin, C. M. & Azrin, N. H. (1988). Behavioral and cognitive treatments of geriatric insomnia. *Journal of Consulting and Clinical Psychology*, 56: 748–53.

Morin, C. M. & Gramling, S. E. (1989). Sleep patterns and aging: Comparison of older adults with and without insomnia complaints. *Psychology & Aging*, 4: 290–4.

Morin, C. M., Bastien, C. & Savard, J. (2003). Current status of cognitive-behavior therapy for insomnia: Evidence for treatment effectiveness and feasibility. In M. L. Perlis & K. L. Lichstein (eds), *Treating Sleep Disorders: Principles and Practice of Behavioral Sleep Medicine*, pp. 262–85. New York: John Wiley & Sons Inc.

Morin, C. M., Culbert, J. P. & Schwartz, S. M. (1994). Nonpharmacological interventions for insomnia: A meta-analysis of treatment efficacy. *American Journal of Psychiatry*, 151: 1172–80.

Morin, C. M., Mimeault, V. & Gagne, A. (1999). Nonpharmacological treatment of late-life insomnia. *Journal of Psychosomatic Research*, 46: 103–16.

Moul, D. E., Nofzinger, E. A., Pilkonis, P. A. *et al.* (2002). Symptom reports in severe chronic insomnia. *Sleep*, 25: 553–63.

Moussavian, H. (2001). Improvement of acne in depressed patients treated with paroxetine. *Journal of the American Academy of Childhood and Adolescent Psychiatry*, 40: 505–6.

Mowrer, O. H. (1947). On the dual nature of learning: A reinterpretation of 'conditioning' and 'problem solving'. *Harvard Educational Review*, 17: 102–48.

Murray, C. J. L. & Lopez, A. D. (1996) *The Global Burden of Disease.* Geneva: World Health Organization/Harvard School of Public Health/World Bank.

Murtagh, D. R. & Greenwood, K. M. (1995). Identifying effective psychological treatments for insomnia: A meta-analysis. *Journal of Consulting and Clinical Psychology*, 63: 19–89.

National Institute of Health (1996). Technology assessment panel on integration of behavioral and relaxation approaches into the treatment of chronic pain and insomnia. *Journal of the American Medical Association*, 276: 313–18.

National Sleep Foundation (1991). *Sleep in America.* Princeton, NJ: The Gallup Organization.

Needleman, L. D. (2003). Case conceptualization in preventing and responding to therapeutic difficulties. In R. L. Leahy (ed.), *Roadblocks in Cognitive-Behavioral Therapy: Transforming Challenges into Opportunities for Change* (pp. 3–23). New York: Guilford Press.

Nezu, A. M., Nezu, C. M. & Lombardo, E. (2004). *Cognitive-Behavioral Case Formulation and Treatment Design: A Problem-Solving Approach.* New York: Springer.

Nolen-Hoeksema, S. (1991). Responses to depression and their effects on the duration of depressive episodes. *Journal of Abnormal Psychology,* 100: 569–82.

Nolen-Hoeksema, S. (2002). Gender differences in depression. In I. H. Gotlib & C. C. Hammen (eds), *Handbook of Depression.* New York: Guilford Press.

Nolen-Hoeksema, S. (2004). *Abnormal Psychology,* 3rd edn. New York: McGraw-Hill.

Norcross, J. C. & Goldfried, M. R. (eds) (1992). *Handbook of Psychotherapy Integration.* New York: Basic Books.

Norcross, J. C. & Newman, C. (1992). Psychotherapy integration: Setting the context. In Norcross, J. C. & Goldfried, M. R. (eds) *Handbook of Psychotherapy Integration* (pp. 3–46). New York: Basic Books.

Norcross, J. C. & Thomas, B. L. (1988). What's stopping us now? Obstacles to psychotherapy integration. *Journal of Integrative and Eclectic Psychotherapy,* 7: 74–80.

Nowell, P. D., Mazumdar, S., Buysse, D. J. *et al.* (1997). Benzodiazepines and zolpidem for chronic insomnia: A meta-analysis of treatment efficacy. *Journal of American Medical Association,* 278: 2170–77.

O'Donnell, B. F., Lawlor, F., Simpson, J. *et al.* (1997). The impact of chronic urticaria on the quality of life. *British Journal of Dermatology,* 136: 197–201.

O'Leary, K. D. & Wilson, G. T. (1987). *Behavior Therapy: Application and Outcome,* 2nd edn. Engelwood Cliffs, NJ: Prentice-Hall.

O'Sullivan, R. L., Christensen, G. A. & Stein, D. J. (1999). Pharmacotherapy of trichotillomania. In D. J. Stein, G. A. Christenson & E. Hollander (eds), *Trichotillomania* (pp. 93–124). Washington, DC: American Psychiatric Publishing.

Ohayon, M. M. (2002). Epidemiology of insomnia: What we know and what we still need to learn. *Sleep Medicine Review,* 6, 83–96.

Ohayon, M. M., Caulet, M., Priest, R. G. & Guilleminault, C. (1997). DSM-IV and ICSD-90 insomnia symptoms and sleep dissatisfaction. *British Journal of Psychiatry,* 171: 382–8.

Olesen, J. & Goadsby, P. J. (2006). The migraines: Introduction. In J. Olesen, P. J. Goadsby, N. M. Ramadan. P. Tfelt-Hansen & K. M. A. Welch (eds), *The Headaches,* 3rd edn, pp. 231–3. Philadelphia: Lippincott, Williams & Wilkins.

Olesen, J. & Lipton, B. L. (2006). Classification of headache. In J. Olesen, P. J. Goadsby, N. M. Ramadan. P. Tfelt-Hansen & K. M. A. Welch (eds), *The Headaches,* 3rd edn (pp. 9–15). Philadelphia: Lippincott, Williams & Wilkins.

Olsen, E. A. (1999). Disorders of epidermal appendages and related disorders. In I. M. Freedberg, A. Z. Eisen, K. Wolff *et al.* (eds), *Fitzpatrick's Dermatology in General Medicine,* 5th edn (pp 729–51). New York, McGraw-Hill.

Orr, S. P., Lasko, N. B., Shalev, A. Y. & Pitman, R. K. (1995). Physiological responses to loud tones in Vietnam veterans with post-traumatic stress disorder. *Journal of Abnormal Psychology,* 104: 75–82.

Oster, M. I. (2006). Treating treatment failures: Hypnotic treatment of posttraumatic stress disorder. In R. Chapman (ed.), *The Clinical Use of Hypnosis with Cognitive Behavior Therapy: A Practitioner's Casebook* (pp. 213–41). New York: Springer.

Ozer, E., Best, S., Lipsey, T. & Weiss, D. S. (2003). Predictors of posttraumatic stress disorder symptoms in adults: A meta-analysis. *Psychological Bulletin,* 129: 52–73.

Packard, R. C. (1987). Differing expectations of headache patients and their physicians. In C. S. Adler, S. M. Adler & R. C. Packard (eds), *Psychiatric Aspects of Headache* (pp. 29–33). Baltimore: Williams & Wilkins.

Patterson, D. R. & Jensen, M. P. (2003). Hypnosis and clinical pain. *Psychological Bulletin*, 129: 495–521.

Paykel, E. S. & Priest, R. G. (1992). Recognition and management of depression in general practice: Consensus Statement. *British Medical Journal*, 305: 1198–202.

Pearlstein, T., Stone, A., Lund, S. *et al.* (1997). Comparison of fluoxetine, bupropion, and placebo in the treatment of premenstrual dysphoric disorder. *Journal of Clinical Psychopharmacology*, 17: 261–6.

Perelman, M. A. (2001). Integrating sildenafil and sex therapy: Unconsummated marriage secondary to ED and RE. *Journal of Sex Education and Therapy*, 26: 13–21.

Perelman, M. A. (2003). Sex coaching for physicians: Combination treatment for patient and partner. *International Journal of Impotence Research*, 15(Suppl 5): S67–74.

Perelman, M. A. (2005). Psychosocial evaluation and combination treatment of men with erectile dysfunction. *Urologic Clinics of North America*, 32: 441–5.

Persons, J. B. (1989). *Cognitive Therapy in Practice: A Case Formulation Approach*. New York: Norton.

Persons, J. B. & Davidson, J. (2001). Cognitive-behavioral case formulation. In K. Dobson (ed.), *Handbook of Cognitive-Behavioral Therapies* (pp. 86–110). New York: Guilford Press.

Persons, J. B., Davidson, J. & Tompkins, M. A. (2001). *Essential Components of Cognitive-Behavior Therapy for Depression*. Washington, DC: American Psychological Association.

Philips, C. (1978). Tension headache: Theoretical problems. *Behavior Research and Therapy*, 16: 249–61.

Phillips, K. A. (1996) Body dysmorphic disorder: Diagnosis and treatment of imagined ugliness. *Journal of Clinical Psychiatry*, 57: 61–5.

Phillips, K. A. & Dufresne, Jr., R. G. (2003). Body dysmorphic disorder. In J. Y. M. Koo & C. S. Lee (eds), *Psychocutaneous Medicine* (pp. 153–67). New York: Marcel Dekker.

Phillips, K. A. & Najjar, F. (2003). An open-label study of citalophram in body dysmorphic disorder. *Journal of Clinical Psychiatry*, 64: 715–20.

Phillips, K. A., Albertini, R. S. & Rasmussen, S. A. (2002) A randominzed placebo-controlled trial of fluoxetine in body dysmorphic disorder. *Archives of General Psychiatry*, 59: 381–8.

Phillips, K. A., Dufresne, R. G., Wilkel, C. S. *et al.* (2000). Rate of body dysmorphic disorder in dermatology patients. *Journal of the American Academy of Dermatology*, 42: 436–41.

Pilowsky, I. (1969). Abnormal illness behaviour. *British Journal of Medical Psychology*, 42: 347–51.

Pincus, H. A. & Pettit, A. R. (2001). The societal costs of chronic major depression. *Journal of Clinical Psychiatry*, 62(Suppl. 6): 5–9.

Pinnell, C. A. & Covino, N. A. (2000). Empirical findings on the use of hypnosis in medicine: A critical review. *International Journal of Clinical and Experimental Hypnosis*, 48: 170–94.

Pitman, R. K. (1993). Biological findings in posttraumatic stress disorder: Implications for DSM-IV classification. In E. B. Foa (ed.), *Posttraumatic Stress Disorder: DSM-IV and Beyond*. Washington, DC: American Psychiatric Press.

Pitman, R. K., Orr, S. P., Shalev, A. *et al.* (1999). Psychophysiologic alterations in posttraumatic stress disorder. *Seminars in Clinical Neuropsychiatry*, 4: 234–41.

Plakun, E. M. & Shapiro, E. R. (2000). Psychodynamic psychotherapy for PTSD. *Journal of Clinical Psychiatry*, 61: 787–8.

Price, V. (1991). Alopecia areata: Clinical aspects. *Journal of Investigative Dermatology*, 96: 68.

Prigerson, H. G., Maciejewski, P. K. & Rosenheck, R. A. (2002). Population attributable fractions of psychiatric disorders and behavioral outcomes associated with combat exposure among US men. *American Journal of Public Health*, 92: 59–63.

Pryse-Phillips, W. E. M., Dodick, D. W., Edmeads, J. G. *et al.* (1997). Guidelines for the diagnosis and management of migraine in clinical practice. *Canadian Medical Association*, 156: 1273–87.

Rachman, S. J. (1977). The conditioning theory of fear acquisition: A critical examination. *Behaviour Research and Therapy*, 15: 375–87.

Rademaker, M., Garioch, J. J. & Simpson, N. B. (1989). Acne in school children: No longer a concern for dermatologists. *British Medical Journal*, 298: 1217–19.

Rauch, S. L., Whalen, P. J., Shin, L. M. *et al.* (2000). Exaggerated amygdala response to masked facial stimuli in posttraumatic stress disaorder: A functional MRI study. *Biological Psychiatry*, 47: 769–76.

Resick, P. A. & Schnicke, M. K. (1992). Cognitive processing therapy for sexual assault victims. *Journal of Consulting and Clinical Psychology*, 60: 748–56.

Resnick, H. S., Kilpatrick, D. G., Dansky, B. S., Saunders, B. E. & Best, C. L. (1993). Prevalence of civilian trauma and posttraumatic stress disorder in a representative national sample of women. *Journal of Consulting and Clinical Psychology*, 61: 984–91.

Reynolds, B. S. (1981). Erectile dysfunction: A review of behavioral treatment approaches. In R. J. Daitzman (ed.), *Clinical Behavior Therapy and Behavior Modification*, Vol. 2. New York: Garland.

Reynolds, C. F., Kupfer, D. J., Hoch, C. C. *et al.* (1986). Two-year follow up of elderly patients with mixed depression and dementia: Clinical and EEG sleep findings. *Journal of the American Geriatrics Society*, 34: 793–9.

Riedel, B. W., Lichstein, K. L. & Dwyer, W. (1995). Sleep compression and sleep education for older insomniacs: Self-help versus therapist guidance. *Psychology of Aging*, 10: 54–63.

Rief, W., Shaw, R. & Fichter, M. M. (1998). Elevated levels of psychophysiological arousal and cortisol in patients with somatization syndrome. *Psychosomatic Medicine*, 60: 198–203.

Riggs, D. S., Rothbaum, B. O. & Foa, E. B. (1995). A prospective examination of symptoms of post-traumatic stress disorder in victims of non-sexual assault. *Journal of Interpersonal Violence*, 2: 201–14.

Robins, L. N. & Regier, D. A. (eds) (1991). *Psychiatric Disorders in America: The Epidemiologic Catchment Area Study*. New York: Free Press.

Rosen, C. R. (2001). Psychogenic erectile dysfunction: Classification and management. In T. F. Lue (ed.), *Urologic Clinics of North America: Erectile Dysfunction* (pp. 269–78). Philadelphia: W. B. Saunders.

Rosen, C. R. (2007). Erectile dysfunction: Integration of medical and psychological approaches. In S. R. Leiblum (ed.), *Principles and Practice of Sex Therapy*, 4th edn (pp. 277–310). New York: Guilford Press.

Rosen, R. C., Fisher, W. A., Eardley, I. *et al.* (2004). The Multinational Men's Attitudes of Life Events and Sexuality (MALES) study: Prevalence of erectile dysfunction and related health concerns in the general population. *Current Medical Research and Opinion*, 20: 607–17.

Rosen, R. C., Leiblum, S. R. & Spector, I. (1994). Psychologically based treatment for male erectile disorder: A cognitive-interpersonal model. *Journal of Sex and Marital Therapy*, 20: 67–85.

Rosen, R. C., Wing, R., Schneider, S. & Gendrano, N., III. (2005). Epidemiology of erectile dysfunction: The role of medical comorbidities and lifestyle factors. *Urologic Clinics of North America*, 32: 403–17.

Rosenbaum, M. S. & Ayllon, T. (1981). The behavioral treatment of neurodermatitis through habit-reversal. *Behaviour Research and Therapy*, 19: 313–18.

Rosenzweig, S. (1936). Some implicit common factors in diverse methods of psychotherapy. *American Journal of Orthopsychiatry*, 6: 412–15.

Rost, K. M., Akins, R. N., Brown, F. W. *et al.* (1992). The comorbidity of DSM-III-R personality disorders in somatization disorder. *General Hospital Psychiatry*, 14: 322–6.

Rothe, M. J. & Grant-Kels, J. M. (1996). Atopic dermatitis: An update. *Journal of American Academy of Dermatology*, 35: 1–13.

Rothner, A. D. (2001). Differential diagnosis of headaches in children and adolescents. In P. A. McGrath & L. M. Hillier (eds), *The Child with Headache: Diagnosis and Treatment* (pp. 57–76). Seattle, IL: IASP Press.

Sadeh, A. & Acebo, C. (2002). The role of actigraphy in sleep medicine. *Sleep Medicine Reviews*, 6: 113–24.

Safran, J. D. & Messer, S. B. (1997). Psychotherapy integration: A postmodern critique. *Clinical Psychology: Science and Practice*, 4: 140–52.

Sanders, D. & Wills, F. (2005). *Cognitive Therapy: An Introduction*, 2nd edn. London: Sage.

Saral, T. B. (2003). Mental imagery in sex therapy. In A. A. Sheikh (ed.), *Healing Images: The Role of Imagination in Health* (pp. 272–3). New York: Baywood.

Sataeia, M. J. (2002). Epidemiology, consequences, and evaluation of insomnia. In T. L. Lee-Chiong, M. J. Staeia & M. A. Carskadon (eds), *Sleep Medicine* (pp. 151–60). Philadelphia: Hanley & Belfus.

Satcher, D. (2000). Mental health: A report of the Surgeon General – Executive summary. *Professional Psychology: Research and Practice*, 31(1): 5–13.

Scher, A. I. (2006). Progressive headache: Epidemiology, natural history, and risk factors. In R. B. Lipton & M. E. Bigal (eds), *Migraine and Other Headache Disorders* (pp. 37–44). New York: Taylor & Francis.

Schnuff, N., Neylan, T. C., Lenoci, M. A. *et al.* (2001). Decreased hippocampal N-acetylaspartate in the absence of atrophy in posttraumatic stress disorder. *Biological Psychiatry*, 50: 952–9.

Schoenberger, N. E. (2000). Research on hypnosis as an adjunct to cognitive-behavioral psychotherapy. *International Journal of Clinical and Experimental Hypnosis*, 48: 154–69.

Schoenberger, N. E., Kirsch, I., Gearan, P., Montgomery, G. & Pastyrnak, S. L. (1997). Hypnotic enhancement of a cognitive-behavioral treatment for public speaking anxiety. *Behavior Therapy*, 28: 127–40.

Schultz, K. D. (1978). Imagery and the control of depression. In J. L. Singer & K. S. Pope (eds), *The Power of Human Imagination: New Methods in Psychotherapy* (pp. 281–307). New York: Plenum Press.

Schultz, K. D. (1984). The use of imagery in alleviating depression. In A. A. Sheikh (ed.), *Imagination and Healing* (pp. 129–58). New York: Baywood.

Schultz, K. D. (2003). The use of imagery in alleviating depression. In A. A. Sheikh (ed.), *Healing Images: The Role of Imagination in Health* (pp. 343–80). New York: Baywood.

Schwartz, G. (1984). Psychophysiology of imagery and healing: A systems perspective. In A.A. Sheikh (ed.), *Imagination and Healing* (pp. 35–50). New York: Baywood.

Schwartz, G., Fair, P. L., Salt, P., Mandel, M. R. & Klerman, G. L. (1976). Facial muscle patterning in affective imagery in depressed and non-depressed subjects. *Science*, 192: 489–91.

Schwartz, L. S. (1990). A biopsychosocial treatment approach to post-traumatic stress disorder. *Journal of Traumatic Stress*, 3: 221–38.

Scott, M. J. (1960). *Hypnosis in Skin and Allergic Diseases*. Springfield, IL: Charles C. Thomas.

Seagraves, R. T. (1982). *Marital Therapy: A Combined Psychodynamic-Behavioral Approach*. New York: Plenum Press.

Segal, Z. V., Williams, J. M. G. & Teasdale, J. D. (2002). *Mindfulness-Based Cognitive Therapy for Depression: A New Approach to Preventing Relapse*. New York: Guilford.

Segraves, R. T. & Althof, S. (2002). Psychotherapy and pharmacotherapy for sexual dysfunctions. In P. E. Nathan & J. M. Gorman (eds), *A Guide to Treatments that Work*, 2nd edn (pp. 497–524). New York: Oxford University Press.

Shaw, J. A. (1987). Unmasking the illusion of safety: Psychic trauma in war. *Bulletin of Menninger Clinic*, 51: 49–63.

Sheftell, F. & Cady, R. (2006). Migraine without aura. In R. B. Lipton & M. E. Bigal (eds), *Migraine and Other Headache Disorders* (pp. 173–87). New York: Taylor & Francis.

Shenefelt, P. D. (2000). Hypnosis in dermatology. *Archives of Dermatology*, 136: 393–9.

Shertzer, C. L. & Lookingbill, D. P. (1987). Effects of relaxation therapy and hypnotizability in chronic urticaria. *Archives of Dermatology*, 123: 913–16.

Shin, L. M., McNally, R. J., Kosslyn, S. M. *et al.* (1999). Regional cerebral blood flow during script-driven imagery in childhood sexual abuse-related PTSD: A PET investigation. *American Journal of Psychiatry*, 156: 575–84.

Sierra, M. & Berrios, G. E. (1999). Flashbulb memories and other repetitive images: A psychiatric perspective. *Comprehensive Psychiatry*, 40: 115–25.

Silberstein, S. D. (2000). Practice parameter: Evidence-based guidelines for migraine headache (an evidence-based review). *Neurology*, 56(1): 142.

Simon, G. E. & Gureje, O. (1999). Stability of somatization disorder and somatization symptoms among primary care patients. *Archives of General Psychiatry*, 56: 90–95.

Simon, G. E. & Von Korff, M. (1991). Somatization and psychiatric disorder in the NIMH Epidemiologic Catchment Area Study. *American Journal of Psychiatry*, 148: 1494–500.

Smith, G. R., Monson, R. A. & Ray, D. C. (1986). Patients with multiple unexplained symptoms: Their characteristics, functional health, and health care utilization. *Archives of Internal Medicine*, 146: 69–72.

Smith, M. T., Perlis, M. L., Park, A. *et al.* (2002). Comparative meta-analysis of pharmacotherapy and behavior therapy for persistent insomnia. *American Journal of Psychiatry*, 159: 5–11.

Smucker, M. R. (1997). Post-traumatic stress disorder. In R. L. Leahy (ed.), *Practicing Cognitive Therapy: A Guide to Interventions* (pp. 193–220). Northvale, NJ: Jason Aronson.

Smucker, M. R. & Dancu, C. V. (1999). *Cognitive Behavioral Treatment for Adult Survivors of Childhood Trauma: Imagery Rescripting and Reprocessing*. New York: Jason Aronson.

Smucker, M. R. & Niederee, J. (1995). Treating incest-related PTSD and pathogenic schemas through imaginal exposure and rescripting. *Cognitive and Behavioral Practice*, 2: 63–93.

Smucker, M. R., Dancu, C. V., Foa, E. B. & Niederee, J. (1995). Imagery rescripting: A new treatment for survivors of childhood sexual abuse suffering from posttraumatic stress. *Journal of Cognitive Psychotherapy*, 9: 3–17.

Smucker, M. R., Weis, J. & Grunert, B. (2002). Imagery rescripting therapy for trauma survivors with PTSD. In A. A. Sheikh (ed.), *Handbook of Therapeutic Imagery Techniques* (pp. 85–97). Amityville, NY: Baywood.

Sokel, B., Christie, D., Kent, A., Lansdown, R. & Atherton, D. (1993) a comparison of hypnotherapy and biofeedback in the treatment of childhood atopic eczema, *Contemporary Hypnosis*, 10: 145–54.

Soldatos, C. R., Dikeos, D. G. & Whitehead, A. (1999). Tolerance and rebound insomnia with rapidly eliminated hypnotics: A meta-analysis of sleep laboratory studies. *International Clinical Psychopharmacology*, 14: 287–303.

Soldatos, C. R., Allaert, F. A., Ohta, T. & Dikeos, D. G. (2005). How do individuals sleep around the world? Results from a single-day survey in ten countries. *Sleep Medicine*, 6: 5–13.

Solomon, D. A., Keller, M. B., Leon, A. C. *et al.* (2000). Multiple recurrences of major depressive disorder. *American Journal of Psychiatry*, 157(2): 229–33.

Soter, N. A. (1999) Urticaria and angioedema. In I. M. Freedberg, A. Z. Eisen, K. Wolff et al. (eds), *Fitzpatrick's Dermatology in General Medicine*, 5th edn, pp. 1409–18. New York: McGraw-Hill.

Spanos, N. P. & Barber, T. X. (1974). Toward a convergence in hypnosis research. *American Psychologist*, 29: 500–11.

Spanos, N. P. & Barber, T. X. (1976). Behavior modification and hypnosis. In M. Hersen, R. M. Eisler & P. M. Miller (eds), *Progress in Behavior Modification*. New York: Academic.

Spanos, N. P., Radtke-Bodorik, H. L., Ferguson, J. D. & Jones, B. (1979). The effects of hypnotic susceptibility, suggestions for analgesia and the utilization of cognitive strategies on the reduction of pain. *Journal of Abnormal Psychology*, 88: 282–92.

Spiegel, D. (1981). Vietnam grief work using hypnosis. *American Journal of Clinical Hypnosis*, 24: 33–40.

Spiegel, D. (1993). Hypnosis in the treatment of posttraumatic stress disorder. In J. W. Rhue, S. J. Lynn & I. Kirsch (eds), *Handbook of Clinical Hypnosis* (pp. 493–508). Washington, DC: American Psychological Association.

Spiegel, D. & Albert, L. (1983). Naloxone fails to reverse hypnotic alleviation of chronic pain. *Psychopharmacology*, 81: 140–43.

Spiegel, D. & Spiegel, H. (1990). Hypnosis techniques with insomnia. In D. C. Hammond (ed.), *Handbook of Hypnotic Suggestions and Metaphors*, p. 255. New York: W. W. Norton.

Spiegel, D., Hunt, T. & Dondershine, H. E. (1988). Dissociation and hypnotizability in post-traumatic stress disorder. *American Journal of Psychiatry*, 145: 301–5.

Spielberger, C. D., Gorsuch, R. L. & Lushene, R. E. (1970). *Manual for the State-Trait Anxiety Inventory*. Palo Alto, CA: Consulting Psychologists Press.

Spielman, A. J., Caruso, L. S. & Glovinsky, P. B. (1987). A behavioral perspective on insomnia treatment. *Clinics of North America*, 10: 541–53.

Stanton, H. (1990a). Visualization for treating insomnia. In D. C. Hammond (ed.), *Handbook of Hypnotic Suggestions and Metaphors*, pp. 254–5. New York: W.W. Norton.

Stanton, H. E. (1990b). Dumping the 'rubbish'. In D. C. Hammond (ed.). *Handbook of Hypnotic Suggestions and Metaphors* (p. 313). New York: W. W. Norton.

Stanton, H. E. (1997). Adoring the clenched fist technique. *Contemporary Hypnosis*, 14: 189–94.

Stanton, H. E. (1999). Hypnotic relaxation and insomnia: A simple solution? *Sleep and Hypnosis*, 1: 64–7.

Stein, C. (1963). Clenched-fist as a hypnobehavioral procedure. *American Journal of Clinical Hypnosis*, 2: 113–19.

Stein, D. J. & Hollander, E (1992). Dermatology and conditions related to obsessive-compulsive disorder. *Journal of the American Academy of Dermatology*, 26: 237–42.

Stein, D. J., Vythilingum, B., Seedat, S. & Harvey, B. H. (2003). Trichotillomania. In J. Y. M. Koo & C. S. Lee (eds), *Psychocutaneous Medicine* (pp. 203–13). New York: Marcel Dekker.

Stepanski, E. J. (2000). Behavioral therapy for insomnia. In M. H. Kryger, T. Roth & W. C. Dement (eds), *Principles and Practice of Sleep Medicine*, 3rd edn. Philadelphia: W. B. Saunders.

Stewart, A. C. & Thomas, S. E. (1995) Hypnotherapy as a treatment for atopic dermatitis in adults and children. *British Journal of Dermatology*, 132: 778–83.

Stewart, W. F. Lipton, R., Celentano, D. D. & Reed, M. L. (1991). Prevalence of migraine headache in the United States: Relation to age, income, race, and other sociodemographic factors. *Journal of the American Medical Association*, 267: 64–9.

Stewart, W. F., Lipton, R. B., Kolodner, K., Liberman, J. N. & Sawyer, J. (1999). Reliability of the migraine disability assessment score in a population-based sample of headache sufferers. *Cephalalgia*, 19: 107–13.

Stewart, W. F., Ricci, J. A., Chee, F. & Lipton, R. (2002). Employer burden of headache in the United States: Results from the North American Productivity Audit (Abstract). *Cephalalgia*, 22: 600.

Stewart, W. F., Ricci, J. A., Chee, F. *et al.* (2003). Lost productive time and cost due to common pain conditions in the US workforce. *Journal of the American Medical Association*, 290: 2443–54.

Stoller, M. (1994). Economic effects of insomnia. *Clinical Therapeutics*, 16(Disc. 854): 873–97.

Strauss, J. S. & Thiboutot, D. M. (1999). Diseases of the sebaceous glands. In I. M. Freedberg, A. Z. Eisen, K. Wolff, *et al.* (eds) *Dermatology in General Medicine, 5th Edition* (pp. 769-84). New York: McGraw- Fitzpatrick's Hill.

Stricker, G. & Gold, J. R. (eds) (1993). *Comprehensive Handbook of Psychotherapy Integration*. New York: Plenum Press.

Stricker, G. & Gold, J. (eds) (2006). *A Casebook of Psychotherapy Integration*. Washington, DC: American Psychological Association.

Stutman, R. K. & Bliss, E. L. (1985). Posttraumatic stress disorder, hypnotisability, and imagery. *American Journal of Psychiatry*, 142: 741–3.

Taylor, F. R. & Martin, V. T. (2004). Migraine headache. In E. W. Loder & V. T. Martin (eds), *Headache: A Guide for the Primary Care Physician*. Philadelphia: American College of Physicians.

Taylor, S. (2004). *Advances in the Treatment of Posttraumatic Stress Disorder: Cognitive-Behavioral Perspectives*. New York: Springer.

Taylor, S. (2006). *Clinician's Guide to PTSD: A Cognitive-Behavioral Approach*. New York: Guilford Press.

Taylor, S., Thordarson, D. S., Maxfield, L. *et al.* (2003). Comparative efficacy, speed, and adverse effects of three treatments for PTSD: Exposure therapy, EMDR, and relaxation training. *Journal of Consulting and Clinical Psychology*, 71: 330–38.

Teasdale, J., Segal, Z. V., Williams, J. M. G. *et al.* (2000). Prevention and relapse/recurrence in major depression by mindfulness-based cognitive therapy. *Journal of Consulting and Clinical Psychology*, 68: 615–23.

Thomassen, R., van Hemert, A. M., Huyse, F. J. *et al.* (2003). Somatoform disorders in consultation-liaison psychiatry: A comparison with other mental disorders. *General Hospital Psychiatry*, 25: 8–13.

Thompson, I. M., Tangen, C. M., Goodman, P. J. *et al.* (2005). Erectile dysfunction and subsequent cardiovascular disease. *Journal of the American Medical Association*, 294: 2996–3002.

Thornton, E. M. (1976). *Hypnotism, Hysteria and Epilepsy: A Historical Synthesis*. London: William Heinemann.

Toone, B. K. (1990). Disorders of hysterical conversion. In C. Bass (ed.), *Somatization: Physical Symptoms and Psychological Illness* (pp. 207–34). Boston: Blackwell Scientific.

Tosi, D. J. & Baisden, B. S. (1984). Cognitive-experiential therapy and hypnosis. In W. C. Wester & A. H. Smith (eds), *Clinical Hypnosis: A Multidisciplinary Approach* (pp. 155–78). Philadelphia: J. B. Lippincott.

Trabert, W. (1995). 100 years of delusional parasitosis: Meta-analysis of 1,223 case reports. *Psychopathology*, 28: 238–46.

Turkdogan, D., Cagirici, S., Soylemez, D. *et al.* (2006). Charactersitic and overlapping features of migraine and tension-type headache. *Headache*, 46: 461–8.

Ursano, R. J., Bell, C., Eth, S. *et al.* (2006). Practice guideline for the treatment of patients with acute stress disorder and posttraumatic stress disorder. In J. S. McIntyre (Chair) (ed.), *American Psychiatric Association Practice Guidelines for the Treatment of Psychiatric Disorders Compendium* (pp. 1003–95). Arlington, VA: American Psychiatric Association.

Van Moffaert, M. (2003). The spectrum of dermatological self-mutilation and self-destruction including dermatitis artefacta and neurotic excoriations. In J. Y. M. Koo & C. S. Lee (eds), *Psychocutaneous Medicine* (pp. 169–89). New York: Marcel Dekker.

Van Ommeren, M., Sharma, B., Sharma, G. K. *et al.* (2002). The relationship between somatic and PTSD symptoms among Bhutanese refugee torture survivors: Examination of comorbidity with anxiety and depression. *Journal of Traumatic Stress*, 15: 415–22.

Veale, D., De Haro, L. & Lambrou, C. (2003). Cosmetic rhinoplasty in body dysmorphic disorder. *British Journal of Plastic Surgery*, 56: 546–51.

Vijselaar, J. & Van der Hart, O. (1992). The first report of hypnotic treatment of traumatic grief: A brief communication. *International Journal of Clinical and Experimental Hypnosis*, 40: 1–6.

Vythilingum, B. & Stein, D. J. (2001). Trichotillomania. *Primary Care Psychiatry*, 8: 58–63.

Wachtel, P. L. (1977). *Psychoanalysis and Behavior Therapy: Toward an Integration*. New York: Basic Books.

Wachtel, P. L. (1997). *Psychoanalysis, Behavior Therapy, and the Representational World*. Washington, DC: American Psychological Association.

Wade, T. J. & Cairney, J. (2000). Major depressive disorder and marital transition among mothers: Results from a national panel study. *Journal of Nervous and Mental Disease*, 188: 741–50.

Wagstaff, G. F. & Royce, C. (1994). Hypnosis and the treatment of nail biting: A preliminary trial. *Contemporary Hypnosis*, 11: 9–13.

Waldinger, M. D. (2002). The neurobiological approach to premature ejaculation. *Journal of Urology*, 168: 2359–67.

Waldinger, M. D., Zwinderman, A. H., Olivier, B. *et al.* (2005). Proposal for a definition of lifelong premature ejaculation based on epidemiological stopwatch data. *Journal of Sexual Medicine*, 2: 498–507.

Wall, P. D. (1993). Pain and the placebo response. In J. Marsh (ed.), *Ciba Foundation Symposium: Vol. 174. Experimental and Theoretical Studies of Consciousness* (pp. 187–216). Chichester: John Wiley & Sons Ltd.

Walsh, J. K. (2004). Drugs used to treat insomnia in 2002: Regulatory-based rather than evidence-based medicine. *Sleep*, 27: 1441–2.

Walsh, J. K. & Schweitzer, P. K. (1999). Ten-year trends in the pharmacological treatment of insomnia. *Sleep*, 22: 371–5.

Watkins, H. (1990). The door of forgiveness. In D. C. Hammond (ed.). *Handbook of Hypnotic Suggestions and Metaphors* (pp. 313–15). New York: W. W. Norton.

Weaver, D. B. & Becker, P. M. (1996). Treatment of insomnia with audiotaped hypnosis. *38th Annual Scientific Meeting & Workshops on Clinical Hypnosis*, Orlando: American Society of Clinical Hypnosis.

Weiss, D. S. & Marmar, C. R. (1997). The Impact of Event Scale – Revised. In J. P. Wilson & T. M. Keane (eds), *Assessing Psychological Trauma and PTSD* (pp. 399–428). New York: Guilford Press.

Weissman, A. N. & Beck, A. T. (1978). Development and validation of the Dysfunctional Attitude Scale: A preliminary investigation. Paper presented at the meeting of the Association for the Advancement of Behavior Therapy, Chicago.

Weitzenhoffer, A. (2000). *The Practice of Hypnotism*. New York: John Wiley & Sons Inc..

Welkowitz, L. A., Held, J. L. & Held, A. L. (1989). Management of neurotic scratching with behavioral therapy. *Journal of the American Academy of Dermatology*, 21: 802–4.

Wenzlaff, R. M. (2004). Mental control and depressive rumination. In C. Papageorgiou & A. Wells (eds), *Depressive Rumination: Nature, Theory and Treatment* (pp. 59–77). Chichester: John Wiley & Sons Ltd.

White, C. A. (2001). *Cognitive Behavior Therapy for Chronic Medical Problems: A Guide to Assessment and Treatment in Practice*. Chichester: John Wiley & Sons Ltd.

Whiting, P., Bagnall, A. M., Snowden, A. J., Cornell, J. E., Mulrow, C. D. & Ramirez, G. (2001). Interventions for the treatment and management of chronic fatigue syndrome: A systematic review. *Journal of the American Medical Association*, 286: 1360–8.

Wincze, J. P. & Carey, M. P. (2001). *Sexual Dysfunction: A Guide for Assessment and Treatment*, 2nd edn. New York: Guilford Press.

Wirtz, P. W. & Harrell, A. V. (1987). Effects of postassault exposure to attack-similar stimuli on long-term recovery of victims. *Journal of Consulting and Clinical Psychology*, 55: 10–16.

Wolpe, J. (1958). *Psychothearpy by Reciprocal Inhibition*. Stanford, CA: Stanford University Press.

Woolfolk, R. L. & Allen, L.A. (2007). *Treating Somatization*, New York: Guilford Press.

Woolfolk, R. L., Allen, L. A., Gara, M. A. & Escobar, J. I. (1998). *The Somatic Symptom Questionnaire*. Unpublished manuscript.

World Health Organization (1994). *Composite International Diagnostic Interview (CIDI)*. Washington, DC: American Psychiatric Press.

World Health Organization (1998). *Well-being Measures in Primary Healthcare/The Depcare Project*. Copenhagen: WHO Regional Office for Europe.

Yapko, M. D. (1992). *Hypnosis and the Treatment of Depressions: Strategies for Change.* New York: Brunner/Mazel.

Yapko, M. D. (2001). *Treating Depression with Hypnosis: Integrating Cognitive-Behavioral and Strategic Approaches.* Philadelphia: Brunner/Routledge.

Yapko, M. D. (2003). *Trancework: An Introduction to the Practice of Clinical Hypnosis,* 3rd edn. New York: Brunner-Routledge.

Yapko, M. D. (2006). Utilizing hypnosis in addressing ruminative depression-related insomnia. In M. D. Yapko (ed.), *Hypnosis and Treating Depression: Applications in Clinical Practice* (pp. 141–59). Routledge: New York.

Yehuda, R. (2002). Status of cortisol findings in PTSD. *Psychiatric Clinics of North America,* 25: 341–68.

Yehuda, R. & Wong, C. M. (2002). Etiology and biology of post-traumatic stress disorder: Implications for treatment. *Psychiatric Clinics of North America,* 8: 109–34.

Yehuda, R., McFarlane, A. C. & Shalev, A. Y. (1998). Predicting the development of posttraumatic stress disorder from acute response to a traumatic event. *Biological Psychiatry,* 44, 1305–13.

Yehuda, R., Marshall, R., Penkower, A. & Wong, C. M. (2002). Pharmacological treatments for posttraumatic stress disorder. In P. E. Nathan & J. M. Gorman (eds), *A Guide to Treatments That Work,* 2nd edn (pp. 411–45). New York: Oxford University Press.

Yehuda, R., Resnick, H., Kahana, B. & Giller, E. L. (1993). Long-lasting hormonal alterations in extreme stress in humans: Normative or maladaptive? *Psychosomatic Medicine,* 55: 287–97.

Yehuda, R., Giller E. L. J., Southwick, S. M. *et al.* (1991). Hypothalamic-pituitary-adrenal dysfunction in posttraumatic stress disorder. *Biological Psychiatry,* 30: 266–74.

Yosipovitch, G., Tang, M., Dawn, A. G. *et al.* (2007). Study of psychological stress, sebum production and acne vulgaris in adolescents. *Acta Dermato-Venereologica,* 87(2): 135–9.

Youngren, M. A. & Lewinshon, P. M. (1980). The functional relation between depression and problematic interpersonal behavior. *Journal of Abnormal Psychology,* 89: 333–41.

Zachariae, R., Oster, H., Bjerring, P. & Kragballe, K. (1996). Effects of psychologic intervention on psoriasis: A preliminary report. *Journal of the American Academy of Dermatology,* 34: 1008–15.

Zane, L. T. (2003). Psychoneuroendocrinimmunodermatology. In J. Y. M. Koo & C. S. Lee (eds), *Psychocutaneous Medicine* (pp. 65–95). New York: Marcel Dekker.

Zarren, J. & Eimer, B. (2001). *Brief Cognitive Hypnosis: Facilitating the Change of Dysfunctional Behavior.* New York: Springer.

Zayfert, C. & Becker, C. B. (2007). *Cognitive-Behavioral Therapy for PTSD: A Case Formulation Approach.* New York: Guilford Press.

Zilbergeld, B. (1992). *The New Male Sexuality.* New York: Bantam Books.

Zilbergeld, B. & Hammond, D. C. (1988). The use of hypnosis in treating desire disorders. In S. R. Leiblum & R. C. Rosen (eds), *Sexual Desire Disorders* (pp. 192–225). New York: Guilford Press.

INDEX